The SAC Classification in Implant Dentistry

The SAC Classification in Implant Dentistry

SECOND EDITION

The SAC Classification in Implant Dentistry

SECOND EDITION

A. DAWSON, W. MARTIN, W. D. POLIDO

QUINTESSENCE PUBLISHING

Berlin | Chicago | Tokyo
Barcelona | London | Milan | Mexico City | Moscow | Paris | Prague | Seoul | Warsaw
Beijing | Istanbul | Sao Paulo | Zagreb

German National Library CIP Data

The German National Library has listed this publication in the German National Bibliography. Detailed bibliographical data are available at http://dnb.ddb.de.

QUINTESSENCE PUBLISHING

Ifenpfad 2–4, 12107 Berlin, Germany
www.quintessence-publishing.com

Illustrations:	Ute Drewes, Basel (CH), www.drewes.ch
Editing:	Quintessence Publishing Co, Inc, Batavia (US)
Layout and Production:	Quintessenz Verlags-GmbH, Berlin (DE)
Printing:	Grafički zavod Hrvatske, Zagreb (HR), www.gzh.hr

Printed in Croatia

ISBN 978-1-78698-110-3

The tooth identification system used in The SAC Classification in Implant Dentistry is that of the FDI World Dental Federation.

Foreword

The SAC Classification in Implant Dentistry

Almost 20 years ago, the International Team for Implantology – ITI – formalized the SAC classification to categorize oral implant treatment procedures into three levels of difficulty: Straightforward, Advanced, and Complex. *The SAC Classification in Implant Dentistry* was published in 2009, and it immediately became clear that this approach to classifying treatment risk when planning patient treatment was a tool many dentists had been waiting for. Applying the SAC approach to the evaluation of patient-related risk factors and treatment modifiers has since become a standard procedure for many practitioners, contributing to a higher degree of predictability in the execution and outcome of proposed treatment. The SAC classification has been recognized by dental professionals as an objective, evidence-based framework, also making it an invaluable educational tool for both predoctoral and postgraduate training programs.

As dental materials, technology, and clinical techniques have evolved in the intervening years, the ITI decided to review the SAC classification and present it to clinicians in an updated form: a digital book that can be accessed from any device or computer as needed. With its mission to promote and disseminate knowledge covering all aspects of implant dentistry and related tissue regeneration, the ITI recommends this SAC Assessment Tool to all professionals in the field.

Charlotte Stilwell
ITI President

Daniel Wismeijer
Chairman, ITI Education Committee

Acknowledgments

It may be trite, but it is true: projects such as this do not succeed without the commitment and hard work of a large team of people. Consequently, we would like to acknowledge the following people and groups.

The ITI Board of Directors trusted us to update one of the ITI's crown jewels – the SAC Classification. This is a heady responsibility, as we know that the SAC Classification is widely used and respected by clinicians in implant dentistry. We thank the Board for their trust and support.

The staff at the ITI Headquarters have supported us throughout the project. From the events team that organized our meetings, to the Communications and Education teams for providing material, all have worked cheerfully and willingly to help us. Of special note: many thanks to Kati Benthaus and Katalina Cano, our project managers, who have guided us through the process.

Thanks must go to Stefan Keller and his fellow IT wizards at FERN who have turned our dreams of what we would like to do with the online tool into reality.

Thanks also to Änne Kappeler and the team at Quintessence. Their professionalism and patience have allowed us to produce something that we can all be truly proud of.

Of course, we could not have done anything without the support of our colleagues on the Consensus Group who met in Zurich and Berlin and who toiled tirelessly to develop the framework for the new tool. Thanks also to the members of the ITI Education Committee and all the others who acted as our beta testers, and to those who have contributed material to this book. The quality of the group-achieved outcome is much, much more than the sum of the contributing parts.

And finally, but most importantly, we must thank our wives, children and families for their understanding and support. We could not have done this without you.

Anthony Dawson William C. Martin Waldemar D. Polido

Editors / Authors

Anthony Dawson, BDS, MDS, FRACDS
Associate Professor in Prosthodontics
School of Dentistry and Medical Sciences
Charles Sturt University
346 Leeds Parade
Orange, New South Wales 2800
Australia
Email: tdawson@csu.edu.au

William C. Martin, DMD, MS, FACP
Clinical Professor and Director
Center for Implant Dentistry
Department of Oral and Maxillofacial Surgery
College of Dentistry
University of Florida
1395 Center Drive, Rm D7-6
Gainesville, Florida 32610
United States of America
Email: wmartin@dental.ufl.edu

Waldemar D. Polido, DDS, MS, PhD
Clinical Professor, Department of Oral and
Maxillofacial Surgery and Hospital Dentistry
Co-Director, Center for Implant, Esthetic and
Innovative Dentistry
Indiana University School of Dentistry
1121 W Michigan St, DS 109C
Indianapolis, Indiana 46202
United States of America
Email: wdpolido@iu.edu

Contributors

Daniel Buser, DMD, Dr med dent
Professor Emeritus
University of Bern

Buser & Frei Center for Implantology
Werkgasse 2
3018 Bern
Switzerland
Email: danbuser@mac.com

Paolo Casentini, DDS, DMD
Private practice
Studio Dr Paolo Casentini
(Implantology, Oral Surgery, Periodontology, Esthetic Dentistry)
Via Anco Marzio 2
20123 Milano MI
Italy
Email: paolocasentini@fastwebnet.it

Vivianne Chappuis, PhD, DMD
Professor
Department of Oral Surgery and Stomatology
School of Dental Medicine
University of Bern
Freiburgstrasse 7
3010 Bern
Switzerland
Email: vivianne.chappuis@zmk.unibe.ch

Stephen Chen, MDSc, PhD
Faculty of Medicine, Dentistry and Health Sciences
Melbourne Dental School
The University of Melbourne
720 Swanston Street
Carlton, Victoria 3053
Australia
Email: schen@periomelbourne.com.au

Matteo Chiapasco, MD
Professor
Unit of Oral Surgery
Department of Biomedical, Surgical, and Dental Sciences
University of Milan
Via della Commenda 10
20122 Milano MI
Italy
Email: matteo.chiapasco@unimi.it

Anthony J. Dickinson, OAM, BDSc, MSD, FRACDS
1564 Malvern Road
Glen Iris, Victoria 3146
Australia
Email: ajd1@i-pros.com.au

Luiz H. Gonzaga, DDS, MS
Clinical Associate Professor
Center for Implant Dentistry
Department of Oral and Maxillofacial Surgery
College of Dentistry
University of Florida
1395 Center Drive, Rm D7-6
Gainesville, Florida 32610-0434
United States of America
Email: lgonzaga@dental.ufl.edu

Stefan Keller Babotai, Dr sc nat
FERN Media Solutions GmbH
Weiherallee 11B
8610 Uster
Switzerland
Email: stefan.keller@fern.ch

Johannes Kleinheinz, MD, DDS
Professor
Department of Cranio-Maxillofacial Surgery
University Hospital Münster
Albert-Schweitzer-Campus 1
48149 Münster
Germany
Email: johannes.kleinheinz@ukmuenster.de

Wei-Shao Lin, DDS, FACP, PhD
Associate Professor
Interim Chair, Department of Prosthodontics
Program Director, Advanced Education Program in Prosthodontics
Indiana University School of Dentistry
1121 W Michigan St, DS-S406
Indianapolis, Indiana 46202
United States of America
Email: weislin@iu.edu

Dean Morton, BDS, MS, FACP
Professor
Department of Prosthodontics
Director, Center for Implant, Esthetic, and Innovative Dentistry
Indiana University School of Dentistry
1121 W Michigan St
Indianapolis, Indiana 46202
United States of America
Email: deamorto@iu.edu

Ali Murat Kökat, DDS, PhD
Prosthodontist
Private Practice
Valikonağı St 159/5
Nisantasi 34363 Sisli
Istanbul
Turkey
Email: alimurat@outlook.com

Mario Roccuzzo, DMD
Lecturer in Periodontology
Division of Maxillofacial Surgery
University of Turin
Corso Bramante 88
10126 Torino
Italy
and
Adjunct Clinical Assistant Professor
Department of Periodontics and Oral Medicine
University of Michigan
1011 N University Avenue
Ann Arbor, Michigan 48109-1078
United States of America
and
Private Practice Limited to Periodontology
Corso Tassoni 14
10143 Torino
Italy
Email: mroccuzzo@icloud.com

Charlotte Stilwell, DDS
Specialist Dental Services
94 Harley Street
London W1G 7HX
United Kingdom
Email: charlotte.stilwell@iti.org

Alejandro Treviño Santos, DDS, MSc
Postdoctoral and Research Division
Faculty of Dentistry
Department of Prosthodontics and Implantology
National Autonomous University of Mexico
Prolongación Reforma 1190
05349, Santa Fe
Ciudad de México
Mexico
Email: aletresan@hotmail.com

Daniel Wismeijer, PhD, DMD
Private Practice
Zutphensestraatweg 26
6955 AH Ellecom
Netherlands
Email: Danwismeijer@gmail.com

Table of Contents

CHAPTER 1:

Introduction to the Updated SAC Classification

A. DAWSON, W. MARTIN, W. D. POLIDO

1.1 Introduction

Implant dentistry is an integral part of modern dental practice, providing a strong evidence-based option for the rehabilitation of partially and completely edentulous patients. Clinical and technologic advancements in this field have increased the level of confidence that clinicians have in this form of therapy and have also led to a broader base of incorporation into daily practice. What was once the domain of specialist practice is now a common treatment modality in many, if not most, general practices. This has increased the need for all clinicians involved with the field of implant dentistry, irrespective of specialty, to be able to provide therapy at an appropriate level of care.

It has long been recognized that clinical situations present with different levels of difficulty and with different degrees of risk for esthetic, restorative, and surgical complications. Despite the advances in knowledge and improved techniques, implant dentistry is not free from risks of complications or suboptimal outcomes. Over the last decade, research in this field has increasingly provided information regarding the risks associated with this treatment option. The successful osseointegration of an implant is no longer the primary focus of treatment. Rather, the range of potential problems with implants and their related prostheses has come into sharper focus. It is in this environment that the SAC classification has evolved to assist practitioners in recognizing risk factors and providing appropriate levels of care.

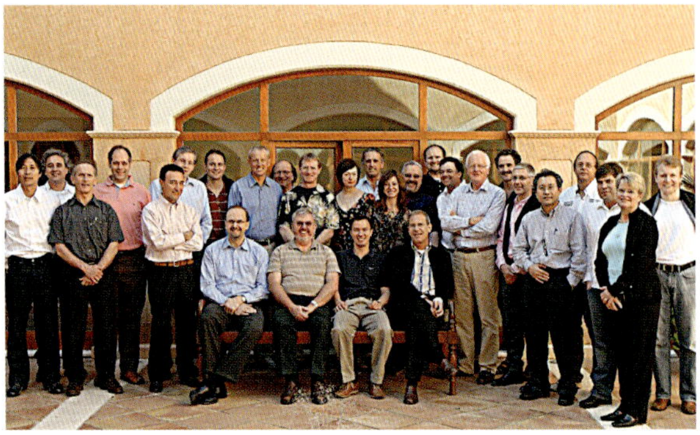

Fig 1. The participants of the SAC Consensus Conference held by the ITI in Palma de Mallorca in March 2007. (Source: The SAC Classification in Implant Dentistry, 2009).

1.2 Historical Background

The concept of assessing risk factors in implant dentistry has attracted considerable attention since the early 1990s, when the number of clinicians placing and restoring implants increased significantly. With this increase in use, the number of associated complications also increased.

Renouard and Rangert (1999) published a classification system that addressed the risk factors involved with the surgical and restorative phases of implant rehabilitation. At that time, they affirmed that some risk factors are relative, while others are absolute. The distinction between the two is not as clear as it might appear. However, several relative contraindications or one absolute contraindication should lead to a reevaluation of the original treatment plan. Although they were using terms like "OK," "Caution," and "Danger," and using the green, yellow, and red colors associated with increased risk factors, an integrated decision tree was not present.

The term *SAC*, with the associated risk factor classification and color scheme, was first used by its two creators, Sailer and Pajarola (1999), in an atlas of oral surgery, with the intent to classify risk factors for general dentists practicing dentoalveolar surgery. The authors described in detail various clinical situations for procedures in oral surgery, such as the removal of third molars, and proposed the classification S = *Simple*, A = *Advanced*, and C = *Complex*. This concept was then adopted in 1999 by the Swiss Society of Oral Implantology (SSOI) during a 1-week congress on quality guidelines in dentistry. The working group of the SSOI developed this SAC classification from a surgical and prosthetic point of view for various clinical situations in implant dentistry. This SAC classification was then adopted by the International Team for Implantology (ITI) in 2003 during the ITI Consensus Conference in Gstaad, Switzerland. The surgical SAC classification was presented in the proceedings of this conference (Buser et al, 2004). The ITI Education Core Group decided in 2006 to slightly modify the original classification by changing the term *Simple* to *Straightforward*.

In March 2007, the ITI held a consensus conference in Palma de Mallorca in Mallorca, Spain aimed at improving on the SAC classification (Figure 1). In its initial form, the SAC classification tended to be subjective, as it related the perceived difficulty of the treatment to the individual practitioner. The Mallorca meeting sought to develop a classification scheme that was more structured and objective. The results of this conference were published in an adjunct to the ITI Treatment Guide series in 2009 (Dawson & Chen, 2009). Later in 2009, the ITI developed an SAC Assessment Tool that clinicians could use to determine the normative classification for a case type that they were treating and identify any additional modifying factors that might apply to their own patient's clinical situation.

The participants in the first SAC Conference were as follows: Urs Belser (Switzerland), Daniel Botticelli (Italy), Daniel Buser (Switzerland), Stephen Chen (Australia), Luca Cordaro (Italy), Anthony Dawson (Australia), Anthony Dickinson (Australia), Javier G. Fabrega (Spain), Andreas Feloutzis (Greece), Kerstin Fischer (Sweden), Christoph Hämmerle (Switzerland), Timothy Head (Canada), Frank Higginbottom (USA), Haldun Iplikcioglu (Turkey), Alessandro Januario (Brazil), Simon Jensen (Denmark), Hideaki Katsuyama

(Japan), Christian Krenkel (Austria), Richard Leesungbok (South Korea), Will Martin (USA), Lisa Heitz-Mayfield (Australia), Dean Morton (USA), Helena Rebelo (Portugal), Paul Rousseau (France), Bruno Schmid (Switzerland), Hendrik Terheyden (Germany), Adrian Watkinson (UK), and Daniel Wismeijer (Netherlands).

The 2009 version of the SAC classification scheme has received widespread acceptance in the dental profession and in the realm of dental education (Mattheos et al, 2014), where it has formed the basis of implant dentistry teaching in many predoctoral and postgraduate dental programs.

From its initial release in 2009, clinical techniques, materials, and technology have continued to evolve and, in early 2017, the ITI recognized that there was a need to review the SAC classification to ensure that it was still consistent with contemporary implant practice. A review group met in Zurich in October 2018, and again in Berlin in April 2019, to develop an updated SAC classification scheme. The primary aim of this review was to develop an updated SAC Assessment Tool, as this had been found to be clinicians' favored way of determining the classification of their patients' treatment needs. The publication of this book satisfies the secondary goal of the review: to document the rationale for this SAC Assessment Tool and the evolution of the SAC classification.

1.3 The Review Team

This text documents the proceedings of consensus meetings held by the ITI in 2018 and 2019. The following individuals contributed to the findings of this conference and the content of this publication (Figure 2):

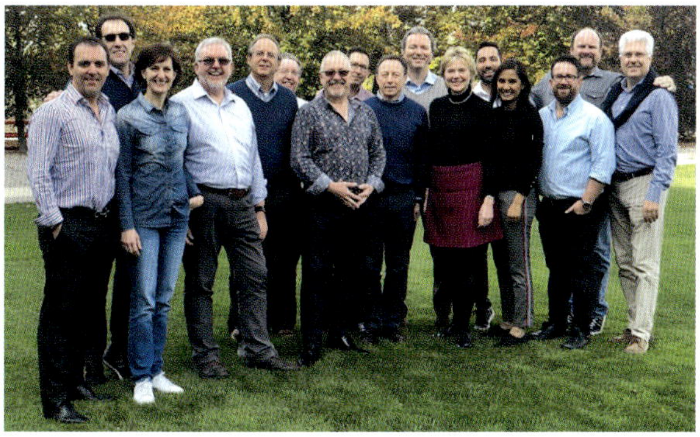

Fig 2. Review team members.

Paolo Casentini	*Italy*	Dean Morton	*USA*
David Cochran	*USA*	Waldemar Polido	*USA*
Anthony Dawson	*Australia*	Lira Rahman	*Switzerland*
Luiz Gonzaga	*USA*	Mario Roccuzzo	*Italy*
Stefan Keller	*Switzerland*	Irena Sailer	*Switzerland*
Thomas Kiss	*Switzerland*	Charlotte Stilwell	*UK*
Johannes Kleinheinz	*Germany*	Mauro Tosta	*Brazil*
Ali Kökat	*Turkey*	Alejandro Treviño Santos	*Mexico*
William Martin	*USA*	Daniel Wismeijer	*Netherlands*

1.4 Potential Roles for the SAC Classification

On its surface, the SAC classification provides an assessment of the potential difficulty and risk of an implant-related treatment for a given clinical situation and serves as a guide for clinicians in both patient selection and treatment planning. In addition, it can also fulfill several additional roles.

Primarily, the classification scheme is aimed at providing clinicians with an objective and evidence-based framework against which they can assess clinical cases regarding the complexity of the planned treatment. This can then be used to assist them in deciding if they possess the necessary skills and knowledge to complete the treatment themselves, or whether referral to a more experienced clinician is indicated. With this capacity, they can build their experience in implant dentistry incrementally and minimize potential risk to their patients. Recently, the current SAC Assessment Tool validity was tested in regard to the agreement level between users, confirming its role as a clinical decision-making tool, as well as a valuable tool for the education of less experienced clinicians (Correia et al, 2020).

The SAC classification can also act as a checklist for more experienced clinicians to help them ensure that all relevant risks have been considered in the patient assessment and treatment planning phases of care.

Communication is a vital part of any step of patient management. In this regard, the SAC classification can aid in communication between clinicians as well as between them and their patients. The classification facilitates communication between colleagues by providing a known framework to exchange information: a shorthand that all involved clinicians are familiar with. When dealing with patients, clinicians can use the SAC classification of their situation to illustrate to patients the complexity and risks associated with their care. As such, it becomes an important tool not only in treatment planning but in the informed consent process as well.

Finally, the SAC classification can aid educators in developing training programs that gradually introduce increasingly more complex cases to their students, allowing an incremental development of knowledge and skill.

1.5 Using this Book

This book is intended to support your use of the SAC Assessment Tool that can be found at www.iti.org. Many sections of this publication are also supported by additional online information from the ITI Academy, the ITI's e-learning platform, including learning modules and assessments, congress lectures, clinical cases, and Consensus Conference papers.

To view this additional material in full and for free, you need to be an ITI Member and logged in at www.iti.org.

Are you an ITI Member?
Please click here to log in to the ITI Academy or scan the QR code below:

Would you like to sign up for ITI membership?
Please click here or scan the QR code below:

Would you like to create a free ITI Academy account? Please click here or scan the QR code below. Please note that only selected items featured in this publication will be available to view on the ITI Academy free of charge.

As soon as you have logged in or have created your free ITI Academy account, and if you are reading the print version of this publication, you can scan QR codes like the one below and will be taken to the corresponding item in the ITI Academy.

If you are an ITI Member and reading the online version of the book on the ITI Academy, you can also click on the link in the text that accompanies each QR code:

The SAC Assessment Tool distills the content of this book in an easy-to-use process that takes you through each step necessary to identify the degree of complexity and potential risk involved in individual clinical cases. To start your assessment, scan the QR code to the left or click on the link.

CHAPTER 2:

The Rationale Behind the Updated SAC Classification

A. DAWSON, C. STILWELL

Please refer to chapter 1, section 1.5 for information on the prerequisites for accessing the additional online information from the ITI Academy via the QR-codes and links provided in this chapter.

Please note that to view this additional material in full and for free, you need to be an ITI Member and logged in at www.iti.org.

2.1 Definitions

Case type: A class of implant-supported prostheses that share similar defining characteristics. For example, implant-supported crowns for single-tooth replacements, or short-span implant-supported fixed dental prostheses replacing three or four teeth and supported by two implants.

Process: The implant dentistry "process" is defined as the full range of issues pertaining to assessment, planning, management of treatment, and subsequent maintenance of the implant and prosthetic reconstruction; it does not merely refer to the clinical treatment procedures that are involved.

Normative classification: In this context, "normative" relates to the classification that conforms to the norm, or standard, for a given clinical situation in implant dentistry. The normative classification relates to the most likely classification of a case type. The final classification of a specific case may differ from the normative classification for the case type as a result of individual risk factors.

Timing of implant placement and loading: Loading and placement protocols have been investigated by the ITI at its last four Consensus Conferences. Hämmerle and coworkers (Hämmerle et al, 2004) defined the timing of implant placement relative to the event of tooth removal in a site, relating this to healing events rather than a specific time frame. This classification is detailed in Table 1.

Table 1 Implant placement protocols (Hämmerle et al, 2004).

Classification	Definition
Type 1	Implant placement immediately following tooth extraction and as part of the same surgical procedure
Type 2	Complete soft tissue coverage of the socket (typically 4 to 8 weeks)
Type 3	Substantial clinical and/or radiographic bone fill of the socket (typically 12 to 16 weeks)
Type 4	Healed site (typically more than 16 weeks)

Review article from the 3rd ITI Consensus Conference on the Placement of Implants in Extraction Sockets by Hämmerle and coworkers (2004).

Implant loading protocols were also the subject of consensus conference reviews. At the Fourth ITI Consensus Conference, Weber and coworkers (Weber et al, 2009) defined the timing of implant loading relative to its placement. These descriptions are summarized in Table 2.

Table 2 Implant loading protocols (Weber et al, 2009).

Classification	Definition
Conventional loading	Greater than 2 months subsequent to implant placement
Early loading	Between 1 week and 2 months subsequent to implant placement
Immediate loading	Earlier than 1 week subsequent to implant placement

Review article from the 4th ITI Consensus Conference on Loading Protocols by Weber and coworkers (2009).

Most recently, the relationships between the timing of implant placement (relative to the time that the tooth in the placement site was extracted) and the timing of loading of the implant with a provisional or definitive prosthesis in partially dentate patients were addressed by Gallucci et al (Gallucci et al, 2018). The outcomes of this review, correlating the evidence for the various combinations of placement and loading protocol, are summarized in Table 3. Protocols that had multiple high-quality studies were deemed scientifically and clinically validated (SCV) and could be seen as suitable for routine use by appropriately trained and experienced clinicians. Clinically documented (CD) approaches had less support in the published literature but did possess reasonable long-term clinical documentation to allow their use in specific situations. Finally, clinically insufficiently documented (CID) protocols lacked sufficient scientific evidence and clinical documentation to be recommended for use. This review built on previous consensus meetings where definitions of the placement and loading protocols were developed.

Table 3 Summary of placement and loading protocols (Gallucci et al, 2018).

	Loading protocol		
	Immediate restoration/loading (Type A)	Early loading (Type B)	Conventional loading (Type C)
Implant placement protocol			
Immediate placement (Type 1)	Type 1A CD	Type 1B CD	Type 1C SCV
Early placement (Type 2–3)	Type 2–3A CID	Type 2–3B CID	Type 2–3C SCV
Late placement (Type 4)	Type 4A CD	Type 4B SCV	Type 4C SCV

Review article from the 6th ITI Consensus Conference on Implant Placement and Loading Protocols in Partially Edentulous Patients by Gallucci and coworkers (2018).

Risk factors: This term refers to any preexisting condition, treatment option, or material choice that may have an adverse effect on the outcome of treatment. These factors have the potential to influence the final SAC classification of a clinical situation.

2.2 Assumptions

This classification assumes that appropriate training, preparation, and care are devoted to the planning and implementation of treatment plans. No classification can adequately address cases or outcomes that deviate significantly from the norm. In addition, it is assumed that clinicians will be practicing within the bounds of their clinical competence and abilities. Thus, within each classification, the following general and specific assumptions are implied:

- Treatment will be provided in an appropriately equipped dental office with an appropriate aseptic technique.
- Adequate clinical and laboratory support is available.
- Patients' medical conditions are appropriately addressed.
- The surgical procedures are planned and provided following recognized protocols.
- The prosthesis is designed, manufactured, and managed correctly.

ITI Learning Module Surgical Setup for Office-Based Implant Surgery by Waldemar Daudt Polido.

2.3 Is the Clinician a Risk Factor?

With the increasing popularity of dental implant treatments with both patients and dental practitioners, the risks associated with the clinician are often overlooked. Derks and coworkers (Derks et al, 2016) described a situation where implant complications from peri-implantitis were significantly correlated with the level of experience of the dentist who was completing the restorative part of the treatment. In this study of real-world treatments, general dentists were 4.3 times more likely to be associated with a peri-implantitis problem than were restorative specialists. While this result may relate to confounding biases in the data set used in this study, which could not be controlled due to the nature of the data, it is still a somewhat disconcerting statistic.

It is also a concern in connection with the incidence of complaints and medicolegal claims relating to implant treatments that are increasing in many jurisdictions. In some regions, professional indemnity insurers are charging additional premiums for particular groups of practitioners who are participating in implant dentistry. These insurance companies do so on the basis of their own actuarial research, which indicates additional risk associated with these treatments in the hands of specific cohorts of practitioners.

2.3.1 Factors impacting the clinician as a risk factor

2.3.1.1 EXPERIENCE

It is a widely held truism in the surgical disciplines in medicine that a surgeon needs to complete between 50 and 100 procedures to be considered competent. The real evidence for this is somewhat less clear. Jerjes and Hopper (2018) described a number of investigations into the relationship between experience and postoperative outcomes in both medical and dental surgical disciplines. Their review found no consistent relationship between these factors. However, it did find evidence that there was often a threshold level of experience below which surgeons could be expected to have greater incidence of problems, indicating that there was a "learning curve" related to most surgical procedures. This threshold value varied between disciplines and studies.

In a systematic review of the relationship between surgeon experience and implant failure rates, Sendyk and others (Sendyk et al, 2017) noted that this relationship did not correlate with the surgeon's specialty but was significantly related to the number of implants that the surgeon had placed. In an earlier study, Lambert and coworkers (Lambert et al, 1997) found similar outcomes, noting that implant failure rates were two times higher for inexperienced surgeons (ie, who had placed less than 50 implants) compared to those of surgeons who had placed 50 or more implants. They also noted that the first nine implants placed by a surgeon under training where at the greatest risk of failure. These findings could be reasonably accepted as showing a relationship between experience and outcomes in implant treatments.

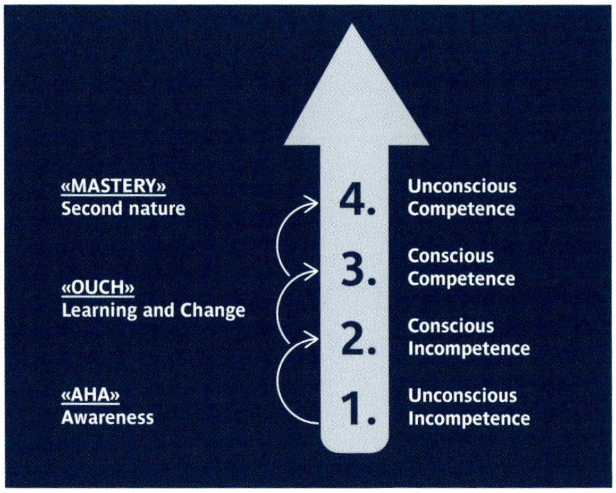

Fig 1. The Conscious Competence Learning Model.

2.3.1.2 TRAINING

Training is another area of consideration. The Conscious Competence Learning Model (Curtiss & Warren, 1973) is an accepted description of how people learn new skills. In this model (Figure 1), four stages of learning are described:

1. **Unconsciously incompetent:** Here the person knows little about what they are doing. They cannot comprehend the potential difficulties involved in a process, and they often feel that they are performing the task to a high standard. They do not know what they do not know, and this is a major impediment to learning.
2. **Consciously incompetent:** The learner comprehends that they fall short of ideal performance and understands their knowledge deficit. Making mistakes at this stage is often a key part of learning.
3. **Consciously competent:** The person at this level of learning can perform the task to an acceptable standard, but this requires concentration and attention to detail.
4. **Unconsciously competent:** The individual at this level has had so much practice that they can perform this task without conscious effort. These people can be good teachers in the technique but can also make the task appear "too easy" to casual observers.

Congress lecture Surgical Treatment of Esthetic Disasters by Waldemar Daudt Polido.

Training in implant dentistry needs to address each of these learner levels. For the *unconsciously incompetent*, clinical training must address their knowledge deficit and stress best-practice approaches to treatment provision. Simulations of treatment provision, and mentoring by more experienced clinicians, can assist the *consciously incompetent* practitioner to pass through this level without endangering patients under their care. Mentoring will also benefit the *consciously competent* clinician by supporting their incremental development of skills. Finally, for the unconsciously competent clinician, training must support their focus on practicing in a reflective and consistent manner. The unconsciously competent clinician is at some risk of complacency and overconfidence and must make a conscious effort to remain focused on current best practices and the evolution of techniques in implant dentistry. They are also something of a risk to less knowledgeable and less skillful colleagues who might observe them providing patient care and conclude that these treatments are more straightforward than they really are.

2.3.1.3 SELF-ASSESSMENT OF ABILITY

Another way of considering this journey of skill development is the so-called "Dunning-Kruger Effect" (Kruger & Dunning, 1999). This describes a form of cognitive bias that leads to individuals overestimating their own ability because they lack sufficient knowledge and understanding of what they are doing to realistically measure their level of skill. It is only through painful discovery of the limitations of their ability that they can begin to learn. This correlates well with the unconsciously incompetent level described above. It is also a potentially dangerous issue with a novice clinician involved in providing a potentially complex treatment to a patient.

2.3.1.4 SHARED LEARNING

Training in implant dentistry is provided at a number of levels. At its simplest, clinicians learn from each other as they progress along the learning curve. This is the process by which most of today's acknowledged "experts" learned these skills in the period during which implant treatments were evolving.

With implant dentistry now an established discipline, learning from shared experience is valuable for clinicians who have a sound understanding of implant treatments. Here, the consciously and unconsciously competent clinicians can benchmark their understanding against that of others.

However, this approach is unlikely to be effective if the individuals (eg, those in the unconsciously incompetent group) sharing their experiences do not fully understand the significance of what these experiences represent. This model is often popular today with younger practitioners who learn from colleagues via online forums, but this represents a real risk of being "the blind leading the blind."

2.3.1.5 SHORT TRAINING COURSES

Similar observations might be made about the short, company-led programs. Often the aim of this training is to make practitioners aware of the processes needed to handle that company's componentry, and thus these programs often focus on the "how" rather than the "why" or "why not." Also, due to the brevity of these courses, the biologic and biomechanical principles involved in implant treatments must be greatly abbreviated or are simply not covered at all. Unfortunately, this method can be fraught with danger to patients and cannot allow for a focus on best-practice protocols, as these concepts may be unknown to those learning.

2.3.1.6 STRUCTURED EDUCATION AND TRAINING

The most effective training comes from structured programs that provide a sound basis for patient selection and treatment. These courses address the basic sciences that underpin successful treatment, introduce protocols for patient assessment and selection and treatment planning, and then provide candidates with the opportunity to perform actual treatment and patient maintenance with assistance and guidance from more experienced mentors. Given the breadth of the topics to be covered, these programs must extend over longer periods compared with other approaches. Thus, these programs can be expensive in terms of time and money and difficult to fit in alongside daily practice, leading to under-utilization of this type of education and training.

Intuitively, one might expect that better-quality training would result in fewer complications or failure. While this is generally accepted in health care, little evidence is available to support these conclusions. Certainly, patients and regulators see this connection as true, and this forms that basic assumption that underpins mandated continuing professional development requirements.

2.3.2 Reducing clinician-related risk

2.3.2.1 RECOGNIZING "HUMAN FACTOR" RISKS

What have been described as "human factors" are becoming recognized as sources of error in health care provision. Much of the research in this area comes from the commercial aviation industry, but these findings are beginning to permeate into health care safety considerations.

A second edition of Renouard and Rangert's book about risk factors was published in 2008 (Renouard & Rangert, 2008) and brought the topic of experience and human factors to the discussion.

In a recent review of these factors and their influence in dental implantology, Renouard and coworkers (Renouard et al, 2017) described five hazardous attitudes or behaviors that are potentially detrimental to safe practice. Originally identified in aviation, these types are:

1. **Impulsiveness:** The urge to get things done quickly, without necessarily considering potential dangers.
2. **Anti-authority:** The attitude held by some practitioners that rules, regulations, and protocols are for others, and do not pertain to them.
3. **Invulnerability:** Practitioners who believe that adverse outcomes only happen to others, and not to them.
4. **Macho:** The belief that a practitioner must be constantly demonstrating their superiority over others. While this is mostly a male trait, it can affect women as well.
5. **Resignation:** The belief that no matter what a practitioner does, it will not have any effect on the outcome.

2.3.2.2 STRESS AS A RISK FACTOR

Renouard and coworkers also discuss stress as a potential problem. While the stress response is adaptive (ie, it is protective against external threats), it can have negative effects in a health care setting where the stress is mostly self-induced. Stress factors such as time pressures, staff problems, and interpersonal frictions between the dentist and the patient can all have a negative effect on performance. Stress tends to reduce the practitioner's ability to rationally think through a problem and rather promotes the use of automatic responses, which may be incorrect or unhelpful. These factors are well studied in the medical literature as well, as it relates to many daily issues, like less sleep, financial problems, and health or family issues (West et al, 2006).

2.3.2.3 MITIGATING THE HUMAN FACTOR ISSUES

To counter these "human factor" issues, Renouard recommends using techniques that have been developed for the airline industry to address safety problems: so-called "crew resource management." The concept of the "sterile cockpit" where all extraneous activity is banned during high-risk periods, such as take-off and landing, can be transferred to the dental implantology setting for use during critical periods of treatment provision. Strict division of responsibilities between team members also reduces stress and "information overload." Additionally, checklists can be very useful in concentrating attention on critical steps, especially in highly procedural tasks such as those seen in medicine and dentistry. This approach has also been promoted by other authors (Gawande, 2009; Pinsky et al, 2010). Here the SAC classification can be used as a checklist to ensure that all factors relevant to the patient's presentation are assessed and incorporated into treatment plans.

2.3.2.4 CLINICIAN RISK FACTOR IN RELATION TO OTHER SOURCES OF RISKS

The clinician is central to most decisions and their practical application in implant treatment. Risks in implant dentistry can be attributed to four main sources: the patient, the treatment approach, the biomaterials, and the clinician. This relationship between the clinician, the materials, and the patient factors was first described by Chen and Schärer in 1993 (Chen & Schärer, 1993). Further, Buser and Chen (Buser & Chen, 2008), published on a model that also illustrates the potential interactions between these factors, as shown in Figure 2.

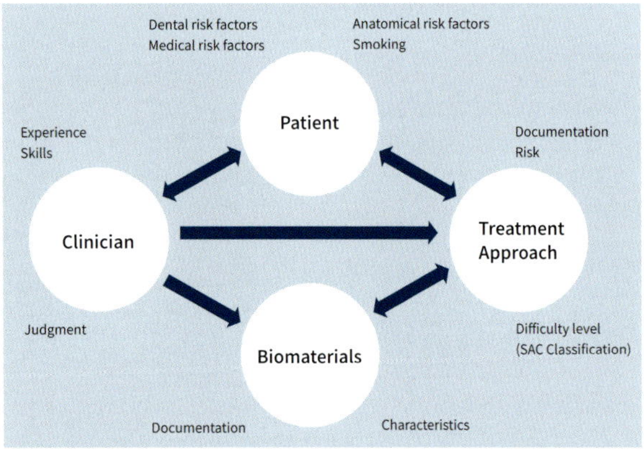

Fig 2. Potential sources of risk (Source: ITI Treatment Guide Vol. 3 "Implant Placement in Post-Extraction Sites")

In this model, the clinician has a potentially disproportionate influence: they select the patient, the treatment approach, and the biomaterials, and they subsequently carry out the treatment on the patient. Thus, a flaw or shortcoming in their knowledge or skills will put their patient at greater risk of adverse outcomes. Therefore, in answer to the question posed earlier, we must conclude that the clinician has the potential to be a significant risk factor.

Can the SAC classification assist in reducing risk? By focusing the attention of the clinician on potential risk factors, it should ensure that the clinician-related risk is mitigated. However, the review group did not believe that the clinician could be considered as a factor in determining the SAC classification for a case, as they were not confident that all clinicians could accurately self-assess their ability. Nonetheless, discussions such as this may assist individuals in progressing along their own learning journey and improve their ability to control this potential risk.

2.4 Classification Rationale

In the 2009 version of the SAC classification (Dawson & Chen, 2009) the main determinants of the classification were:

- The esthetic risk
- The complexity of the process
- The risks of complications

These factors were considered for each of the treatments considered in this publication, and a normative SAC classification was derived for each of these case types. Further modifiers were considered that might increase or decrease the level of complexity or risk, but these did not change the normative classification for the case type.

In this update, the normative classifications have been reviewed, but they have not altered greatly. These are still based on the factors above, with an increased emphasis on the SAC classification as a risk management instrument.

The updated SAC Assessment Tool now allows users to derive a SAC classification for their specific case based on the pattern of risk factors that they report. Risks are considered in four broad areas:

- **General risks:** These are the issues normally identified during anamnesis and the initial clinical assessment and are mostly patient related.
- **Esthetic risk:** Esthetic issues are often the patient's only way of measuring the treatment outcome. This is more than a consideration of "is the treatment site visible during function and/or smiling, and are the peri-implant mucosal tissues visible?" but also includes other factors described by Martin and coworkers (Martin et al, 2017) in their discussion of the esthetic risk assessment for single-tooth implant prostheses. Esthetic risk assessment for more extensive tooth replacement situations have also been considered.
- **Edentulous esthetic risk:** When patients undergo complete loss of teeth, several unique clinical factors specific to this patient subset can have a significant influence on esthetic outcomes. The edentulous esthetic risk assessment will highlight these factors as they influence particular case types.
- **Surgical risk:** Factors influencing the complexity and risk of the surgical phase of treatment.
- **Prosthetic risks:** Factors relating the implant-supported prosthesis; for example, the clinical processes involved, the mode of manufacture, the materials used, and the design employed.

Each of these areas will be considered in more detail later in this book.

CHAPTER 3:

Risks in Implant Dentistry

A. DAWSON, W. MARTIN, W. D. POLIDO

Please refer to chapter 1, section 1.5 for information on the prerequisites for accessing the additional online information from the ITI Academy via the QR codes and links provided in this chapter.

Please note that to view this additional material in full and for free, you need to be an ITI Member and logged in at www.iti.org.

3.1 Principles of Risk Management

All interventions in health care carry some risk of failure, complications, or other suboptimal outcomes. Implant treatments are no different.

The risk management cycle is a term used to define a process aimed at limiting the incidence of adverse outcomes, and their impact.

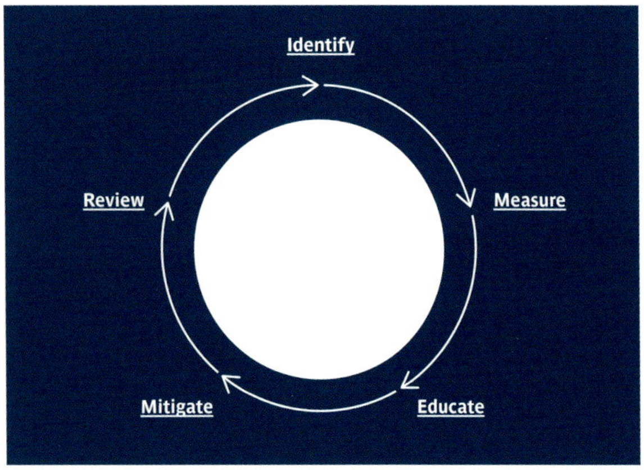

Fig 1. The risk management cycle.

In general, this cycle aims to:

- **Identify** potential problems
- **Measure** the incidence of these adverse outcomes and the impact that they have
- **Educate** users about these potential problems
- Develop strategies to **mitigate** the incidence or effect of these problems
- **Review** the effectiveness of these mitigation strategies

As indicated in Figure 1, this is a continuous process where outcomes are monitored, and refinements are made to mitigation strategies to incrementally improve process outcomes.

In implant dentistry, the users refer to patients and clinicians. However, the process remains the same. Although it is not usually referenced in such terms, effective practice in most areas of health care, including implant dentistry, follow the basic principles of risk management. A common dental practice example of this might be the management of dental caries. Here, our modern preventive approach to caries management centers on identifying risk factors (eg, patient behavior/diet, salivary function, oral microflora, plaque retentive restorations, etc) and measuring their impact. We then can focus on reducing risk by attempting to mitigate these risks through patient education and risk-reduction focused treatments. We then continue to monitor our patient's progress and the success of our interventions.

The importance or severity of a risk can be considered in terms of the likelihood of that risk being realized and the impact or significance associated with the outcome that follows. These situations are often tabulated in a risk matrix, an example of which can be seen in Table 1.

While we often concentrate our efforts on mitigating the risks of high-impact outcomes, like implant failure, it must also be noted that less dire outcomes that are more common, such as peri-implant disease, may be more important.

Table 1 An example of a risk matrix.

LIKELIHOOD \ IMPACT	Negligible	Minor	Moderate	Significant	Severe
Verly Likely	Low Med	Medium	Med Hi	High	High
Likely	Low	Low Med	Medium	Med Hi	High
Possible	Low	Low Med	Medium	Med Hi	Med Hi
Unlikely	Low	Low Med	Low Med	Medium	Med Hi
Very Unlikely	Low	Low	Low Med	Medium	Medium

3.2 The SAC Classification as a Risk Management Tool

The SAC classification is essentially a tool that assists practitioners to identify risks so that they can educate their patients about these potential problems as part of the informed consent process. Clinicians then use their understanding of these risks to plan treatments that minimize risk. Patients are then monitored after the completion of treatment to identify problems that might arise as early as possible, thus allowing intervention to minimize the impact of the problem on the ongoing quality of treatment outcomes.

This review of the SAC classification system incorporated this risk-management focus on risk identification, the likelihood of this problem arising, and the potential impacts of these risks on treatment outcome. Three subgroups in the review team each looked at one major area of risk factors. A "Systems" group reviewed general patient-related risk factors and worked to develop concepts in the SAC Assessment Tool workflow and algorithm. The "Surgical" and "Prosthetic" groups looked at surgical and restorative risk factors respectively, concentrating on risks associated with the treatment approach and technologies. The results from the deliberations of these groups represent a consensus opinion of the risk factors most likely to influence dental implant treatments.

3.3 General Risks

A. DAWSON, J. KLEINHEINZ, A. MURAT KÖKAT, D. WISMEIJER

A structured approach to patient assessment and treatment planning aims to identify all factors that have the potential to have some impact or influence on our treatment. Such a structured approach has been promoted by the ITI in its Academy Learning Module "Structured Assessment and Treatment Planning" (Weber, 2015), and the sequence and steps in this process are illustrated in Figure 2.

ITI Learning Module Structured Assessment and Treatment Planning by Hans-Peter Weber.

Identification of potential risk factors occurs relatively early in this process—during the information-gathering phase that incorporates anamnesis, clinical examination, imaging, and other investigations.

Identification of general risk factors is almost always done in the anamnesis and clinical examination. These factors relate to potential problems arising out of the patient's medical and dental history and their presenting condition. These general factors fall into three main clusters:

- Patient medical factors
- Patient-related attitudinal/behavioral factors
- Site-related factors

3.3.1 Patient medical factors

Most implant patients present with a range of historical and ongoing medical issues that may have an impact on implant treatment. The following were considered the most significant.

3.3.1.1 MEDICAL FITNESS

A patient's current health status has the potential to influence their fitness to undergo treatment, and also how well they will heal after implant surgery.

The American Society of Anesthesiologists (ASA) has developed a physical status classification and risk management tool that is widely used to assess patients' fitness for surgical interventions. The ASA Physical Status classification system (Doyle et al, 2019) is detailed in Table 2.

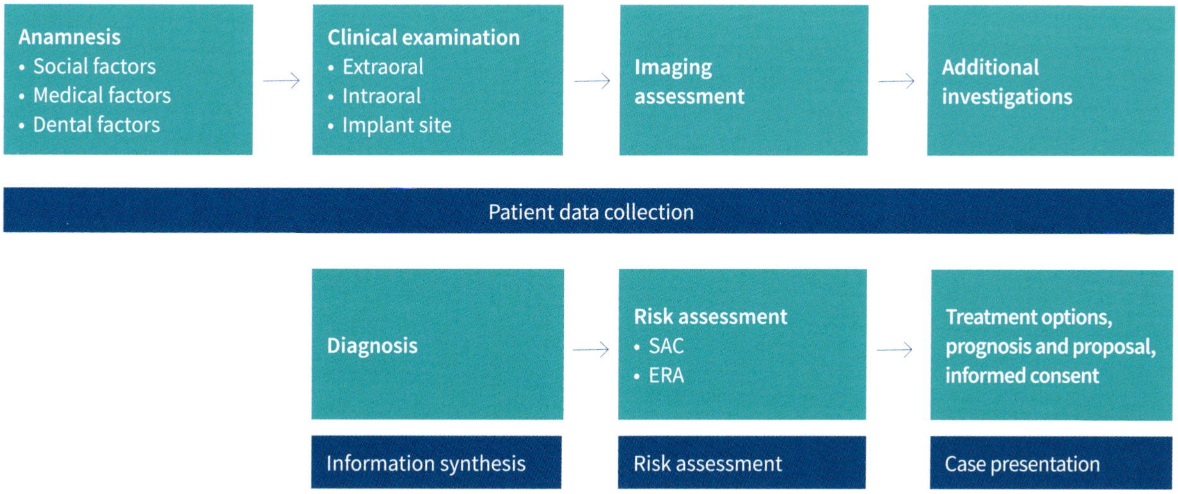

Fig 2. A structured approach to patient assessment and treatment planning.

Table 2 The ASA Physical Status Classification.

ASA PS Classiciation	Definition
ASA I	A normal healthy patient
ASA II	A patient with mild systemic disease
ASA III	A patient with severe systemic disease
ASA IV	A patient with severe systemic disease that is a constant threat to life
ASA V	A moribund patient who is not expected to survive without the operation
ASA VI	A declared brain-dead patient whose organs are being removed for donor purposes

Healthy patients (ASA I) and those with mild, well-controlled systemic disease (ASA II) are generally good candidates for implant surgery. Some patients identified as ASA III (severe systemic disease that may or may not be well controlled) can be treated with care but have higher risk and might best be managed by highly trained and experienced clinicians. While there may be some occasional indications for implant treatment in ASA IV cases, these treatments are high risk and should be restricted to specialist facilities where emergency medical care is readily available, and by highly experienced surgical teams.

ITI Learning Module Patient Medical Factors by Simon Storgård Jensen.

Medical status may also impact the speed of implant healing (usually a slowdown) and the esthetic outcome of treatments. For example, conditions associated with abnormal scarring after surgery, such as the development of keloid scars, may impact esthetic outcomes.

3.3.1.2 MEDICATIONS

Pharmaceutically active substances include prescription medications, over-the-counter medicines, herbal remedies, dietary supplements, and recreational substances. All of these may have an influence on implant treatment either directly through their influence on implant healing and/or peri-implant tissue health, or indirectly through their effects on the patient's behavior.

Review article from the 6th ITI Consensus Conference on Medication-Related Dental Implant Failure by Vivianne Chappuis and coworkers (2017).

ITI Learning Module Pharmacology with Relevance to Dental Implant Therapy by Stephen Barter.

Possibly of most importance relating to implant surgery are the antiresorptive drugs used to manage osteoporosis. These medications have been linked to a condition known as medication-related osteonecrosis of the jaws (MRONJ) that can also arise following surgical interventions involving the facial skeleton (Figure 3). The risk of MRONJ arising is related to the type of medication (usually biphosphonates), the dosage used and the duration of therapy (as some types of antiresorptives accumulate in facial bones). Antiresorptives with higher potency are usually administered via intravenous route, and hence they are associated with greater risk. This condition can be very difficult to treat and is usually associated with significant discomfort and disfigurement. In cases where there is a history of intravenous treatment, such as in patients with metastatic bone disease or Paget's Disease, the risks are such that implant treatment would normally be contraindicated.

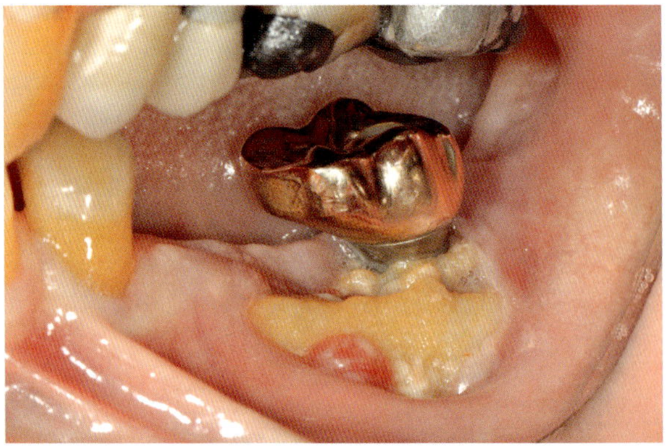

Fig 3. MRONJ associated with an implant in the mandibular left molar region.

3.3.1.3 RADIATION

Radiotherapy can have a dramatically adverse effect on bone healing. Osteoradionecrosis can arise following surgery in irradiated bone due to the reduction in blood supply to affected bone. This effect is dose related. The dosage to the area where implant placement is planned is the significant consideration, rather than the dosage used to treat the cancer. Doses of less than 50 Gray may allow implant placement with care. Doses of greater than 50 Gray to the area of interest would likely contraindicate implant placement. Time after radiation therapy, and presence of other coadjutant factors, such as smoking and oral hygiene can also impact the rate of occurrence of osteoradionecrosis of the jaws (Aarup-Kristensen et al, 2019).

3.3.1.4 GROWTH STATUS

Implants act in a similar way to ankylosed teeth to retard the development of surrounding bone. As such, placement of implants in growing individuals is normally contraindicated. These implant-supported prostheses can become unesthetic and/or nonfunctional due to apparent infraocclusion as a

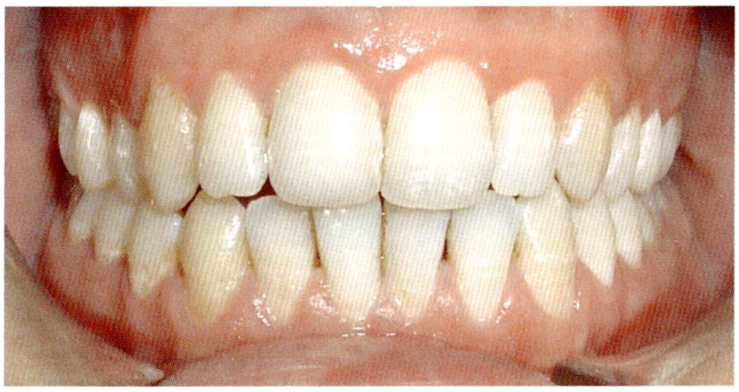

Fig 4. Five-year follow-up of an implant-supported crown replacing the maxillary right central incisor.

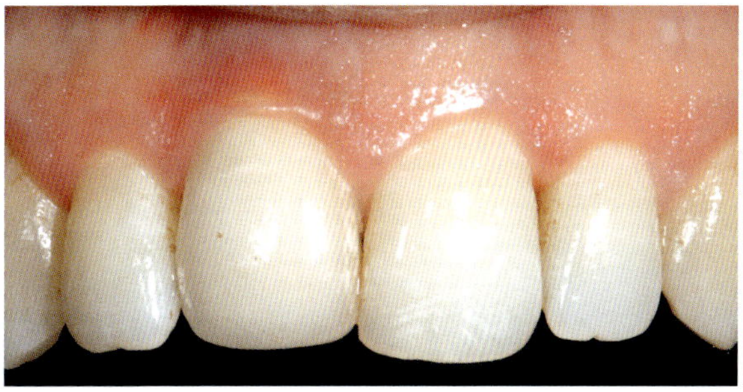

Fig 5. 15-year follow-up. Note the difference in incisal edge between implant-supported crown and adjacent natural teeth, due to continuous growth and extrusion of natural teeth.

result of the continued growth of the alveolar bone supporting adjacent teeth. This issue can also arise in older patients, as facial growth can continue—albeit at a very slow rate—well into maturity. The following case demonstrates the esthetic issues that can arise. An implant-supported crown replacing the maxillary right central incisor 5 years after placement in a 24-year-old male patient is seen in Figure 4. Ten years later, there is a significant difference in incisal edge position between the implant-supported crown and the adjacent natural teeth, due to continuous growth and extrusion of natural teeth. The implant crown remained stable (Figure 5).

3.3.2 Patient attitudes/behaviors

3.3.2.1 SMOKING HABIT

Tobacco smoking is related to increased risks of implant failure and peri-implant disease (Heitz-Mayfield & Huynh-Ba, 2009). There is some evidence of a dose-related effect, and that this is mediated by nicotine and other tobacco-derived chemicals that compromise wound healing, the immune response, and increase the risk of scarring. Ideally, patients should cease smoking prior to implant placement, as there is evidence that reducing their smoking habit acts to reduce risk. There is a paucity of evidence relating cannabis use or vaping (electronic cigarettes) to implant failure, but caution is advised when treating patients practicing these habits.

Review article from the 4th ITI Consensus Conference on History of Treated Periodontitis and Smoking as Risks for Implant Therapy by Lisa J. A. Heitz-Mayfield and Guy Huynh-Ba (2009).

3.3.2.2 COMPLIANCE

A patient's willingness and/or ability to comply with instructions is an important factor in any complex treatment where maintenance is vital to long-term success, and where following instructions is essential for optimal treatment outcomes in the short term. Noncompliant patients are more likely to experience problems with treatment and are less likely to follow the necessary steps to overcome these issues. Poor compliance might best be considered relative contraindication for implant therapy until the patient can become motivated to support their treatment.

3.3.2.3 ORAL HYGIENE

Bacterial biofilm accumulation has been associated with the development of peri-implant mucositis and peri-implantitis (Salvi & Zitzmann, 2014), and measures to regularly remove these deposits are the prime strategy for preventing the development of these biologic complications. If patients are unwilling or unable to perform these oral hygiene procedures, implant therapy should be delayed until they can do so. Alternatively, other forms of prosthetic reconstruction might best be considered.

Review article from the 5th ITI Consensus Conference on the Effects of Anti-infective Preventive Measures on the Occurrence of Biologic Implant Complications and Implant Loss by Giovanni E. Salvi and Nicola U. Zitzmann (2014).

3.3.2.4 PATIENT EXPECTATIONS

Unrealized expectations are often the trigger of patient complaints to statutory bodies, or to initiation of legal proceedings against treating practitioners. This risk is only amplified by the expense and invasiveness of implant treatment.

Communicating realistic expectations to patients, and managing their desired outcomes, is an important part of the ongoing consent process. A patient may have high and realistic expectations due to their social position or employment, and managing these situations can be challenging. Patients may also have unrealistic expectations, and managing these can often be virtually impossible. An extreme example of such a situation might involve a patient with body dysmorphic disorder. Unless these expectations can be managed, it is best not to proceed with implant rehabilitation.

3.3.3 Site-related factors

3.3.3.1 PERIODONTAL STATUS

A history of treated periodontal disease has been associated with an increased risk of biologic complications (Heitz-Mayfield & Huynh-Ba, 2009), as has the presence of active periodontal disease with periodontal pockets greater than 5 mm in depth. As an elective rehabilitative treatment, an implant-supported prostheses should not be considered until all active oral diseases are under control. Where implant treatment is planned, treatment to manage the periodontal disease prior to implant placement is mandatory.

Review article from the 4th ITI Consensus Conference on the History of Treated Periodontitis and Smoking as Risks for Implant Therapy by Lisa J. A. Heitz-Mayfield and Guy Huynh-Ba (2009).

3.3.3.2 ACCESS

Implant treatment involves the use of instruments that can occupy more physical space than conventional handpieces. During surgical procedures, the use of templates in conjunction with the surgical handpiece, twist drills, and drivers can consume more vertical space, requiring a large mouth opening by the patient. If there is insufficient space, treatment cannot proceed without changes to instrumentation. Limited (but adequate) space can make treatment more difficult, but insufficient space will need adjunctive treatment to make more space if implant placement and restoration is still desired. The use of a measuring device (such as the Straumann Diagnostic-T; Figure 6) during the consultation visit can assist in identifying situations where access will be difficult. This device identifies the amount of space needed to fit the head of the handpiece with the shortest Straumann kit twist drill (33 mm) at the site of planned implant placement.

3.3.3.3 PREVIOUS SURGERIES IN THE PLANNED IMPLANT SITE

Previous surgeries in the site of a planned implant can result in hard and soft tissue changes that may complicate implant placement and healing. Scarring from these surgeries (Figures 7 and 8) is also often associated with reduced vascularity that may have a negative influence on healing. While a single previous surgical treatment in a site may only have a small impact, multiple surgeries are likely to significantly increase the risk of problems.

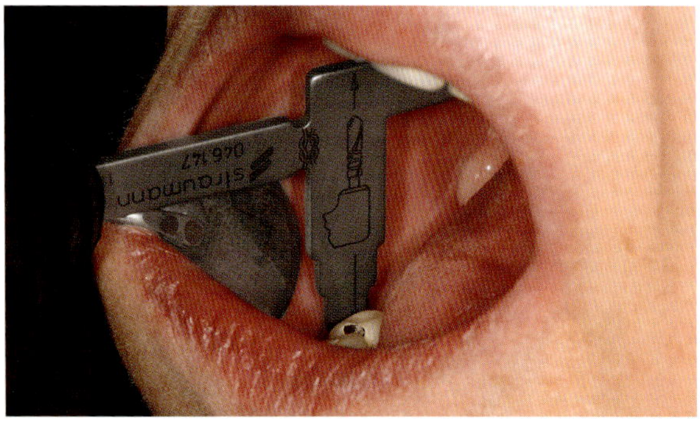

Fig 6. Clinical use of a Diagnostic-T (Straumann, Basel, Switzerland) to assess available space for surgical instrumentation.

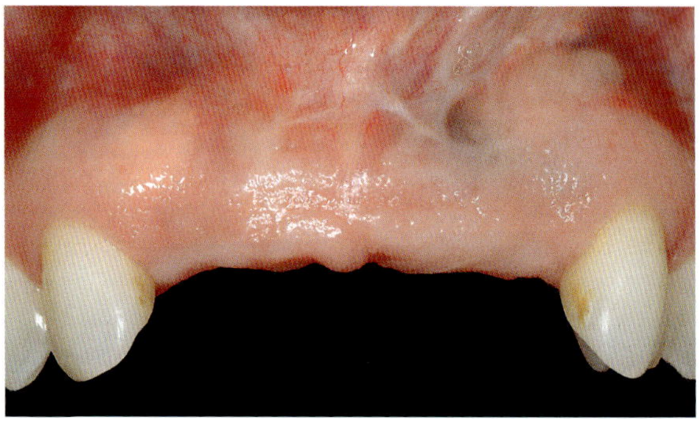

Fig 7. Clinical evaluation of patient missing maxillary central and lateral incisors with evidence of previous surgical procedures.

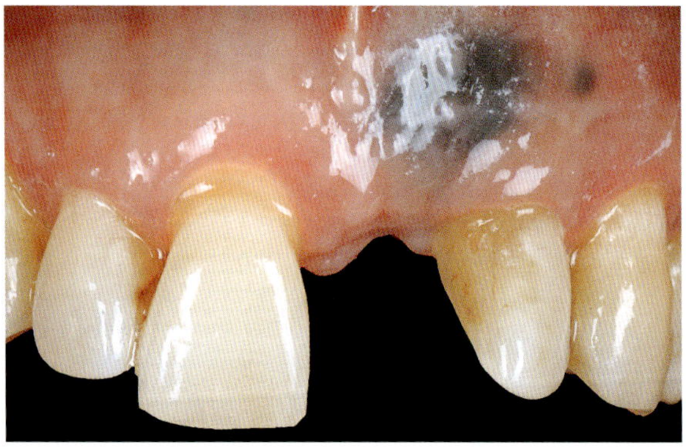

Fig 8. Clinical evaluation of patient missing tooth 21 with evidence of previous surgical procedures.

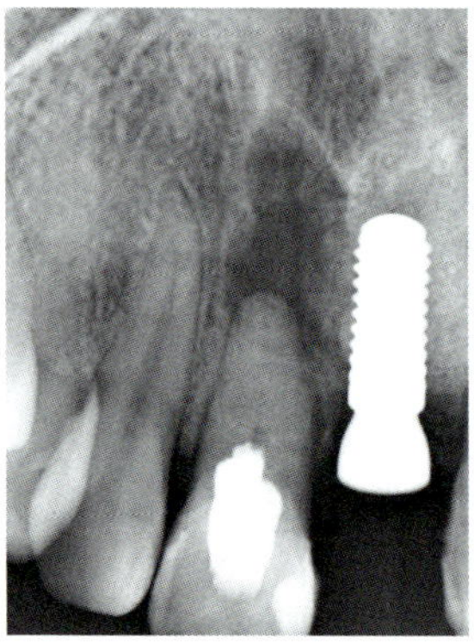

Fig 9. An apical infection adjacent to a recently placed implant can infect this site as well.

3.3.3.4 NEARBY PATHOLOGY

As a general rule, elective treatments such as implant therapy are only provided once all other pathologic conditions have been managed. However, there are situations where this may not be either possible or practical. Notwithstanding this, pathologies that may have an adverse effect on implant healing, or the risk of biologic complications, must be managed before implants are placed. For example, apical periodontitis affecting a tooth in another quadrant might be managed simultaneously with implant treatment. However, apical periodontitis related to a nonvital tooth adjacent to the planned implant site (Figure 9) must be managed prior to implant placement.

3.4 Esthetic Risk

W. MARTIN, V. CHAPPUIS, D. MORTON, D. BUSER

Esthetic issues apply where the implant restoration and the surrounding mucosal margin will be visible during normal functional activity or when the patient smiles. Smiles are as unique to individuals as the treatment necessary to maintain their natural appearance. Implant therapy in the esthetic zone can be a challenging process, as patient demands on esthetics coupled with preexisting deficiencies in the anatomy can present obstacles to obtain ideal results. Failure to achieve esthetic and functional results with dental implants could lead to disastrous situations that would require additional surgical and restorative procedures in an attempt to correct the compromise (Buser et al, 2004; Levine et al, 2014).

Consequently, not all implant treatments will have associated esthetic risk. It is therefore important for clinicians to understand their patient's desires and to perform a thorough initial clinical examination to highlight any potential obstacles that may present as a challenge in achieving an ideal esthetic outcome. Clinicians performing a rehabilitation must have a thorough understanding of tissue biology and the knowledge of all treatment modalities for a given clinical situation, as dental implants may not always be the primary choice. This series of modifiers has been discussed in detail in Chapter 3: "Preoperative Risk Assessment and Treatment Planning for Optimal Esthetic Outcomes" (W. Martin, V. Chappuis, D. Morton, D. Buser) found in "The ITI Treatment Guide, Volume 10: Implant Therapy in the Esthetic Zone: Current Treatment Modalities and Materials for Single-tooth Replacements" (Chappuis & Martin, 2017).

ITI Treatment Guide Vol. 10 Extended Edentulous Spaces in the Esthetic Zone: Current Treatment Modalities and Materials for Single-tooth Replacements by Vivianne Chappuis and Will Martin.

ITI Learning Module Esthetic Risk Assessment by William Christopher Martin.

Table 3 lists the factors that determine esthetic risk in the partially edentulous patient. The esthetic risk assessment (ERA) table was developed to assist clinicians in the diagnosis and planning of treatment in the esthetic zone and to identify clinical situations that could contribute to an esthetic compromise, thus assisting the clinician in determining the SAC classification of the case. It should be noted that, by definition, a case for which there is some esthetic risk (ie, the restoration margin is visible) would have a classification of at least *Advanced*.

Congress Lecture Pre-treatment Analytics to Maximize Longevity of Treatment Outcomes in the Esthetic Zone by William Christopher Martin.

3.4.1 Medical status and smoking habit

The impact of medical issues such as health status and smoking relate primarily to the predictability of the healing process. These issues have been discussed previously.

3.4.2 Gingival display at full smile

The level to which the planned implant restoration and its surrounding mucosal tissue is exposed during function and smiling is a major factor, defining whether the site is considered esthetic or nonesthetic. Special consideration should be given to the assessment of the position of the lip line and subsequent display of teeth, gingival tissues, and papillae and their potential impact on esthetic risk. Greater exposure of this area is associated with increasing esthetic risk. If soft and hard tissue defects exist that cannot be addressed surgically, prosthetic planning for gingival tissue replacement should be initiated before placing the dental implant(s). Situations associated with soft and hard tissue defects show the highest degree of complexity and thus the highest risk of esthetic failure.

Table 3 Esthetic Risk Assessment (ERA; taken from: "ITI Treatment Guide, Volume 10: Implant Therapy in the Esthetic Zone: Current Treatment Modalities and Materials for Single-tooth Replacements" [Chappuis & Martin, 2017])

Esthetic risk factors	Level of risk		
	Low	Medium	High
Medical status	Healthy, uneventful healing		Compromised healing
Smoking habit	Nonsmoker	Light smoker (≤ 10 cigs/day)	Heavy smoker (> 10 cigs/day)
Gingival display at full smile	Low	Medium	High
Width of edentulous span	1 tooth (≥ 7 mm)[1] 1 tooth (≥ 6 mm)[2]	1 tooth (< 7 mm)[1] 1 tooth (< 6 mm)[2]	2 teeth or more
Shape of tooth crowns	Rectangular		Triangular
Restorative status of neighboring teeth	Virgin		Restored
Gingival phenotype	Low-scalloped, thick	Medium-scalloped, medium-thick	High-scalloped, thin
Infection at implant site	None	Chronic	Acute
Soft tissue anatomy	Soft tissue intact		Soft tissue defects
Bone level at adjacent teeth	≤ 5 mm to contact point	5.5 to 6.5 mm to contact point	≥ 7 mm to contact point
Facial bone wall phenotype*	Thick-wall phenotype, ≥ 1 mm thickness		Thin-wall phenotype, < 1 mm thickness
Bone anatomy at alveolar crest	No bone deficiency	Horizontal bone deficiency	Vertical bone deficiency
Patient's esthetic expectations	Realistic expectations		Unrealistic expectations

[1] Standard-diameter implant, regular connection
[2] Narrow-diameter implant, narrow connection
*If 3D imaging is available with the tooth in place

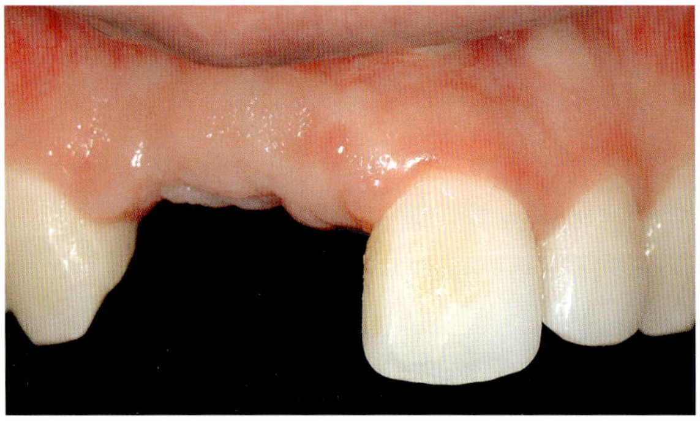

Fig 10. An extended edentulous situation highlighting a deficiency in soft and hard tissue support for implant restorations.

3.4.3 Width of the edentulous space

See also 3.7.1.1. Prosthetic volume.

When evaluating edentulous spaces for restoration, careful attention should be given to the materials planned to replace the missing tooth structure and their space requirements for long-term durability. As the interdental and interroot space decreases, the implant and restorative component options become limited, and the prosthetic volume for ideal restoration emergence and contours suffer, increasing the esthetic risk. When the edentulous space increases to include multiple missing teeth, the esthetic risk also increases due to the unpredictable nature of the interimplant soft and hard tissue support and the increased difficulty to maintain symmetric mucosal contours (Mirtrani et al, 2005; Mankoo, 2008). Esthetic risk can also be influenced by the location of the adjacent missing teeth, as extended spaces lateral to the midline increase the difficulty of maintaining harmonious tissue contours and restoration symmetry. Patients with adjacent missing teeth, including a lateral incisor, present a maximum esthetic risk when adjacent implants are planned (Figure 10).

ITI Learning Module Esthetic Planning for Implant-supported Fixed Dental Prostheses by Daniel S. Thoma.

Congress Lecture How to be Successful in Replacing Multiple Missing Adjacent Teeth in the Esthetic Zone by Hans-Peter Weber.

ITI Treatment Guide Vol. 6 Extended Edentulous Spaces in the Esthetic Zone by Julia-Gabriela Wittneben Matter and Hans-Peter Weber.

When combined with additional risk factors such as high lip line or a thin gingival phenotype, the placement of adjacent implants in extended edentulous areas in the anterior maxilla often represents a maximum esthetic risk. Site development for patients in this category is often mandatory before or during implant placement. The results of such procedures vary, with horizontal augmentation gains often superior to gains achieved in the vertical dimension.

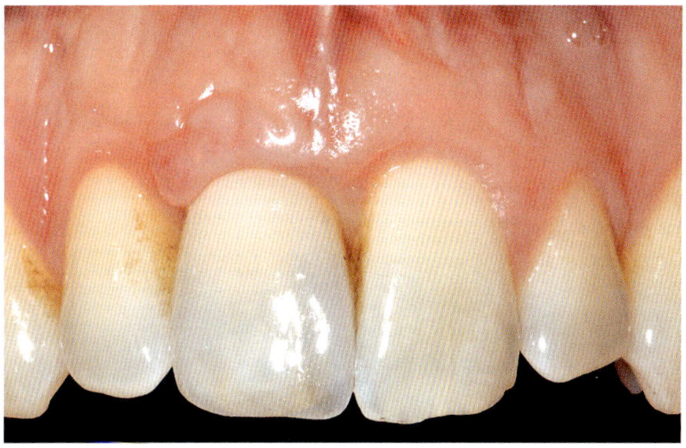

Fig 11. An implant restoration 11 with contours mismatched to those of the adjacent tooth.

3.4.4 Shapes of tooth crowns

One key to clinical outcomes in esthetic dentistry is the symmetry of the restorations and their shape, contours, and textures (Gallucci et al, 2007). If an implant restoration is mismatched with the adjacent tooth, this will greatly influence the appearance and final esthetic outcome (Figure 11). With the esthetic outcome strongly influenced by the symmetry of the final mucosal contours, the risk can often be reduced by the presence of square teeth (and, often, a thick gingival phenotype) (Stellini et al, 2013).

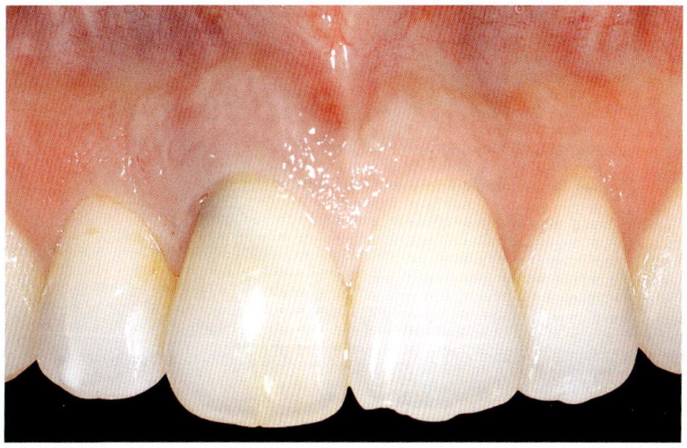

Fig 12. Triangular tooth shape associated with high-scalloped tissue architecture.

There is little question that square-triangular and triangular tooth shapes pose a greater risk, and that risk is most likely associated with the emergence anatomy and tissue support (Takei, 1980; Gobbato et al, 2013) (Figure 12). A high esthetic risk is evident when a triangular tooth shape is associated with localized periodontal defects and the loss of interproximal papillae. These patients will often require a dental implant restoration that is square shaped with broad contact areas, potentially compromising the final appearance. When confronted with this situation, modifying the contours of the adjacent tooth to match those of the implant restoration might be an option to maintain symmetry and avoid black triangles.

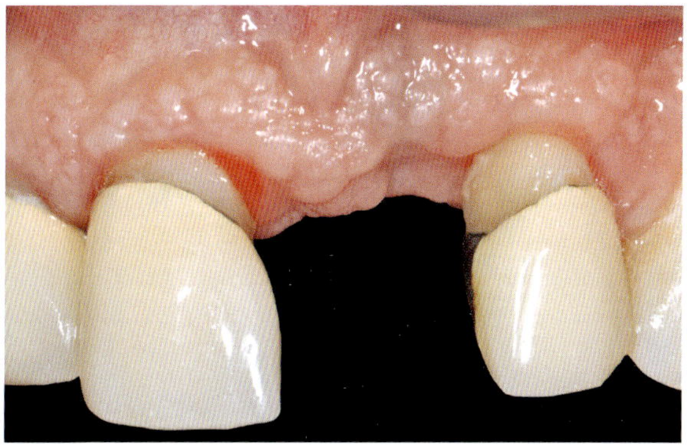

Fig 13. Exposure of crown margins of teeth 11 and 22 subsequent to extraction of tooth 21.

3.4.5 Restorative status of adjacent teeth

The restorative status of teeth surrounding the edentulous space and planned surgical area can have an influence on esthetic outcomes and should be addressed in the treatment plan. If the teeth are virgin (nonrestored), the esthetic risk can vary greatly, as their characteristics (thickness, translucency, optical properties) will play a role in the ability of the laboratory technician to create a restoration that accurately mimics the surrounding teeth. If the adjacent teeth have restorations (crowns or veneers) that extend into the gingival sulcus and surgery is planned in the area, an elevated esthetic risk exists (Richter & Ueno, 1973; Lindhe et al, 1987; Felton et al, 1991; Sanavi et al, 1998). Subgingival margins on adjacent teeth are often associated with recession subsequent to the placement of an implant, and esthetic complications can be associated with exposed restorative margins or an altered gingival architecture (Figure 13).

3.4.6 Gingival phenotype

Phenotypes are the description of physical characteristics of an individual and are considered an expression of their genotype. The characteristics of the gingival phenotype (thick or thin) at an implant site can influence the treatment approach (surgical and restorative) as well as the ability to achieve an acceptable esthetic outcome.

Thick gingival phenotype. A thick gingival phenotype presents a low esthetic risk when replacing single missing teeth in the anterior area. The gingival tissue in these patients is often characterized by a predominance of thick, broad-banded keratinized tissue that is typically resistant to recession after surgical procedures (Chen & Buser, 2014; Chen et al, 2009; Kan et al, 2003; Kois, 2001).

Thin gingival phenotype. A thin gingival phenotype is characterized by a high-scalloped gingival architecture that is often associated with attractive single-tooth implant outcomes. The successful maintenance of the soft tissue architecture depends on the support of facial bone and the periodontal support from the adjacent teeth (Cardaropoli et al, 2004; Kan et al, 2003; Kois, 2001; Weisgold, 1977). The health and proximity of adjacent structures as they traverse the connective tissues and epithelium is important to establishing and maintaining papillae. The thin and friable nature of the soft tissues is conducive to the formation and maintenance of natural and predictable interproximal papillae, but an increased esthetic risk is associated with the possibility of mucosal recession in situations where immediate implants are used (Chen & Buser, 2014; Chen et al, 2009).

3.4.7 Volume of surrounding tissues

Many of the factors in the ERA relate to the volume of the mucosal tissues and supporting bone in the implant site. Their influence on implant placement and restoration in a manner that will allow the development of esthetic symmetry and harmony with surrounding teeth and soft tissues is of critical concern. Issues that might compromise this tissue volume, such as crestal bone resorption and mucosal recession, will increase the esthetic risk and the level of treatment difficulty.

Bony support for peri-implant soft tissues is critical when esthetic risk is present (Belser et al, 1998; Buser & von Arx, 2000). One area where this issue has a great impact is in the support for papillae between teeth and implants (Choquet et al, 2001), or between implants (Tarnow et al, 2000; Tarnow et al, 2003). In a single-tooth case with intact papillae supported by the proximal bone crests on adjacent teeth, it is likely that the papillae can be maintained through proper implant selection and good surgical technique, thus leading to low esthetic risk. However, where bony support for the papilla is reduced by periodontal disease, deep subgingival restoration margins, or active infection, the risk of suboptimal outcomes is much higher. This issue can also arise when the mesiodistal space for implant placement is reduced, allowing crestal remodeling to compromise this supporting bone. Longer spans, involving the replacement of multiple missing teeth, can be very difficult in terms of developing the "natural" appearance of papillae between the prosthetic teeth (Buser et al, 2004), and the use of prosthetic soft tissue replacements may be necessary.

Congress Lecture Hard and Soft Tissue Management in the Esthetic Zone – Part I by Luca Cordaro.

Congress Lecture Hard and Soft Tissue Management in the Esthetic Zone – Part II by Luca Cordaro.

3.4.8 Patient's esthetic expectations

Upon completion of the ERA table, the visual impact of low, medium, and high esthetic risk will educate the clinician and patient on the overall treatment risk for achieving an ideal implant-supported restoration. The esthetic risk factor that can determine whether the treatment should proceed is the patient's expectations. With patients who have high or unrealistic expectations combined with a high esthetic risk, treatment should be avoided, or the patient should be advised of the potential shortcomings in treatment with an attempt to change their expectations to be more realistic. It is not uncommon to have patients presenting a high esthetic risk that understand the limitations to treatment and are willing to accept a compromised esthetic outcome (eg, longer contacts, closed embrasures, pink ceramics) (Figure 14).

When advising patients with high esthetic expectations, informing them of limitations in outcomes before the treatment is considered a risk in itself. However, failure to inform patients of treatment limitations before treatment can lead to compromised esthetic outcomes being interpreted by the patient as a complication and in many situations unacceptable.

ITI Learning Module Principles of Evaluating Esthetic Outcomes by Charlotte Stilwell.

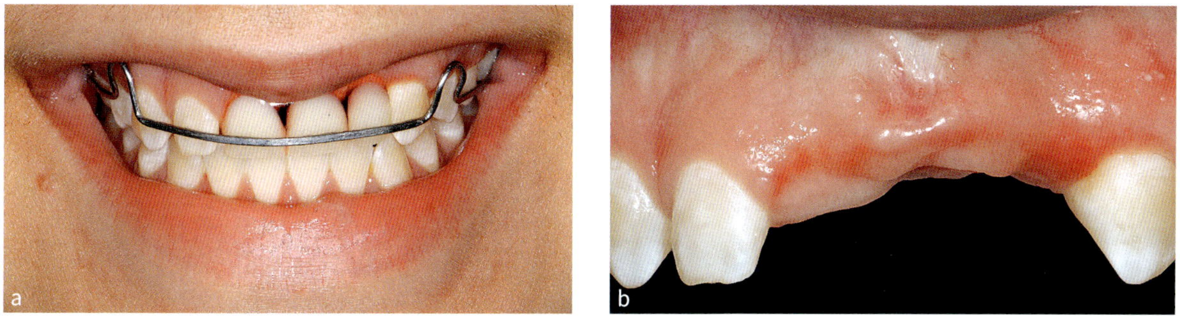

Fig 14 a–b. (a) A patient with missing maxillary anterior teeth and associated high esthetic risk. (b) View of the edentulous area.

3.5 Edentulous Esthetic Risk Assessment (EERA)

L. GONZAGA, W. MARTIN, D. MORTON

In fully edentulous scenarios, esthetic issues occur when implant-supported prostheses inadequately support or blend with the facial structures, teeth, smile line, and residual alveolar ridge. The EERA is a component of the SAC classification. It functions as an independent tool capable of identifying key risk factors that influence esthetic outcomes. These factors are relevant when managing patients with a terminal dentition or when fully edentulous. The systematic use of the EERA checklist during the diagnosis and planning phase can decrease the risk of esthetic as well as technical and biologic complications.

Publications focusing on management of the fully edentulous mandible with prostheses supported by dental implants report high survival and success rates, and low rates of esthetic complications (Polido et al, 2018; Malo et al, 2011). These findings are likely due to the anatomy of the lower two-thirds of the lower one-third of the face, including the lip and its surrounding muscles and the influence of the prosthesis on facial support, the smile line, and phonetics (minimal disruption of speech seal) (Figure 15).

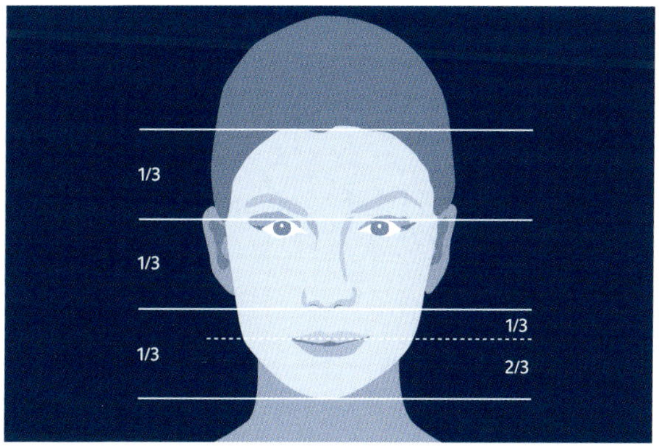

Fig 15. Facial proportions.

Alternatively, the management of the fully edentulous maxilla is more challenging and requires meticulous planning (Desjardins, 1992). The challenges associated with management of the maxilla are well-recognized and can be associated with specific anatomical characteristics, bone resorption patterns, quality of bone, need for prosthetic volume, importance of emergence profile, oral hygiene limitations, influence of the teeth and hard tissue during speech, and the importance of the prosthesis for facial and dental esthetics (Schnitman, 1999; Zitzmann & Marinello, 2000; Taylor, 1991). In 2017, Pollini and coworkers emphasized the challenges associated with management of the edentulous maxilla and developed the lip-tooth-ridge (LTR) classification. The LTR classification offers a guide for treatment planning the edentulous maxilla for fixed or removable prostheses (Figure 16). Utilization of the LTR classification assists clinicians in identifying esthetic risk based on a combination of lip dynamics as well as structural risk based upon prosthetic space availability.

It should be recognized that treatment of the edentulous maxilla will increase esthetic risk due to the need for optimal facial and lip support, the relationship between the ideal tooth position, the lip, and the alveolar ridge, as well as the need for specific prosthesis design to minimize phonetics complications or speech issues.

Congress Lecture The Edentulous Maxilla – Fixed vs. Removable for Esthetic Outcomes by Nicola Ursula Zitzmann.

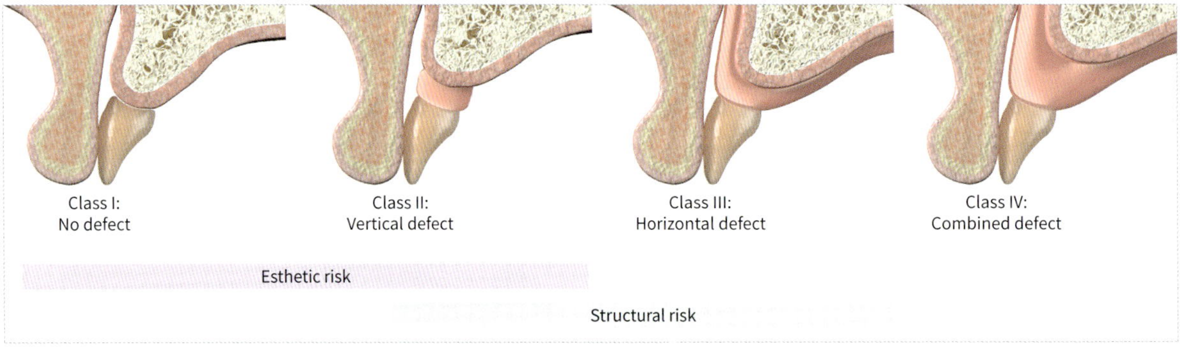

Fig 16. The LTR classification. Visual representation of the four major indications related to the maxillary complete edentulous situation. Note that the classification is based on the defect present between the ridge and the lip horizontally and the prosthetic tooth and ridge vertically. The bone availability for implant placement does not influence the type of indication. (From Pollini et al, 2017, with permission).

The EERA consists of seven clinical risk factors that influence esthetic outcomes when managing fully edentulous arches with implant-assisted prostheses. Table 4 highlights these risk factors. Several factors have been addressed in publications by Zitzmann and Marinello in 1999 and as mentioned previously Pollini and coworkers in 2017. An important key factor when utilizing the EERA is to consider all treatment approaches and options (ie, fixed vs. removable and variations). Doing so will ensure that the clinical and diagnostic findings assist in the identification of information-driven treatment choices. This approach often identifies the need for either an analog (wax try-in) and digital tooth arrangement to determine and review potential treatment outcomes and to effectively utilize the EERA (Figure 17).

Table 4 Edentulous esthetic risk assessment (EERA).

Esthetic risk factors - Edentulous	Level of risk		
	Low	Medium	High
Arch	Mandible		Maxilla
Facial support (fixed)	Alveolar process provides adequate facial support	Minimal changes tolerated by the patient	Flange required for adequate facial support
Facial support (removable)	Flange provides adequate facial support	Minimal changes tolerated by the patient	Insufficient space for a flange
Labial support	Designed tooth position provides satisfactory labial support	Minimal changes tolerated by the patient	Designed tooth position causes unsatisfactory labial support
Upper lip length	Long upper lip (> 20 mm)		Short upper lip (< 20 mm)
Buccal corridor* (atrophic ridge)	Removable prosthesis		Fixed prosthesis
Smile line	No display of the ridge(s) at full smile (maxilla or mandible)		Display of the ridge(s) at full smile (maxilla or mandible)
Maxillomandibular relationship	Class I	Class II	Class III

*Desired narrow corridor in definitive prosthesis.

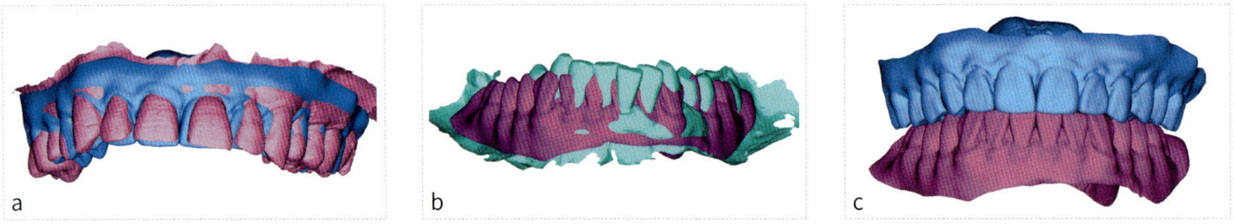

Fig 17 a–c. Example of a digital tooth arrangement for a full-mouth rehabilitation.

3.5.1 Facial support

The determination of optimal or required facial support is a critical factor during the planning process. This is primarily because the facial tissues are supported either by the patient's existing bone and teeth or, in an edentulous scenario, the buccal and labial denture base extensions and the position of the denture teeth. Anatomical factors that influence facial support are residual alveolar ridge, tooth position, and subnasal structures (lip length and thickness, philtrum, nasolabial crease). Facial support is critical because it plays an important role in patients' perception of esthetics and can be specifically associated with both a retrognathic appearance of the maxilla or for compensation of prognathism (Zitzmann & Marinello, 1999). In fully edentulous scenarios, any need for extraoral facial tissue support should be evaluated with and without the existing prosthesis in place from frontal and lateral views (Figure 18).

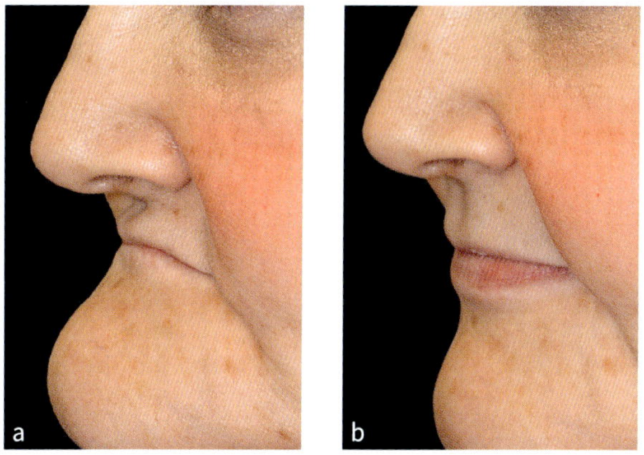

Fig 18 a–b. Pre- and post-placement of maxillary and mandibular overdentures demonstrating improvement in facial support.

3.5.2 Labial support

When evaluating dentate patients, the alveolar ridge shape and cervical crown contour of the central incisors have the greatest influence in labial support (Zitzmann & Marinello, 1999). This influence is altered for the edentulous maxilla due to the absence of tooth support and the resorptive bone pattern after extraction. These factors result in the need for the prosthesis to provide lost support. Other factors that influence buccal and labial tissue support include the musculature (body) of the upper lip, the dry vermilion/vermilion border and tooth length/position. Patients with a thin upper lip should also be considered high esthetic risk as any deficiencies in ridge form, implant position, or type and design of the definitive prosthesis will be magnified and hard to overcome.

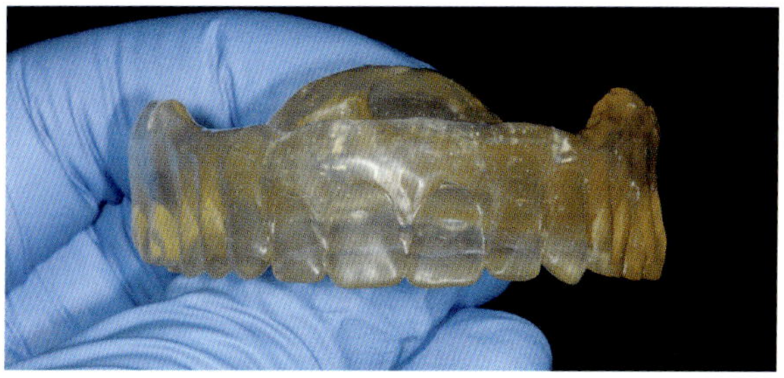

Fig 19. Duplicated denture with labial flange removed.

For edentulous patients planned for implant-supported treatment in the maxilla, the need for prosthesis-provided facial and labial tissue support is a critical component that will assist in the choice of fixed or removable prosthetic solutions. This evaluation should first be performed without the denture in place at full smile. If the residual alveolar ridge is displayed during smiling, the use of a labial flange may be advisable to prevent esthetic problems (Taylor, 1991). In these situations, if a fixed solution is desired, surgical intervention will be necessary, not only to overcome potential esthetic issues, but to create space for the prosthesis and implant components (aka prosthetic volume). The second evaluation would be to determine if the patient can tolerate a "flangeless solution." This can be tested by duplicating the denture, removing the flange, and evaluating labial support (Figures 19 to 21).

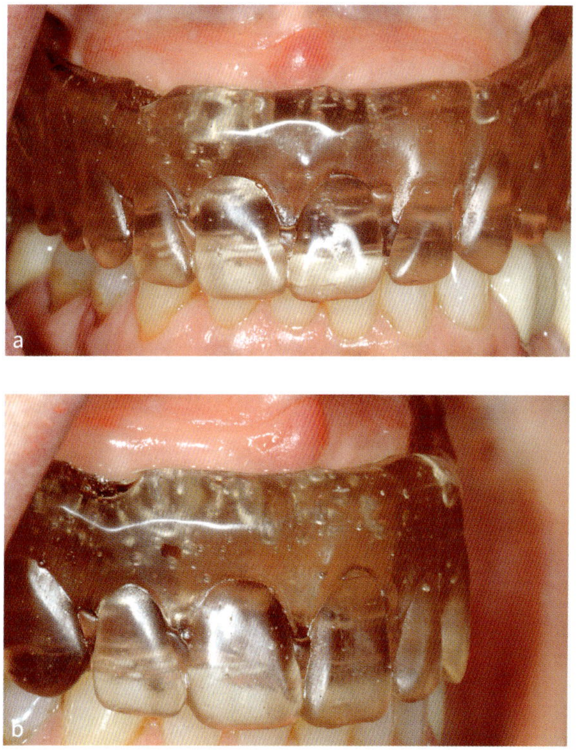

Fig 20 a–b. Try-in of "flangeless" duplicated denture.

Fully edentulous patients that presented with a thin/short lip that are restored with a flangeless prosthetic solution can sometimes demonstrate a transverse upper labial crease during smiling, which can be seen as an esthetic compromise (Figure 22). This transverse labial crease can be influ-

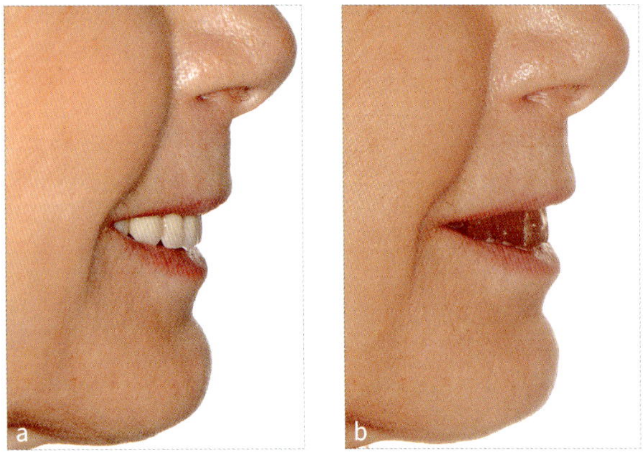

Fig 21 a–b. Labial support evaluation with and without labial flange on prosthesis.

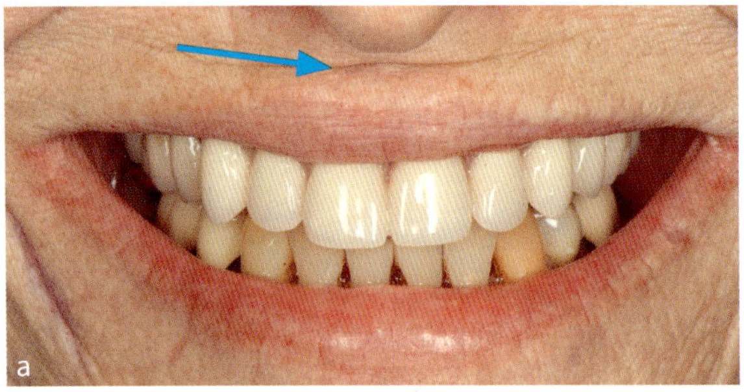

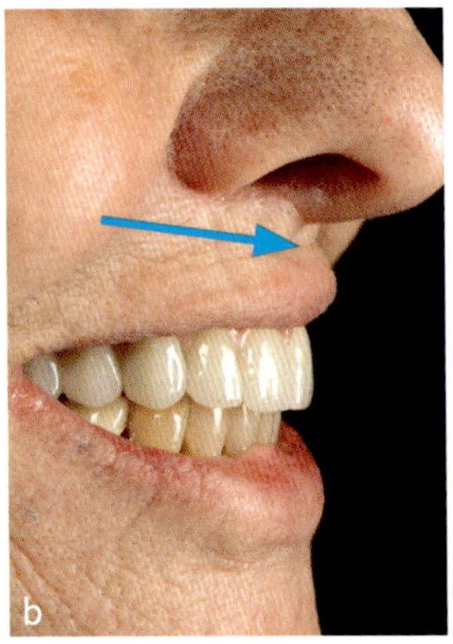

Fig 22 a–b. Presence of transverse labial crease in the definitive fixed full-arch maxillary prosthesis.

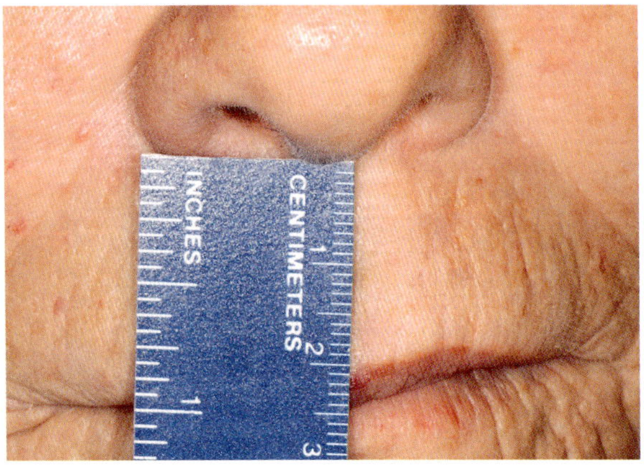

Fig 23. Measurement for upper lip length.

enced by extraoral clinical factors as well. In 2017, Beer and Manestar linked this crease to the presence or hyperactivity of the depressor septi nasi muscle. In their study, they examined 100 consecutive female volunteers, finding that 38% of women older than 40 years presented with an upper labial crease at rest, and 70% presented with a crease during smiling. With this, during the diagnostic phase, the treatment team should evaluate for the presence of a transverse upper labial crease prior to the initiation of care and discuss with the patient possible compromise or need for future cosmetic treatment with botulinum toxin.

3.5.3 Upper lip length

The upper lip position and length is one of the most important elements in anterior esthetics; its static and dynamic assessment will play a crucial role in deciding the type of prosthetic design for the patient (Pollini et al, 2017). For patients with an edentulous maxilla, the position of the lip line at dynamic smile is directly influenced by the length of the upper lip. The length of the upper lip is measured from the base of the column (subnasal) to the philtrum location (Figure 23). The upper lip length will change over the individual's life and continues to strongly influence the display of maxillary teeth. Average lip lengths of 21 to 25 mm were related to 2.2 mm tooth display in the maxilla and 1 mm tooth display in the mandible (Vig & Brundo, 1978). A short upper lip (less than 20 mm measured at rest) represents a higher risk to display the connection or association between the prosthesis and the patient's residual ridge. In patients with a short upper lip, the incisal edges and facial surfaces of the maxillary anterior teeth will be visible in repose, whereas in patients with a long upper lip, the incisal edges and facial surfaces will be covered (Zitzmann & Marinello, 1999).

3.5.4 Buccal corridor

Smile attractiveness is influenced by many additional factors, including the dental midline, smile line and incisal plane convexity, tooth exposure, occlusal plane convexity and cant, buccal corridor, proportion, and symmetry. One of the more controversial aspects of smile attractiveness pertains to buccal corridor size, defined as the negative space between the buccal surfaces of the maxillary teeth and the corners of the mouth during a smile (Martin et al, 2007). In their study, Martin and coworkers reported that laypeople rated smiles with small buccal corridors as significantly ($P < .05$) more attractive than those with large buccal corridors (Figure 24). When evaluating the dentate patient for a tooth/implant combination rehabilitation, the buccal corridor should be evaluated and addressed during the diagnostic phase to determine if orthodontic intervention is necessary or desirable.

In the completely edentulous patient, the pretreatment evaluation of the buccal corridor will play a larger role, as es-

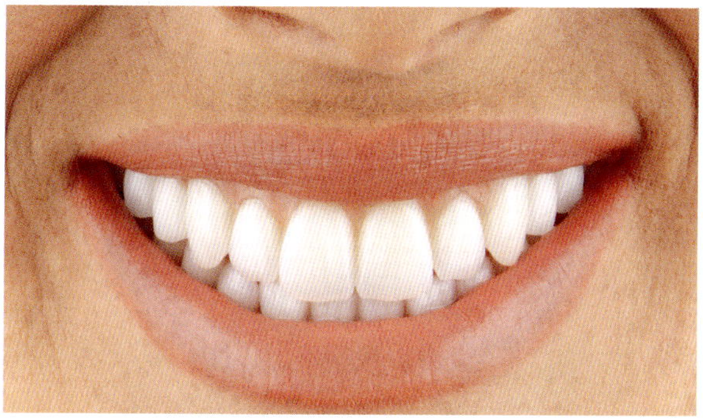

Fig 24. Evaluation of narrow buccal corridor in a maxillary and mandibular hybrid patient.

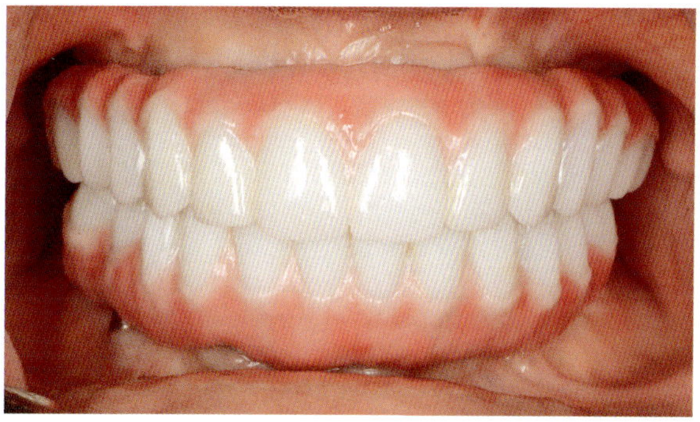

Fig 25. Evaluation of excessive horizontal positioning of teeth in the implant-supported prosthesis to minimize the buccal corridor.

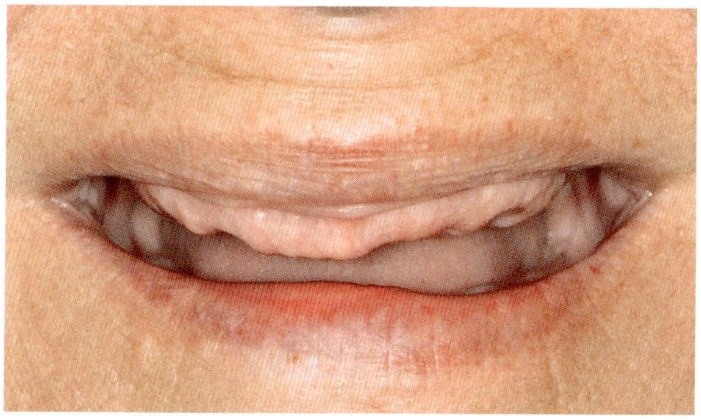

Fig 26. Clinical example of visualization of the residual alveolar ridge at full smile.

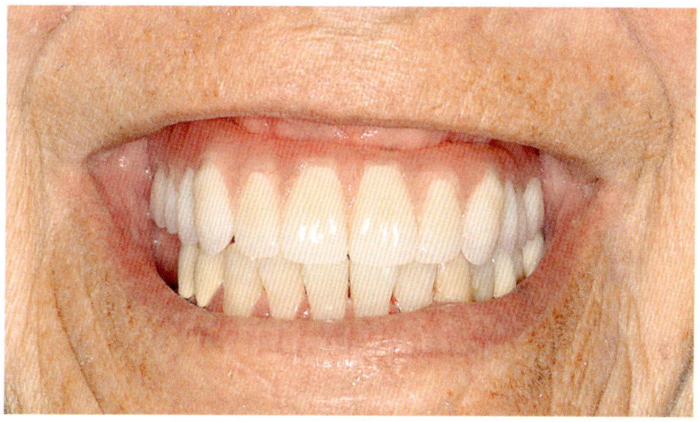

Fig 27. An example of a high smile line and short lip length exposing the transition line, resulting in esthetic compromise.

thetic limitations will be influenced by the position and size of the residual alveolar ridge and its relation to the corners of the mouth at full smile. When the maxillary arch is narrow and the patient desires a fixed solution, the prosthesis will extend horizontally off the ridge, creating the possibility for food entrapment and greater difficulty with maintenance (Figure 25). Depending on the amount of bone resorption and the desired prosthetic design, the residual ridge geometry may need to be surgically modified to ensure a convex emergence profile that will prevent food entrapment and promote appropriate oral hygiene procedures compatible with sustainable oral health (Stein, 1966). In clinical scenarios involving narrow arches, either surgical modification of the ridge prior to implant placement or a removable prosthesis (overdenture) should be considered as an alternative.

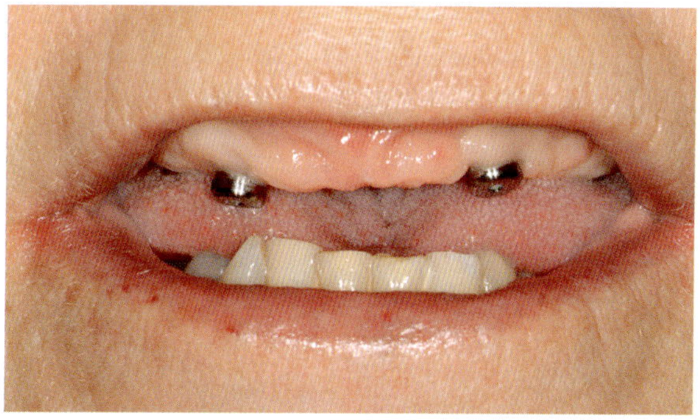

Fig 28. Clinical example of visualization of the residual alveolar ridge with dental implants at full smile in a patient planned for a fixed solution.

3.5.5 Smile line

Based on the upper lip position, Tjan and coworkers (1984) classified the smile for dentate patients as high, medium, or low, with medium and high corresponding to 80% of the population. The smile line is evaluated during a forced smile with and without the prosthesis in place. In edentulous maxillary scenarios, patients that display the residual maxillary ridge when smiling will carry a higher risk of esthetic complications, as the type of prosthesis planned and pre-implant surgical intervention will play a significant role in outcomes (Figure 26). In patients with a high smile line and advanced alveolar ridge resorption, implant-supported overdentures are often preferred due to the added support the labial flange can provide. Extreme esthetic risk is found in patients with a combination of a high smile line and short lip length. Such situations increase the potential for display of the transition line, leading to esthetic compromise (Figure 27). In situations with improper diagnosis and treatment planning, complications can arise that result in unrestorable implants (Figure 28).

3.5.6 Maxillomandibular relationship

Vertical and horizontal bone resorption of the residual alveolar ridges has been described to occur after extraction of the teeth (Carlsson et al, 1967; Tallgren, 1966; Tallgren, 1967). Resorption has been described in complete denture patients after 5 to 25 years (Pollini et al, 2017). The residual ridges undergo a primary resorption that occurs mostly during the first 6 months after extraction, followed by a continuous, steady resorption over the years (Tan et al, 2012; Van der Weijden et al, 2009). Variations in resorption characteristics between the maxilla and the mandible result in altered maxillomandibular relationships. During the diagnostic and planning phase of treatment, the maxillomandibular relationship is evaluated in the clinical setting, often aided by a cephalometric study. Of particular importance during this evaluation is the identification of the proposed or planned tooth position and the relationships between tooth position and the residual ridges. This is mandatory to allow for the evaluation of the skeletal relationship at the correct vertical dimension of occlusion. An ideal setup will show the amount of intermaxillary space, the Angle classification, the need for a denture flange lip support, and the position of the anterior teeth related to potential implant positions.

Discrepancies in interarch relationships, such as crossbites, extreme Angle Class II or III jaw relationships, and an extremely reduced maxillomandibular space can lead to biomechanical risks in the prosthetic phase. It is therefore important to recognize these potential problems at an early stage (Wismeijer et al, 2010).

ITI Treatment Guide Vol. 4 Loading Protocols in Implant Dentistry – Edentulous Patients by Daniel Wismeijer, Paolo Casentini, German Gallucci and Matteo Chiapasco.

Solutions to these problems may include:

- Not placing implants
- Orthognathic surgery prior to implant placement
- Bone grafting procedures
- An alternative prosthetic treatment plan that avoids the anticipated complications (eg, using a removable solution rather than a fixed prosthesis)
- In situations with inadequate intermaxillary space, reduction of the ridge height to allow for greater prosthetic volume

Patients with advanced atrophy of the alveolar ridge will often present in a Class III relationship, which is often due to the alveolar bone remodeling pattern, similar to patients with improper fitting dentures with excessive tooth wear. In severe situations, if a Class I relationship is desired, a removable prosthesis may be necessary.

Congress Lecture Management of Edentulous Arches by Dean Morton.

3.6 Surgical Risks

W. D. POLIDO

Several factors can influence the surgical risk when placing an implant, and they should be identified and addressed as part of the treatment plan. In some instances, they can be individually considered, but in the majority of the clinical presentations, there is an interaction between the different surgical modifying factors, as well as with the general, restorative, and esthetic factors. They can be analyzed in no specific order, but we recommend that all are checked in detail.

An inherent component of any surgical technique is the risk of a complication occurring. The risk of complication is related to a number of factors, including the complexity of the procedure, proximity to anatomical structures, esthetic factors, and the skill and experience of the clinician undertaking the treatment. The risk of complications may range from low to high and must be assessed for each implant site and for the technique(s) selected.

A further consideration is the consequence of a complication. If a complication can be managed without any adverse effect on the implant or restoration, then the complication may be regarded as low risk. If the complication results in adverse bone and/or soft tissue outcomes, the risk of long-term consequences may be medium to high depending upon the nature of the complication.

ITI Learning Module Surgical Complications and Management by Simon Storgård Jensen.

With the purpose of facilitating the decision tree and the risk assessment, we divided the surgical risk factors into four groups, or clusters: *anatomy*, condition of *adjacent teeth*, need for and type of *extractions*, and *surgical complexity*. Each cluster contains different factors that play a role in modifying the risk of a given clinical situation, from a single-tooth replacement to a complete edentulous rehabilitation. Surgical risk factors are classified as either low, medium, or high.

3.6.1 Anatomy

A comprehensive knowledge of oral anatomy is mandatory for anyone practicing implant surgery. Several surgical fac-

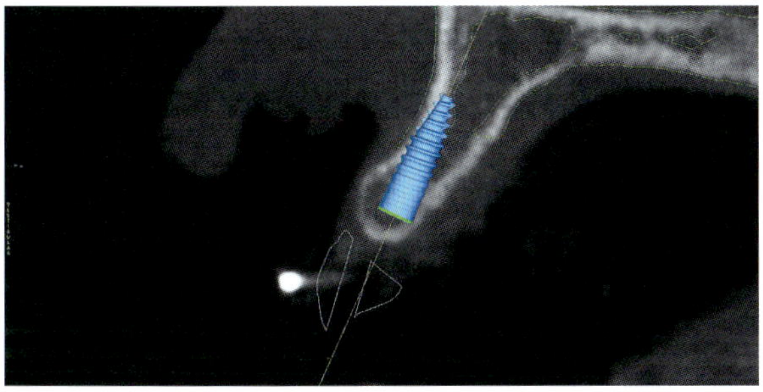

Fig 29. CBCT showing horizontal bone deficiency. Here a narrow ridge still allows placement of a reduced-diameter implant. Use of a regular-diameter implant may require additional grafting procedures.

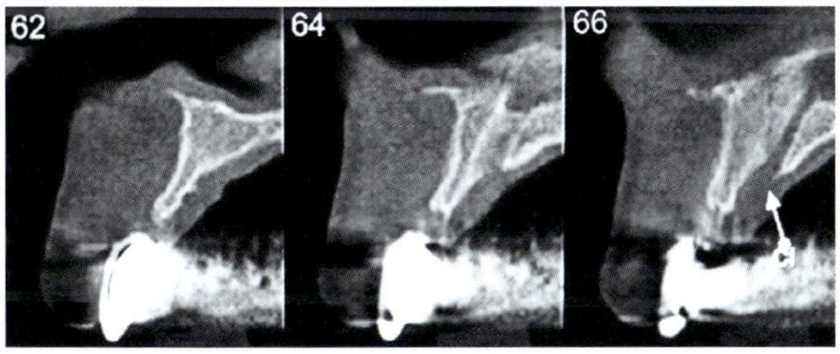

Fig 30. CBCT showing horizontal bone deficiency. A staged bone augmentation is indicated.

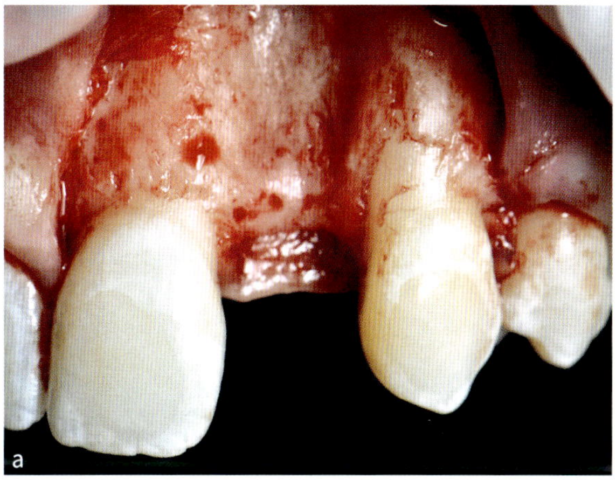

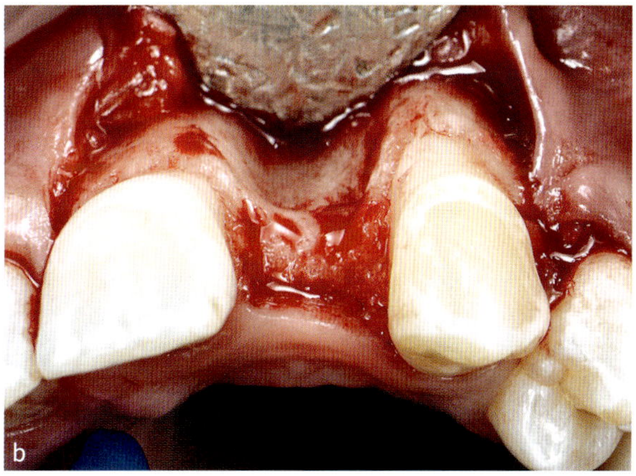

Fig 31 a–b. Clinical intraoperative view showing adequate vertical bone volume (a) and deficient horizontal volume (b) in a maxillary lateral incisor area. This is a high-risk situation requiring staged horizontal bone augmentation.

tors are directly related to the anatomy of a patient, and individual variations may be present.

A basic requirement for implant therapy is bone volume that is sufficient to support an implant of adequate length and width in its ideal restorative position (Buser & von Arx, 2000). Following tooth extraction, resorptive changes result in varying patterns and degrees of bone resorption, leading to reduced horizontal and vertical bone dimensions (Schropp et al, 2003). This in turn may lead to the need for bone augmentation procedures either prior to or at the time of implant placement (Chiapasco et al, 2009). The need for adjunctive bone augmentation procedures increases the difficulty of surgical treatment and requires a more in-depth knowledge of oral and maxillofacial anatomy.

3.6.1.1. BONE VOLUME – HORIZONTAL

When bone volume has adequate width for the planned implant, the risk is considered to be low, since no additional grafting procedures are necessary. Ideally, one should have a minimum of 2 mm of bone surrounding the implant, and a regular-diameter implant (3.5–4.5 mm) should be considered (Benic and Hämmerle, 2014).

With horizontal deficiencies, a simultaneous bone augmentation procedure may be carried out when the anticipated peri-implant defect presents with at least two bone walls (Chiapasco & Casentini, 2018). Small simultaneous horizontal augmentation procedures are regarded as moderately difficult to perform, requiring skill and experience in the use of barrier membranes and/or bone grafts and bone substitutes. In selected situations, the use of reduced-diameter implants (3.0–3.5 mm) can be considered, with simultaneous horizontal augmentation (Figure 29).

In esthetically sensitive sites, there may be a need for a simultaneous bone or soft tissue augmentation to optimize long-term esthetic outcomes (Benic & Hämmerle, 2014; Chiapasco & Casentini, 2018).

If bone is deficient in the horizontal dimension (Figure 30), and the selected implant cannot be placed in the ideal restorative-driven position, a staged grafting approach may be necessary, and the risk is considered to be high. Procedures associated with these types of defects, such as lateral bone augmentation with combinations of block and particulate grafts and/or space-maintaining GBR (guided bone regeneration) procedures (titanium-reinforced membranes, tenting procedures, titanium meshes) have a high degree of difficulty and require additional skill and experience. There is a commensurate increase in the risk of surgical and postoperative complications (Figure 31).

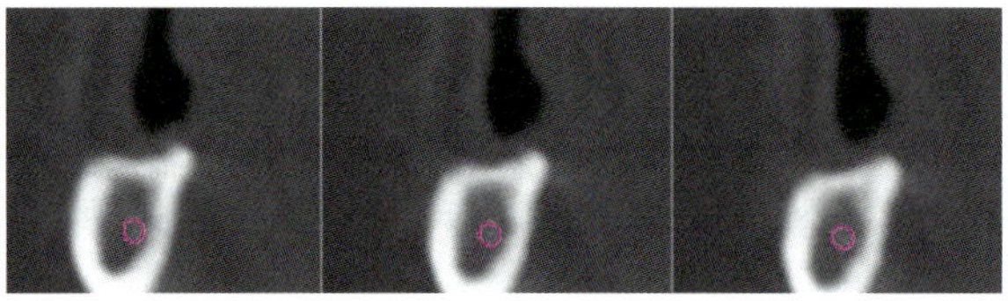

Fig 32. CBCT cross section of posterior mandible site. Note the extreme vertical ridge deficiency. A decision has to be made between short implants vs. staged vertical augmentation.

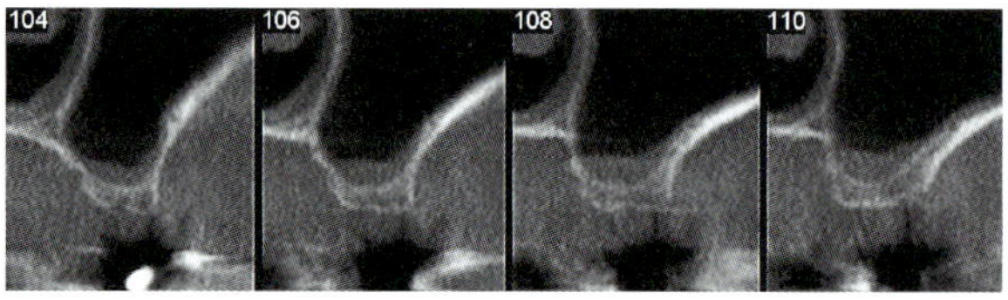

Fig 34. CBCT Illustrating vertical bone deficiency but good horizontal volume in the posterior maxilla. There is a need for a sinus floor augmentation procedure.

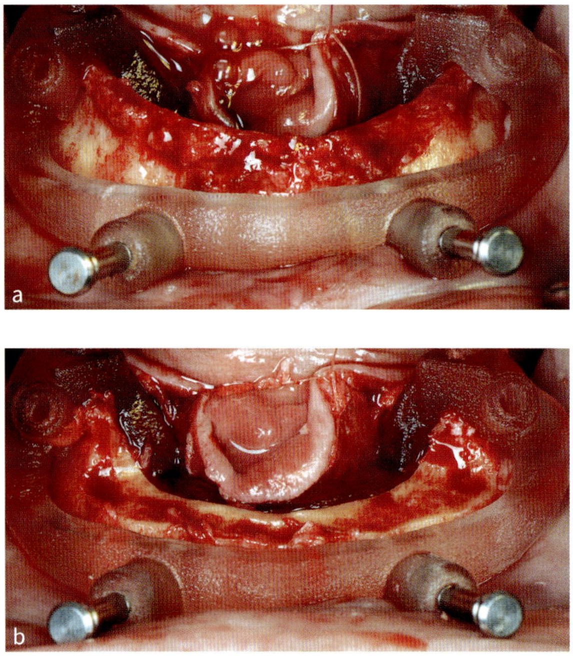

Fig 33 a–b. (a) Completely edentulous ridge, showing need for bone reduction (according to bone reduction guide). (b) Bone reduction performed according to the guide.

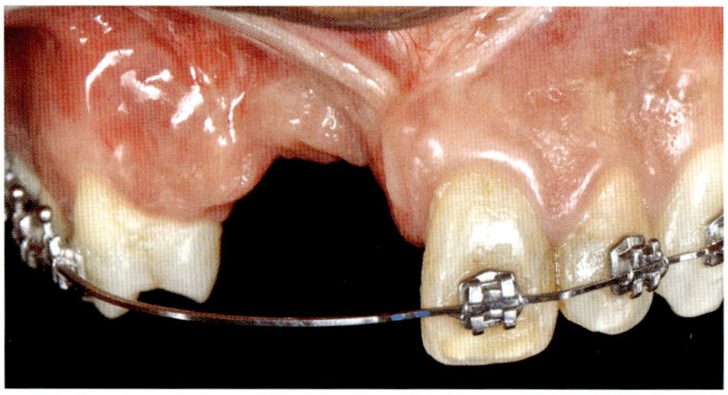

Fig 35. Clinical view of missing maxillary lateral and central incisors. Note large vertical deficiency, presence of soft tissue scars, and low frenulum insertion. Soft tissue management is as important as the management of the bone deficiency.

3.6.1.2 BONE VOLUME – VERTICAL

Adequate bone volume in the vertical dimension is directly related to the outcome of the implant and the restoration. Ideally, an implant with a minimum height of 8 mm should be considered.

Small crestal bone deficiencies may be managed without augmentation. However, the implant shoulder may be deeply positioned in relation to the mucosal margin. This may influence the subsequent restorative procedures and may complicate long-term maintenance of peri-implant tissue health.

If the presence of vital anatomical structures or advanced bone resorption reduces the height of bone in the vertical dimension, implants with shorter lengths may be considered. But the long-term survival of implants with less than 6 mm length is not well documented and may be reduced, although the complexity of placing shorter implants is smaller than staged vertical augmentation techniques (Papaspyridakos et al, 2018). When using short implants, a high crown-to-implant ratio may be expected, and splinting of the implants is recommended. Loading conditions have to be carefully controlled. At sites with reduced bone height, the proximity to vital anatomical structures can increase the risk of surgical complications. For these reasons, sites with small to moderate vertical bone deficiencies allowing placement of shorter implants or simultaneous smaller vertical augmentation should be regarded as having a moderate degree of difficulty (Figure 32).

In certain clinical situations, such as when treating a completely edentulous patient with a hybrid fixed solution, there may be a need for bone reduction in the vertical aspect to create space for the prosthesis. When vertical bone volume allows for implant placement but requires bone reduction, surgical requirements are more extensive, and the risk is considered to be medium (Figure 33).

At sites with significant vertical deficiencies (Figure 34), requiring a separate bone augmentation or a larger bone augmentation simultaneously with implant placement, risk is considered to be high. Techniques for vertical bone augmentation may include sinus and nasal floor grafts, vertical ridge augmentation using block grafts, barrier membranes and/or titanium meshes combined with autogenous bone grafts or bone substitutes, and distraction osteogenesis (Polido & Misch, 2021). These procedures have a high degree of difficulty and an increased risk of surgical complications (Chiapasco & Casentini, 2018). Clinicians are required to have a high level of clinical skill and experience to carry out these procedures successfully. They are particularly challenging and with increased risk in esthetic situations (Figure 35).

3.6.1.3 PRESENCE OF KERATINIZED TISSUE

Adequate volume and quality of gingival soft tissues is essential for the final and long-term stability of the treatment's results.

The presence of an adequate width of keratinized attached mucosa around dental implants may lead to better soft and hard tissue stability, less plaque accumulation, and less soft tissue recession, leading to a lower incidence of peri-implant mucositis and/or peri-implantitis.

The long-term stability of pink esthetics around dental implant prostheses has been strongly correlated with adequate peri-implant soft tissue thickness (Sculean et al, 2014).

Sites with thick (> 4 mm) keratinized tissue are considered to have low risk, whereas sites with 2 to 4 mm of keratinized tissue are considered to be of medium risk. Additional soft tissue procedures may be indicated (Figure 36).

Sites with thin tissue phenotype (< 2 mm) in esthetically important areas are difficult to manage, with elevated risk of esthetic complications (Figure 37). They are at greater risk of recession of the marginal mucosa (Evans & Chen, 2008) and may frequently require adjunctive soft tissue augmentation procedures to prevent this from occurring. When performing bone augmentation procedures, an additional displacement of the mucogingival junction may also occur.

This increases the difficulty of treatment and requires a high level of clinical skill and experience to undertake these procedures with predictable outcomes.

3.6.1.4 QUALITY OF SOFT TISSUES

Adequate soft tissue management is imperative for optimal outcomes. The presence of scars, low muscle insertions, and inflammation can jeopardize healing and compromise surgical flap design and management, vascular supply, and the tissue phenotype.

Absence of scars and inflammation is the ideal situation and provides low-risk situations.

If there is no tissue inflammation but minimal scars are present, usually the soft tissues can be adequately managed during implant placement, creating a medium risk. The clinician needs to have some experience in managing these soft tissues and their potential healing deficiencies.

When scars or strong fibrous tissue attachments are present, they usually require additional staged soft tissue procedures to obtain a better tissue quality (Figure 38). These require more experience and bring additional morbidity, being classified as high risk.

The presence of acute or chronic inflammation, such as fistulas (Figure 39), increases the risk of tearing the tissue and

Fig 36. Thin ridge with less than 2 mm of keratinized tissue in the planned position of the implants. Adjunctive soft tissue management is required.

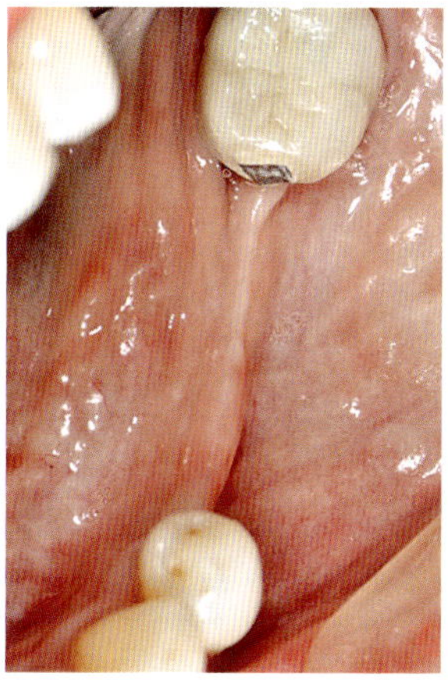

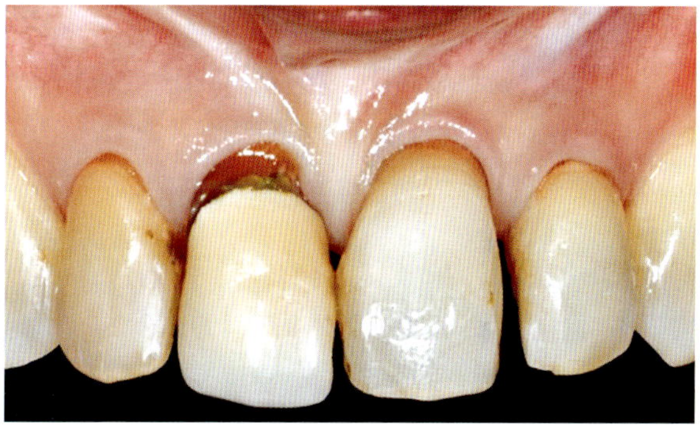

Fig 37. Thin tissue phenotype and recession around central incisors.

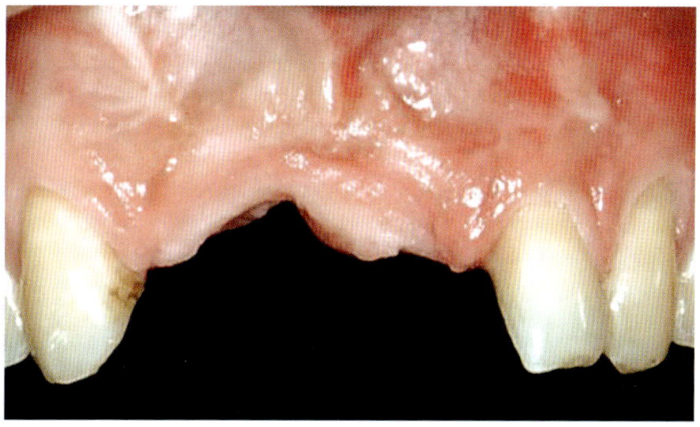

Fig 38. Multiple missing teeth in the anterior area, with soft tissue defects and scars.

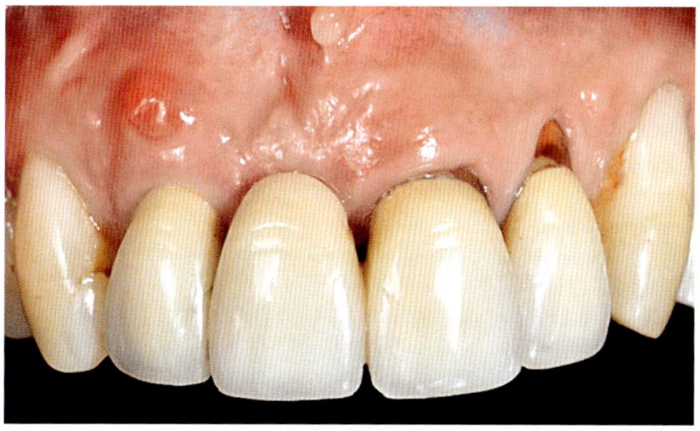

Fig 39. Inflammation on lateral incisor; recession around adjacent canine.

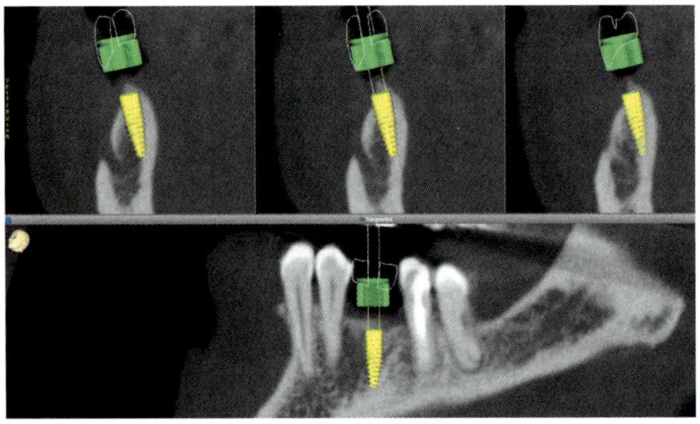

Fig 40. Virtual surgical planning of implant for mandibular premolar region. Note the proximity of planned implant to the mental foramen.

impairing healing, and are also classified as a high risk (Blanco et al, 2019).

3.6.1.5 PROXIMITY TO VITAL ANATOMICAL STRUCTURES

Any implant surgery carries a risk of involvement of nearby anatomical structures such as adjacent roots, neurovascular structures, maxillary sinus, nasal cavity, and perforation of the buccal or lingual/palatal cortical bone. Careful clinical and radiographic preoperative assessment of the bone shape and dimension, as well as the condition of the soft tissues, is required to determine the degree of risk of injuring these structures (Figure 40).

When harvesting bone or soft tissue for grafting, the anatomical risk at the donor site must also be considered. Depending on the clinical situation, the surgical requirements are more complex, and the risk may range from low to high depending on the degree of involvement and proximity to important anatomical structures (Table 5).

ITI Learning Module Anatomy with Relevance to Implant Surgery by Vivianne Chappuis.

Table 5 Surgical modifying factors: Anatomy.

Surgical modifying factors	Risk or degree of difficulty		
	Low	Medium	High
	Site factors		
Anatomy			
Bone volume – horizontal	Adequate	Deficient, but allowing simultaneous augmentation	Deficient, requiring a separate augmentation procedure prior to implant placement
Bone volume – vertical	Adequate	Small deficiency allowing implant placement Small deficiency allowing simultaneous augmentation Adequate for implant placement but requiring bone reduction	Deficient, requiring a separate vertical bone augmentation as a first step of a staged approach Deficient, requiring vertical bone augmentation simultaneously with implant placement
Keratinized tissue	Sufficient (> 4 mm)	Minimal (2–4 mm)	Insufficient (< 2 mm)
Soft tissue quality	No scars or inflammation	Presence of minimal scars/no inflammation	Presence of scars and inflammation
Proximity to vital anatomical structures	Minimal risk of involvement	Moderate risk of involvement	High risk of involvement

3.6.2 Adjacent teeth

When performing surgical procedures, special attention must be paid to the anatomical condition of tissues surrounding the adjacent teeth, especially in the esthetic zone. Even in the posterior region, the presence or absence of healthy tissues surrounding the teeth adjacent to the planned implant site can greatly influence the risk and the final outcome.

3.6.2.1 PAPILLA

The height of the papilla next to dental implants is one of the main parameters affecting the esthetic outcome. The presence or absence of the papilla is influenced by a variety of factors. Compared with natural teeth, the papillae at implant sites are reported to be significantly shorter. Surgical reconstruction of the lost interproximal papilla can be challenging

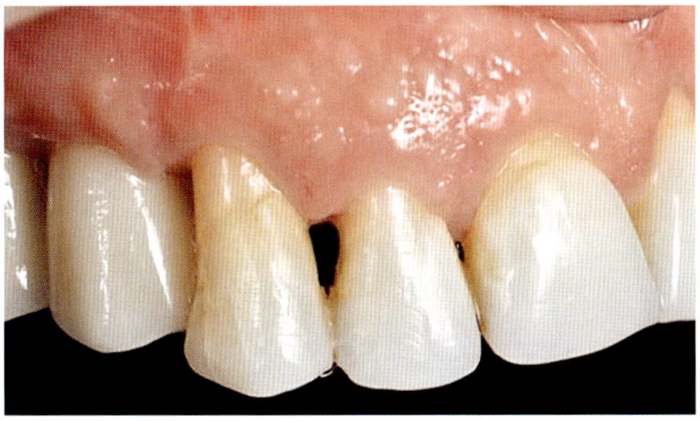

Fig 41. Lack of papilla between the canine and lateral incisor. The canine is periodontally compromised and needs to be extracted.

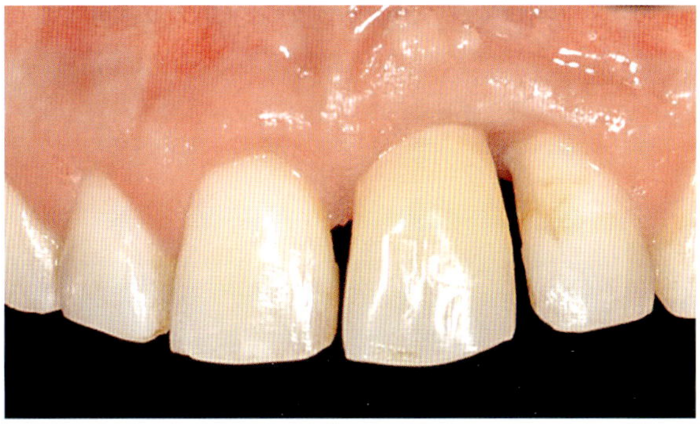

Fig 42. Clinical example of soft tissue recession on teeth adjacent to potential implant site (tooth 21)

and unpredictable. Therefore, the most predictable means to obtain a papilla is to recognize its presence and prevent its loss (Sculean et al, 2014).

The presence of papilla attached to the adjacent tooth brings a low risk. When it is deficient (Figure 41), risk can be medium, depending on the missing tooth site. Absence of a papilla characterizes a high risk.

3.6.2.2 RECESSION

The presence or absence of soft tissue recession in a tooth adjacent to a site where an implant will be placed can influence the outcomes in many aspects. Tooth loss is followed by alveolar bone loss, and in many situations this bone loss can extend to the interproximal bone attached to the adjacent tooth. Previous surgeries, periodontal disease, and trauma are the most common factors associated with recession around teeth on the facial and proximal surfaces adjacent to the missing tooth (Figure 42).

When there is a recession, surgical flaps have to be modified, and grafts over the adjacent tooth roots have to be planned in conjunction with the implant site grafts. The outcomes of grafting procedures around teeth adjacent to edentulous sites are unpredictable (Chackartchi et al, 2019) and can lead to compromised outcomes in the area being treated.

Clinicians must possess expertise in periodontal plastic surgery techniques and have experience in all the factors involved with it.

Absence of recession provides a low risk, whereas presence of recession is considered a high risk.

3.6.2.3 INTERPROXIMAL ATTACHMENT

The presence of interproximal papillae depends on the vertical position of the periodontal and crestal bone attachment of the adjacent tooth. In patients with a vertical distance between the contact point and the bone crest of ≤ 5 mm, complete papilla fill is reported to be obtained.

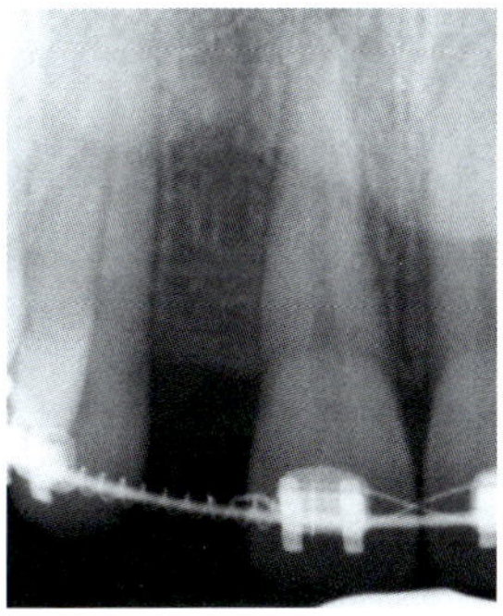

Fig 43. Periapical radiograph illustrating ideal interproximal bone attachment on teeth adjacent to implant site.

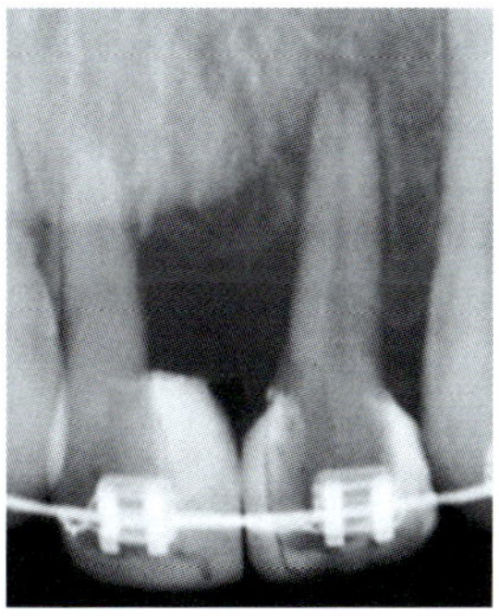

Fig 44. Periapical radiograph illustrating apically positioned bone attachment on teeth adjacent to implant site.

When the distance was > 5 mm, the presence of the papilla was reduced to a frequency of 50% (Sculean et al, 2014).

The amount of bone regenerated in a vertical dimension and the resulting papilla height are limited by the height of the periodontal attachment at the adjacent natural teeth. Preexisting attachment loss at neighboring teeth will therefore result in unfavorable papilla height. No predictable surgical techniques are presently available allowing these biologic limitations to be overcome.

Having the interproximal attachment at the level of the CEJ of the tooth adjacent to where an implant has to be placed brings a low risk for the treatment (Figure 43). The greater the distance between the CEJ and the periodontal attachment (Figure 44), the higher the risk for having adequate tissue around the future implant and restoration, increasing the risk for biologic complications (Table 6).

ITI Learning Module Surgical Assessment of the Implant Site **by Wagner Duarte.**

Table 6 Surgical modifying factors: Adjacent teeth.

Surgical modifying factors	Risk or degree of difficulty		
	Low	Medium	High
	Site factors		
Adjacent Teeth			
Papilla	Complete	Deficient	Absent
Recession	Absent		Present
Interproximal attachment	At cementoenamel junction		Below cementoenamel junction

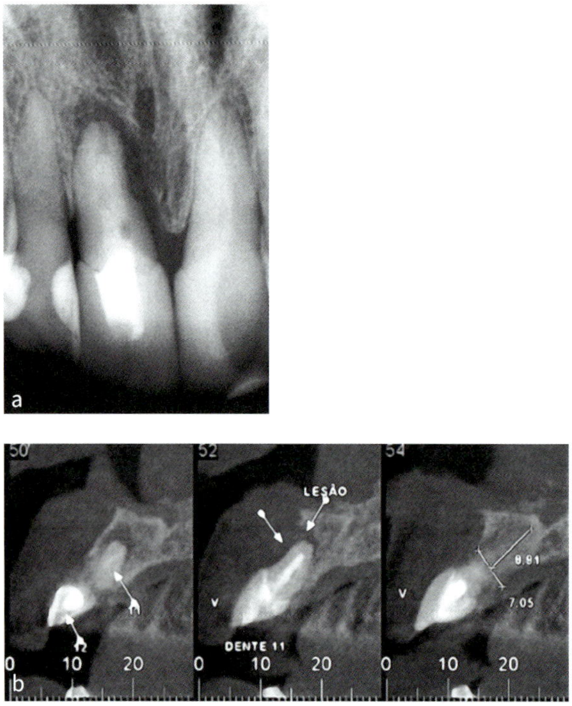

Fig 45 a–b. Periapical radiograph (a) and CBCT (b) prior to extraction of central incisor. Note the significant bone loss in the buccal, mesial, and apical regions. This is a high-risk situation in regard to available alveolar bone after extraction.

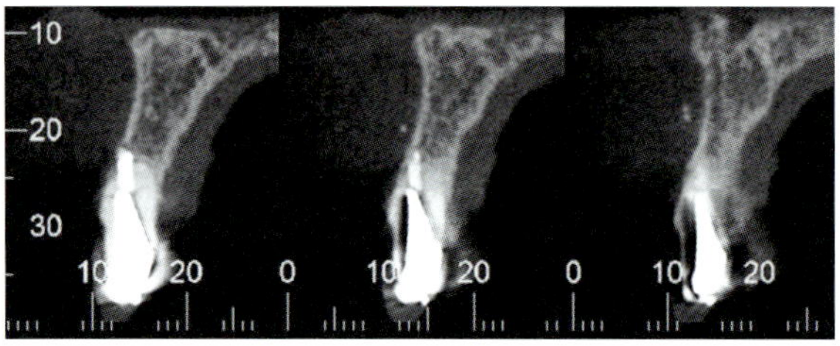

Fig 46. CBCT of maxillary right lateral incisor, showing root that needs removal. Thin labial bone but adequate bone width and height.

3.6.3 Extractions

Risk assessment for implant placement should be done prior to tooth extraction, since tooth extraction is the first step in treatment (Buser et al, 2017). The local anatomy is of great importance for the selection of the treatment option, as bone and root morphology vary in different sites and patients. Three-dimensional bone morphology is best observed through a CBCT image, and it is considered the current standard of care in implant surgery planning (Figure 45).

The decision-making process related to the timing of implant placement (immediate, early, or late) is greatly influenced by factors correlated with radicular morphology, alveolar and basal bone morphology, as well as by the soft tissue quality and quantity around the tooth to be extracted.

All these factors are correlated, and should not be analyzed individually, but yet combined with each other.

3.6.3.1 RADICULAR MORPHOLOGY / INTERRADICULAR BONE

Prosthetic-driven implant planning and good primary stability are mandatory for optimal implant placement. Radicular morphology can influence alveolar bone morphology and the presence or absence of interradicular bone.

Uniradicular teeth in the anterior aspect of the alveolar bone can, when removed, provide adequate remaining alveolar bone for implant placement apically and palatally to the extraction socket (Figure 46). In anterior teeth, due to absence of an interradicular septum, risk of implant placement is considered to be lower than in posterior teeth, when a septum is present. The alveolar bone and basal bone morphology should be observed to confirm the possibility of adequate implant placement. In the esthetic zone, the esthetic risk assessment (Martin et al, 2017) should be utilized (See section 3.4 of this chapter).

In posterior sites, the presence of multiradicular and divergent roots is usually accompanied by large and thick interseptal bone, allowing for implant anchorage. This is a technique-

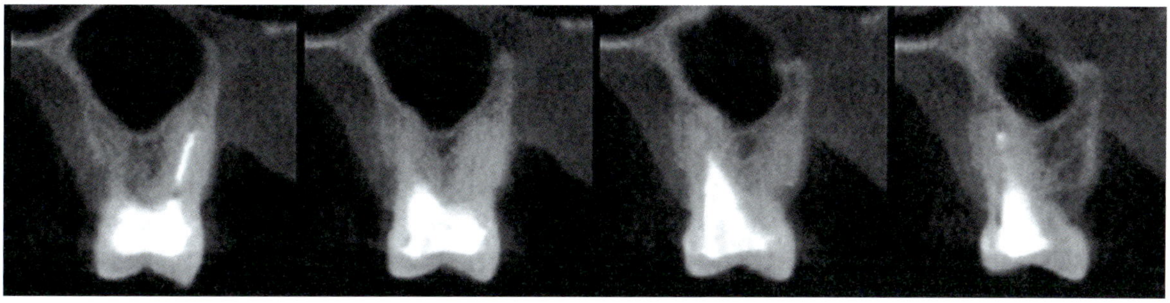

Fig 47. CBCT of maxillary left molar, showing divergent roots, with apex at < 5 mm from sinus floor.

sensitive procedure that requires significant clinical skill and experience. The surgical risk is considered to be medium.

However, if root morphology presents with conical or fused roots, with no interseptal bone, once the tooth has been removed, the resulting socket is wider than the widest implant indicated for the site. Here, the risk is considered to be high. The available alveolar bone apical to the root will dictate if an implant can be anchored (Figure 47).

In situations where there is no bone apical or palatal to the socket after extraction, a ridge preservation procedure (grafting at the time of extraction) may be indicated in an attempt to reduce bone loss. This medium-risk approach leads to an intentional late implant placement, and an additional simultaneous graft may be necessary.

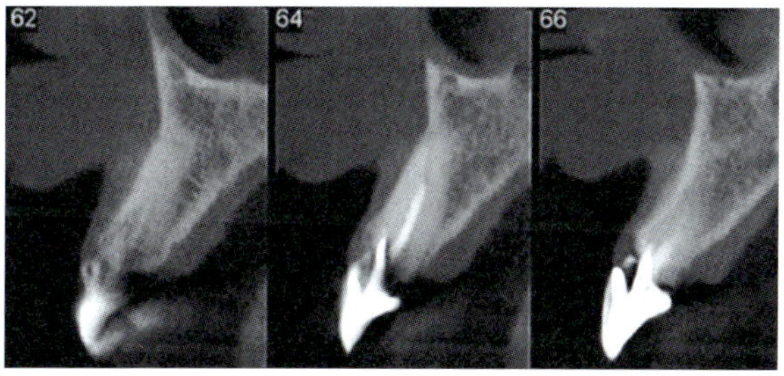

Fig 48. CBCT of the maxillary right lateral incisor. Note thin facial wall thickness, but wide basal bone, potentially allowing for good primary stability.

3.6.3.2 ALVEOLAR AND BASAL BONE MORPHOLOGY

Alveolar bone morphology and the presence or absence of interradicular bone can influence the possibility of obtaining good primary stability.

If alveolar/basal bone after extraction provides sufficient height (> 4 mm) and width (> 2 mm) around the apex of the planned implant, surgical risk is considered to be low, since primary stability can be obtained (Figure 48).

When alveolar/basal bone height is adequate, but width is less than 2 mm around the apex of the planned implant, surgical risk is considered to be medium, since a horizontal augmentation procedure may be necessary, and there is higher risk of not properly achieving primary stability.

If, after tooth extraction, there is insufficient bone height (< 4 mm), due to the proximity to anatomical structures such as the inferior alveolar canal or the maxillary sinus floor, or in the presence of a large periapical pathology, achieving good primary stability may be impossible. Therefore, these situations are considered of high risk. A socket preservation procedure may be indicated in an attempt to reduce bone loss and increase the chance of a straightforward late implant placement.

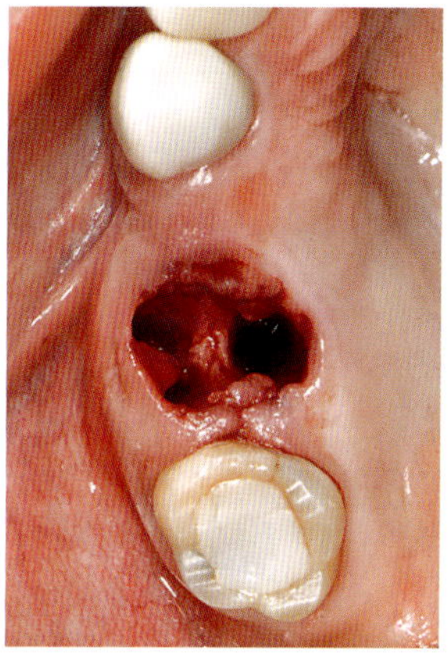

Fig 49. Clinical image after extraction of maxillary molar; socket walls are intact.

3.6.3.3 SOCKET WALLS

Presence or absence of socket walls may facilitate the surgical procedures, since they provide support for the surrounding soft tissues and serve as a housing for bone graft materials (Buser et al, 2017). Careful and minimally invasive extraction procedures are always recommended when implant placement is planned, irrespective of timing.

When all socket walls are intact after tooth extraction, risk is considered to be low (Figure 49).

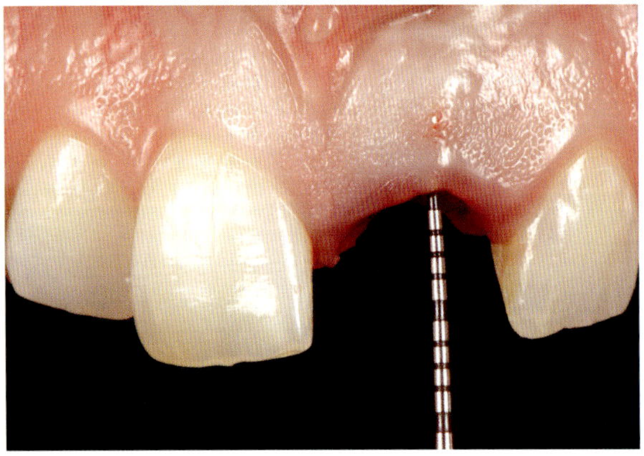

Fig 50. Clinical image after extraction of maxillary central incisor. Probe shows missing buccal wall.

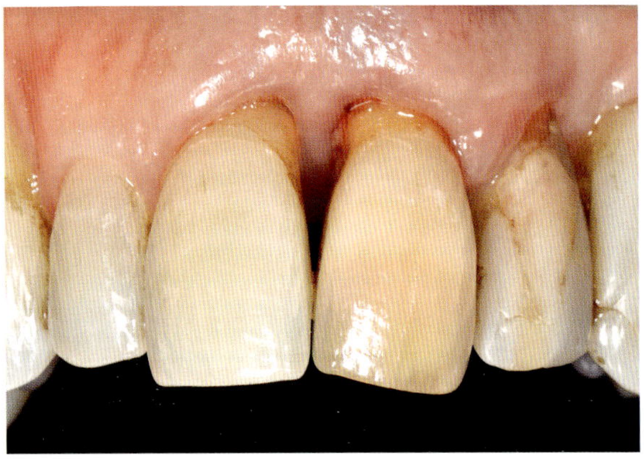

Fig 51. Gingival recession around central incisors and left lateral incisor, to be extracted due to advanced periodontal disease.

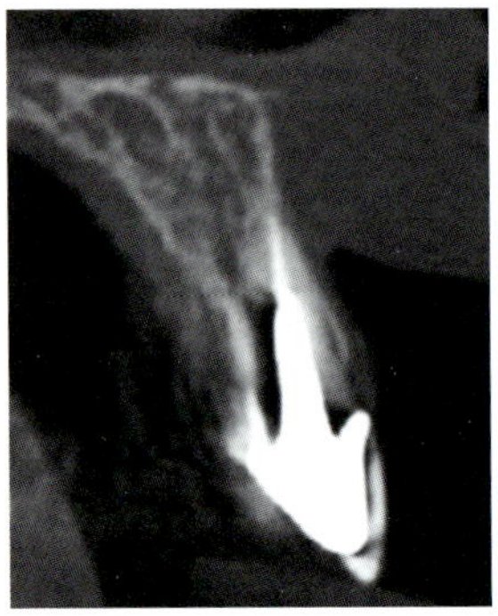

Fig 52. CBCT of central incisor to be extracted due to root fracture. A thin facial wall can be seen.

If socket walls are partially missing due to roots with associated bone defects, or extraction results in small residual defects or dehiscence, risk is considered to be medium. Smaller grafts can be simultaneously placed, or a socket preservation procedure may be performed (Benic & Hämmerle, 2014; Chiapasco & Casentini, 2018) (Figure 50).

Roots associated with significant bone defects, usually caused by periodontal or endodontic problems, can lead to one or more missing socket walls. Aggressive or more invasive extraction procedures may also cause destruction of the socket walls and compromise implant placement or bone augmentation procedures (Figure 51). Gingival recession seems to be inevitable even in thick tissue phenotypes when dehiscence defects are present (Blanco et al, 2019). These situations are considered of high risk.

3.6.3.4 THICKNESS OF FACIAL WALL

The thickness of the facial wall of the extraction socket is a relevant factor in the pattern of bone resorption and remodeling. It significantly influences not only the amount of horizontal gap fill but also the amount of vertical crestal resorption.

The facial bone wall supports the mucosa on the facial aspect of the implant. Hence, resorption of the facial wall is more significant than that of the lingual or palatal wall.

Implants placed immediately into extraction sockets will not prevent the occurrence of ridge alterations that always take place following tooth loss. Adjunctive hard and soft tissue augmentation procedures are frequently performed to minimize the risk of marginal bone resorption and mucosal recession (Buser et al, 2017).

Sites with facial wall thickness greater than 2 mm are at low risk for immediate implant placement. However, if the facial bone wall is thin (< 1 mm) following placement of the implant, there is an increased risk of horizontal and vertical marginal bone resorption and exposure of the implant surface. This in turn increases the likelihood of marginal tissue recession.

The best way to assess the facial bone wall in the anterior area is by the use of a CBCT scan with lip retraction (Januario et al, 2008) (Figure 52).

Due to the larger esthetic risk, sites with thin facial bone walls (< 1 mm) have a high degree of difficulty.

3.6.3.5 ANTICIPATED RESIDUAL DEFECT AFTER IMPLANT PLACEMENT

The thickness of the facial bone wall, as well as the dimension of the horizontal gap (the space between the inner part of the alveolar wall and the implant surface) are anatomical factors that influence the pattern of resorption and bone modeling/remodeling that occurs following immediate implant placement into extraction sockets.

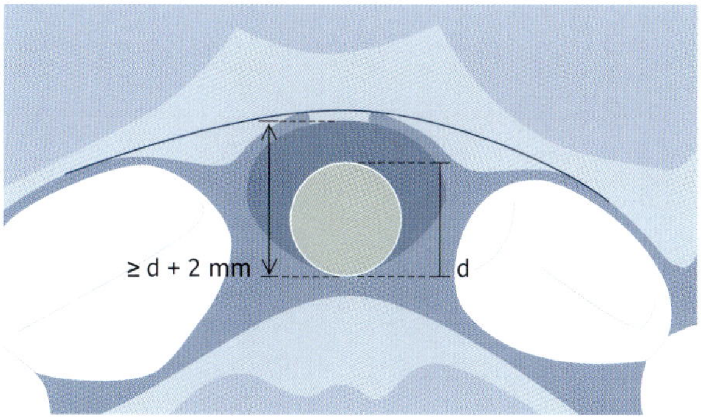

Fig 53 a. Implant placement within the remains of the extraction socket with mostly intact socket walls. (Source: ITI Treatment Guide Vol. 3 "Implant Placement in Post-Extraction Sites.")

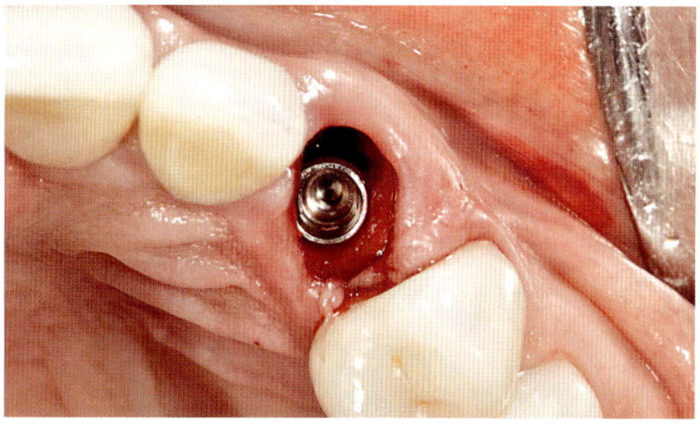

Fig 53 b. Clinical occlusal view of immediate implant placement in a left canine site. Note buccal gap > 2 mm, warranting the use of bone substitutes to support the soft tissues.

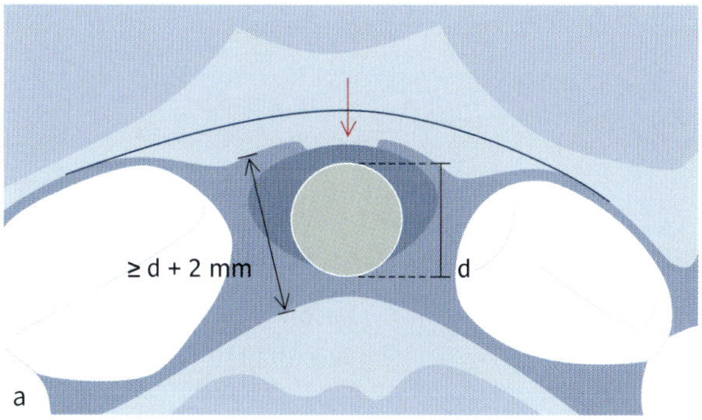

Fig 54 a. Illustration showing implant inside alveolar bone envelope, and flattening of facial bone. This is a typical finding in an early implant placement (Types 2 and 3). (Source: ITI Treatment Guide Vol. 3 "Implant Placement in Post-Extraction Sites.")

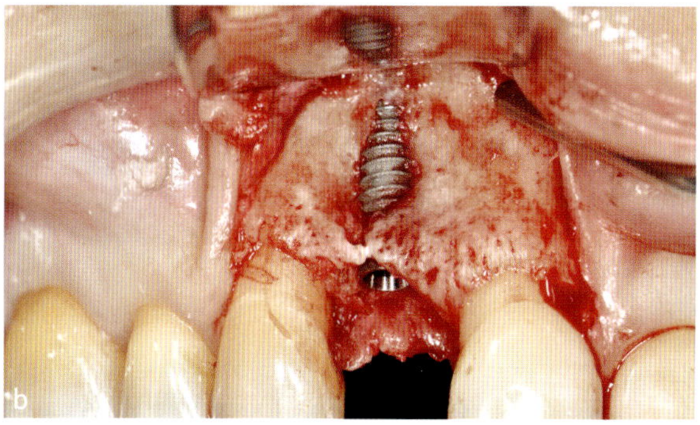

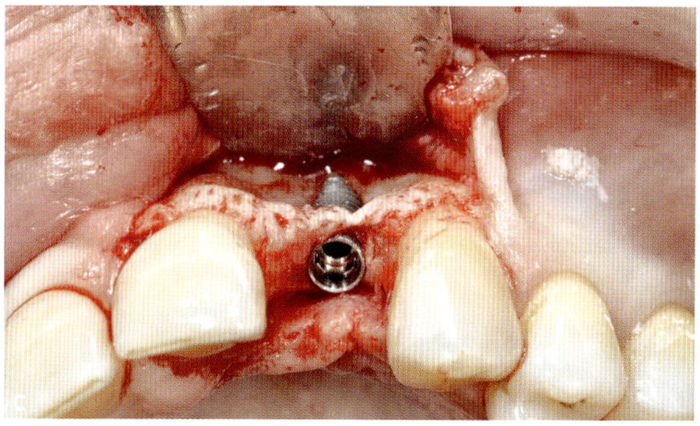

Fig 54 b–c. Clinical view showing implant inside alveolar bone envelope, with flattening of facial bone. Note fenestration with exposed threads, requiring a horizontal bone augmentation procedure.

Considering that a minimum thickness of 2 mm of facial bone wall is needed to avoid collapse after tooth extraction, regeneration techniques and/or soft tissue grafts are important to achieve adequate bony contours around the implants.

If an implant is placed with adequate bone width around it, and no residual defects are expected, it is considered to be at low risk, since no bone augmentation is necessary.

In immediate implant placement, residual defects are usually expected. If there is a one-wall defect (facial bone wall missing or dehiscence of the facial bone wall), the implant is placed inside the alveolar bone envelope (Figure 53). Immediate implant placement is usually considered to be of high esthetic risk.

In an early placement, there is usually a flattening of the facial bone (Figure 54). The implant is still inside the alveolar bone envelope. This situation is considered of medium risk, as there is usually a need for bone augmentation, but it is usually more predictable and a less technique-sensitive procedure.

There may be situations where the implant can be placed in the ideal restoratively driven position, and with good primary stability, but the residual defect is of two or three walls, and the position is considered to be outside of the alveolar envelope (Figure 55). In these instances, the necessary grafting procedures are larger and less predictable, requiring a higher level of expertise from the clinician. The risk factor is considered to be high, and a staged bone augmentation may be indicated.

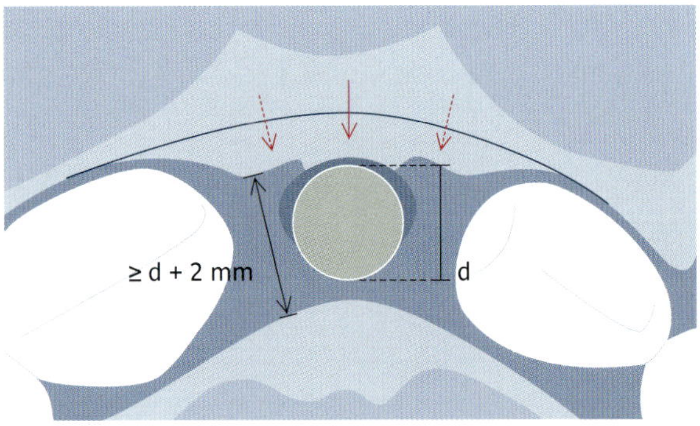

Fig 55 a. Illustration showing implant outside of alveolar bone envelope. (Source: ITI Treatment Guide Vol. 3 "Implant Placement in Post-Extraction Sites."

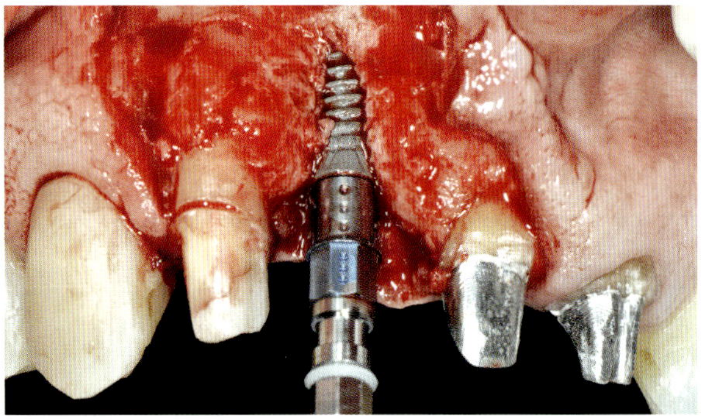

Fig 55 b. Clinical view showing implant outside of alveolar bony envelope. Horizontal bone augmentation is indicated.

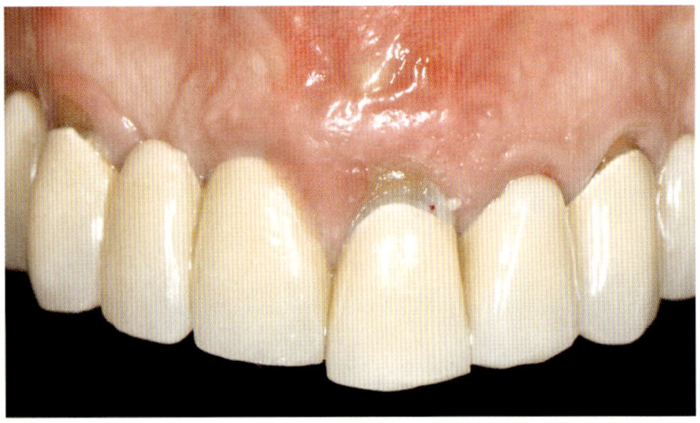

Fig 56. Clinical buccal view, anterior maxilla. Note soft tissue recession on left maxillary incisor.

3.6.3.6 QUALITY AND QUANTITY OF SOFT TISSUES

A thin gingival phenotype around the natural dentition and implants has been correlated with a higher risk of gingival recession than a thick phenotype. A thin phenotype is three times more prone to midfacial recession after immediate implant placement, and this recession tends to be three times larger in thin than in thick gingival biotypes (Sculean et al, 2014).

In areas with a thick tissue phenotype, adequate keratinized tissue, and no recession around the tooth to be extracted, the risk assessment in relation to the soft tissue quality and quantity can be considered low.

When soft tissue recession is present around the tooth to be extracted, it is usually accompanied by a smaller band or a complete absence of keratinized tissue. This classifies it as a high risk in relation to the soft tissue quality and quantity, since the risk of an esthetic complication is increased. Additionally, having inadequate keratinized tissue around the future implant-supported crown may facilitate future biologic complications (Roccuzzo et al, 2016). When recession is present, an early implant placement may be beneficial because, after 6 to 8 weeks of healing, residual bone will have only undergone minimal remodeling, and there will be a significant increase in soft tissue quality and quantity (Chappuis et al, 2017).

Sufficient soft tissue quantity (presence or absence of recession) should always be evaluated in conjunction with the soft tissue quality (amount of keratinized tissue), around the tooth to be extracted (Figure 56; Table 7).

Table 7 Surgical modifying factors: Extractions.

Surgical modifying factors	Risk or degree of difficulty		
	Low	Medium	High
	Site factors		
Extractions			
Radicular morphology/ interradicular bone	Uniradicular	Multiradicular/divergent roots; available interseptal bone allowing implant anchorage	Multiradicular/convergent/wide roots; no available interseptal bone allowing implant anchorage
Alveolar and basal bone morphology	Sufficient bone height (≥ 4 mm) and width (> 2 mm) around apex of planned implant	Sufficient bone height (≥ 4 mm) but deficient bone width (< 2 mm) around apex of planned implant	Insufficient bone height (≤ 4 mm) for apical anchorage of planned implant
Thickness of facial bone wall	≥ 1 mm		< 1 mm
Anticipated residual defect after implant placement	No residual defect	Residual defect with implant position inside alveolar envelope (it can be an immediate or staged placement, but more predictable to graft)	Residual defect with implant position outside the alveolar envelope (less predictable grafting; consider staged grafting)
Soft tissue quality	Adequate keratinized tissue		Inadequate keratinized tissue
Soft tissue quantity	Sufficient (no recession)		Insufficient (recession)
Position in the arch	Not in the esthetic area		Esthetic area

ITI Learning Module Minimally Traumatic Extraction Techniques by Eduardo Lorenzana.

ITI Learning Module Healing of the Extraction Socket by Nikos Mardas.

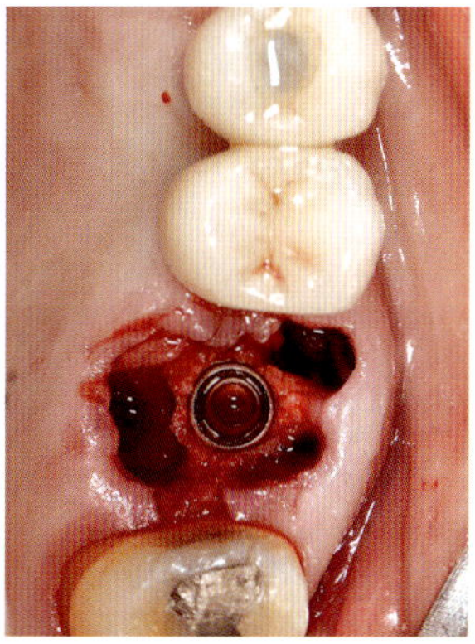

Fig 57. Immediate implant placement in a first molar site. There is need for graft material in the gaps.

3.6.4 Surgical complexity

Surgical complexity factors are those that can individually modify the risk of an implant placement: timing, need for augmentation, and the number of implants. In each of these three situations, other individual factors must be considered and are presented in the following discussion.

ITI Online Academy Learning Pathway on Immediate Placement.

3.6.4.1 TIMING OF PLACEMENT

Immediate implant placement (Type 1) combines tooth extraction and implant placement and reduces the number of surgical procedures that the patient needs to undergo. The peri-implant defect usually presents as a two- or three-walled defect, which is amenable to simultaneous bone augmentation techniques (Figure 57).

In addition, there is an opportunity to attach a provisional restoration to the implant soon after placement so that the patient avoids the need for an interim removable prosthesis.

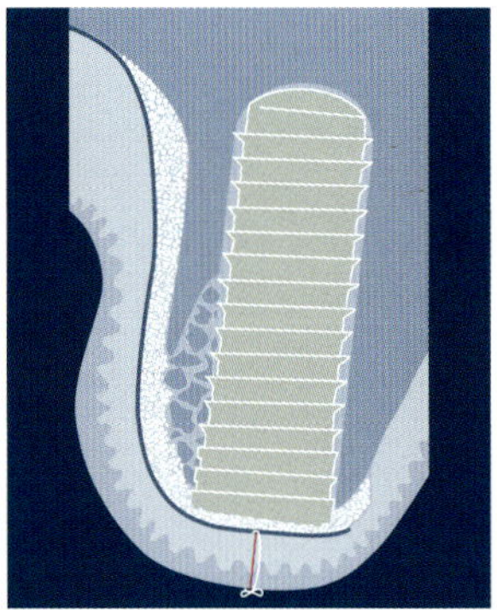

Fig 58. Layered concept of bone augmentation: bone chips, bone substitute, and collagen membrane (blue line). (Source: ITI Treatment Guide Vol. 7 "Ridge Augmentation Procedures in Implant Patients".)

ITI Learning Module Simultaneous Contour Augmentation Using GBR by Daniel Buser, Stephen Chen and Vivianne Chappuis.

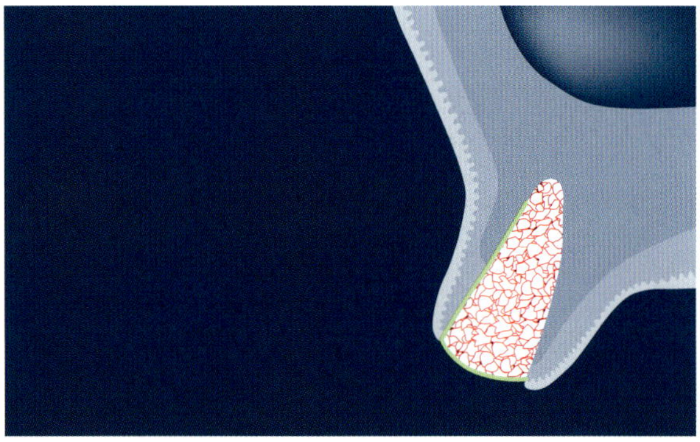

Fig 59. Illustration showing socket preservation procedure. (Source: ITI Treatment Guide Vol. 10 "Implant Therapy in the Esthetic Zone")

Congress Lecture Key Anatomical Factors for Predictable Ridge Preservation and Augmentation by Mauricio Araujo.

However, these advantages are counteracted by the increased technical difficulty of preparing the osteotomy to allow the implant to be placed with initial stability and in a good prosthetic position. There is also an increased risk of mucosal recession, which may compromise soft tissue esthetic outcomes. Additional hard and soft tissue augmentation procedures are usually required to overcome this risk, further increasing the technical demands of the procedure. Although grafting of the peri-implant defect with particulate bone or bone substitutes is readily achieved, grafting of the external surface of the facial bone is more demanding due to the convexity of the bone wall. In immediate placement, the surgery is usually done through a flapless approach, especially in the esthetic zone. If primary soft tissue closure is required, the lack of soft tissue increases the difficulty of attaining tension-free closure. Flap advancement may alter the mucogingival line. The condition of the alveolar and basal bone also has to be considered. Clinicians should be mindful of the fact that bone remodeling following tooth extraction is unpredictable. This may potentially lead to suboptimal bone regenerative outcomes and unpredictable dimensional changes.

In early implant placement (Types 2 and 3), an initial healing period after the extractions allows for several biologic events to take place which are in favor for the clinician and the patient, simplifying the surgical procedure and reducing the risk for postsurgical complications (Buser et al, 2017; Chappuis et al, 2017). Soft tissues spontaneously heal, providing additional thickness of keratinized mucosa, important for covering necessary grafts and to improve the esthetic outcomes. Acute or chronic infection at the site will resolve, reducing the risk of infection. Apical bone formation may enable easier implant bed preparation when compared to a fresh extraction socket. An open-flap procedure is necessary, frequently combined with contour augmentation with guided bone regeneration (Figure 58).

In late implant placement situations (Type 4), bone and soft tissues are completely healed, and hence the surgical risk related to timing is considered to be lower, when bone volume and soft tissue conditions are favorable. It is the least desirable option for the patient, since a longer treatment time is expected, as well as the potential need for multiple procedures, especially in cases of advanced bone remodeling. When an intentional Type 4 placement is planned, socket grafting with a low-substitution-rate bone filler is recommended (Figure 59).

Immediate implant placement (Type 1) is considered to increase technical difficulty of preparing the osteotomy to allow the implant to be placed with initial stability and in a good prosthetic position, when compared to an early (Types 2 and 3) or late (Type 4) placement (Buser et al, 2017). The anatomy of the alveolar socket after extraction can influence the surgical complexity as well and is discussed in more detail in the section about extractions.

When treating a patient who has a compromised dentition, and the treatment involves the extraction of all remaining teeth and simultaneous implant placement, each site planned for implant placement must be looked at individually. However, in the majority of these situations, implants are placed in the remaining basal bone, and the biologic response and influential factors are different than when implants are placed in the alveolar bone (Figure 60).

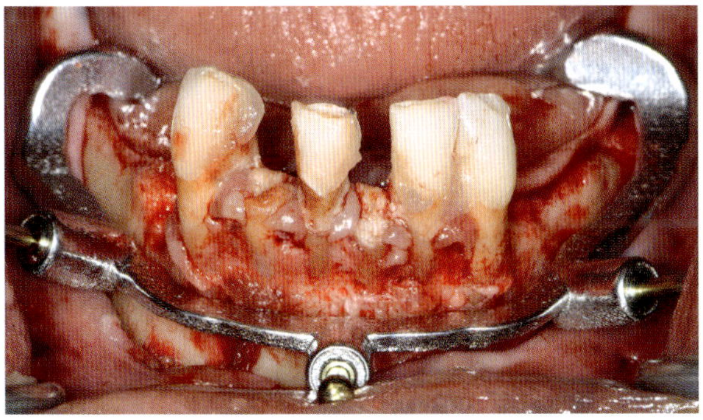

Fig 60. Clinical view of teeth to be extracted for immediate implant placement. Note the alveoloplasty guide showing the level of implant placement. Implants will be mostly in basal bone.

ITI Learning Module Timing of Implant Placement after Tooth Extraction by Stephen Chen.

3.6.4.2 GRAFTING PROCEDURES

Optimal conditions of the alveolar bone and soft tissues are key prerequisites to obtain a good clinical outcome. When these conditions are lacking, the surrounding tissues must be augmented. Augmentation procedures bring increased risk and difficulty to the surgical procedure. Augmentation procedures may have a moderate or high level of difficulty, depending upon the complexity and number of steps involved, and whether a simultaneous or staged approach is indicated (Chiapasco et al, 2009; Chiapasco & Casentini, 2018).

Implant sites that may be managed without adjunctive hard or soft tissue augmentation procedures are regarded as having a low level of difficulty to perform.

Sites that allow implant placement but require small (2 to 4 mm) adjunctive hard and/or soft tissue augmentation procedures have a moderate degree of difficulty, requiring more experience and expertise from the surgeon.

In sites allowing correct 3D positioning and stabilization of the implant but where a large simultaneous horizontal or vertical augmentation is needed, risk is considered to be high. This is also the case for when the site requires a staged augmentation before implant placement.

A wide variety of surgical and augmentation techniques are available to the clinician involved in placing implants. Clinicians must have a sound understanding of the advantages, disadvantages, and clinical evidence supporting the efficacy of techniques they recommend to patients. Augmentation procedures should always be prosthetically driven (Chiapasco & Casentini, 2018).

Congress lecture Predictable Results in Staged Bone Grafts by Waldemar Daudt Polido.

ITI Learning Module Biological Principles of Bone Grafting by Andreas Stavroupoulos.

3.6.4.3 NUMBER OF IMPLANTS

When a single implant is placed, surgical risk is considered to be low, since the surgical procedure is usually simpler and faster, and fewer factors have to be controlled by the clinician.

If two to three implants are placed, risk is considered to be medium, since multiple sites may be involved and the relationship between implants may play a role in the final outcome.

When more than three implants are planned, risk is considered to be high. This is usually the case for fully edentulous treatment or larger partial areas (Polido et al, 2018). The need for accurate spatial relationships between the implants, longer surgical time, increased invasiveness, and multiple surgical sites bring more risk to the procedure (Figure 61).

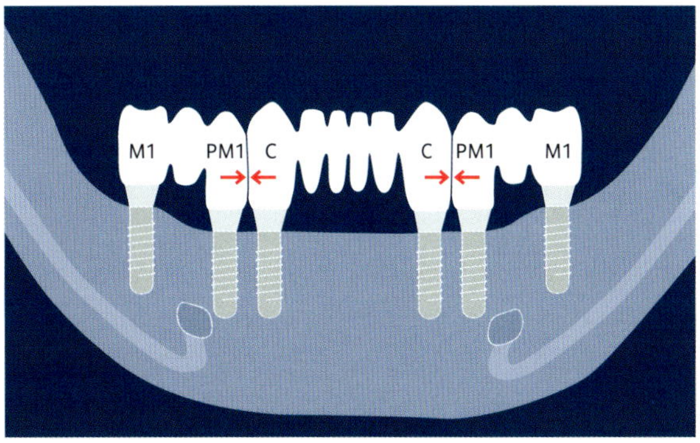

Fig 61. Simultaneous placement of multiple implants is usually associated with high risk. (Source: ITI Treatment Guide Vol. 4 "Loading Protocols in Implant Dentistry.")

Table 8 Surgical modifying factors: Surgical complexity.

Surgical modifying factors	Risk or degree of difficulty		
	Low	Medium	High
	Site factors		
Surgical complexity			
Timing of placement	Healed (late implant placement)	Partially healed (early implant placement)	Immediate implant placement
Grafting procedures	Without adjunct procedures	Simultaneous small hard and/or soft tissue augmentation	Need for large simultaneous horizontal and vertical augmentation; need for staged hard and/or soft tissue procedures
Number of implants	One	Two to three	More than three

Congress lecture Implant Number in the Edentulous Jaw: Practical Considerations for the Fixed Rehabilitation by Waldemar Daudt Polido.

Review article from the 6th ITI Consensus Conference on Number of Implants Placed for Complete-Arch Fixed Prostheses by Waldemar Daudt Polido and coworkers (2017).

In completely edentulous situations, inclination (tilting) of implants may be indicated to avoid more invasive grafting procedures and reduce the cantilever, thus improving implant distribution (Lin & Eckert, 2018). The direct influence of the relationship between multiple implants that need to be splinted adds more complexity to the treatment (Table 8).

3.7 Prosthetic Risks

C. STILWELL, W. MARTIN

The SAC classification includes several modifying factors that have an impact on the level of difficulty and risk of the restorative aspects of implant treatment. They are divided into four groups related to consideration of restorative site factors, occlusal factors, complexity of process, and complicating factors.

Identification of potential restorative risks often requires additional investigations in addition to a comprehensive extraoral, intraoral, and site-specific clinical examination. These additional investigations can be in the form of an analog or digital diagnostic work-up as well as photographic and/or videographic evaluation. These investigations are addressed by the ITI in its Academy Learning Module "Additional Diagnostic Investigations" (Vorster, 2015).

ITI Learning Module Additional Diagnostic Investigations by Christiaan Vorster.

3.7.1 Restorative site factors

Assessment of the restorative site and its characteristics is aimed at determining whether there are any prosthodontic issues with the dimensions and contours of the restorative space. Both can impact treatment complexity and risk for complications. These restorative site factors are highlighted in Table 9 and also addressed by the ITI in its Academy Learning Module "Site-Specific Clinical Examinations" (Shahdad, 2015).

ITI Learning Module Site-Specific Clinical Examination by Shakeel Shahdad.

ITI Treatment Guide Vol. 4 Loading Protocols in Implant Dentistry – Edentulous Patients by Daniel Wismeijer, Paolo Casentini, German Gallucci and Matteo Chiapasco.

ITI Treatment Guide Vol. 10 Implant Therapy in the Esthetic Zone: Current Treatment Modalities and Materials for Single-tooth Replacements by Vivianne Chappuis and William Christopher Martin.

Table 9 Restorative factors.

Restorative factors	Risk or degree of difficulty		
	Low	Medium	High
	Site factors		
Prosthetic volume	**Adequate.** Space available for ideal anatomy of the restoration.	**Compromised.** Can be resolved without adjunctive therapy.	**Inadequate.** Adjunctive therapy will be needed to achieve a satisfactory result.
Interocclusal space	**Adequate.** Possible to create an anatomically and functionally correct planned restoration.	**Compromised.** Can be resolved without adjunctive therapy.	**Inadequate.** Adjunctive therapy will be necessary to achieve sufficient space for the planned restoration.
Volume and characteristics of the edentulous ridge	**Adequate.** No prosthetic soft tissue replacement will be necessary.		**Inadequate.** Prosthetic replacement of soft tissue will be needed for esthetics or phonetics.

3.7.1.1 PROSTHETIC VOLUME

This refers to the 3D space required for the overall prosthesis. The required space will depend on the material planned for the restoration (framework, veneering material, denture teeth, etc) and the associated implant components (abutments, copings, attachments, screws) (Figures 62 and 63). It is described in terms of the mesiodistal, orofacial, and interocclusal space, and where it equates to a volume that is adequate for a restoration with ideal anatomy, it is low risk.

A space that is compromised by being either greater or smaller than ideal will present increased difficulty. If the volume can be rectified without adjunctive therapy, it is regarded as having moderate risk, whereas a case needing significant additional treatment is classified as a high risk.

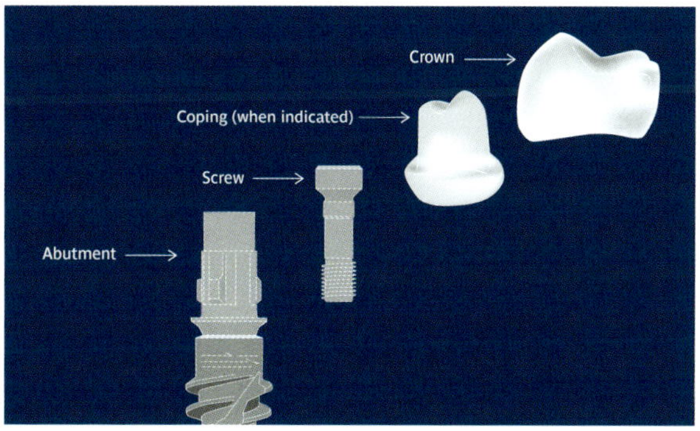

Fig 62. Prosthetic volume for a single-tooth screw-retained implant restoration.

3.7.1.2 INTEROCCLUSAL SPACE

The definition of *interocclusal space* can vary with the resource; authors often use varying reference points: 1) implant platform to opposing occlusal table, 2) abutment level to opposing occlusal table, 3) planned restorative margin to opposing occlusal table, or 4) ridge to opposing occlusal table. It is important to verify these reference points prior to using published numbers in order to prevent potential complications, as a difference of ~3 mm (when utilizing bone-level implants) can exist between reference 1 and 4.

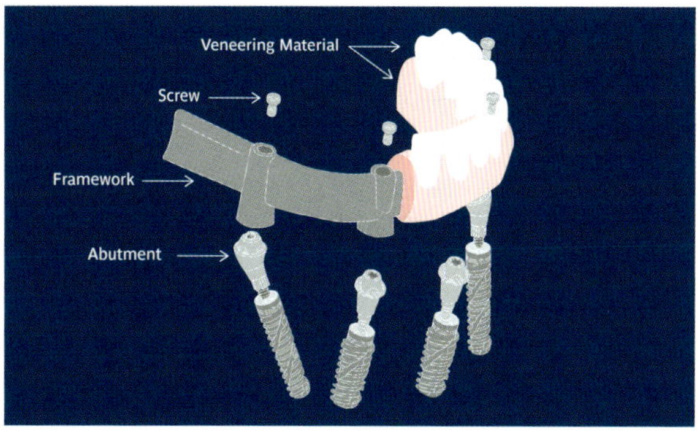

Fig 63. Prosthetic volume for a full-arch screw-retained implant restoration.

Minimum interocclusal space requirements (reference points ridge to opposing occlusal table):

- Crowns: 7 mm (Figure 64)
- Fixed dental prosthesis: 7 mm (Figure 64)
- Overdenture (individual attachment, eg, Locator, Novaloc [Straumann]): 8–11 mm (Figure 65)
- Overdenture (bar with attachment): 14 mm (Figure 66)
- Hybrid (denture tooth, acrylic resin, and framework): 12–15 mm (Figure 67)
- Hybrid (monolithic zirconia): 11–14 mm (Figure 68)

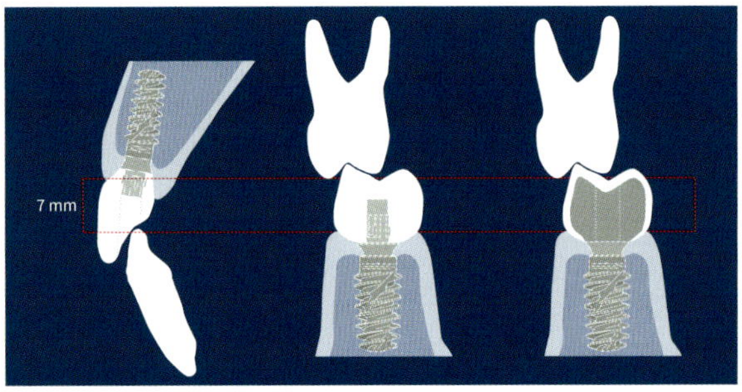

Fig 64. Minimum interocclusal space requirement: Crown (anterior, posterior) and fixed dental prosthesis (FDP).

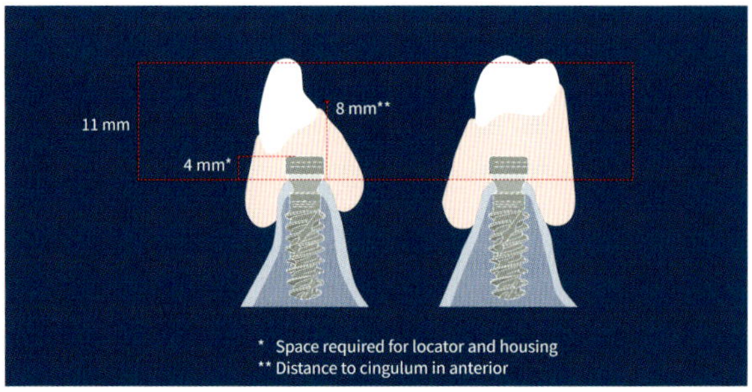

Fig 65. Minimum interocclusal space requirement: Overdenture (individual attachment, eg, Locator, Novaloc).

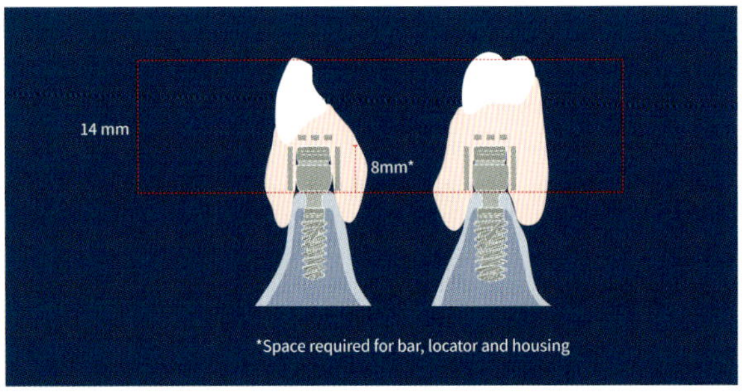

Fig 66. Minimum interocclusal space requirement: Overdenture (bar with attachment).

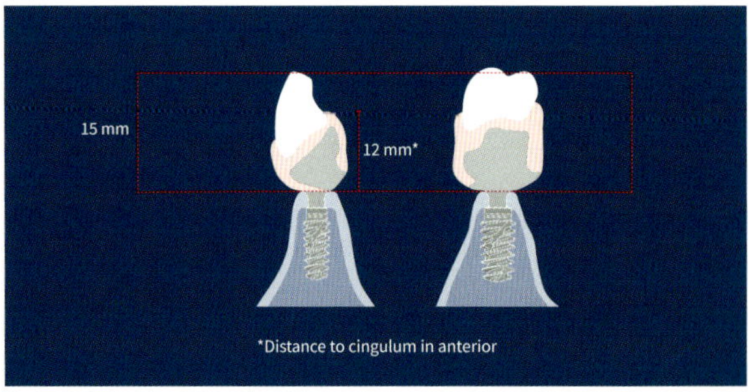

Fig 67. Minimum interocclusal space requirement: Hybrid (denture tooth, acrylic resin, and framework).

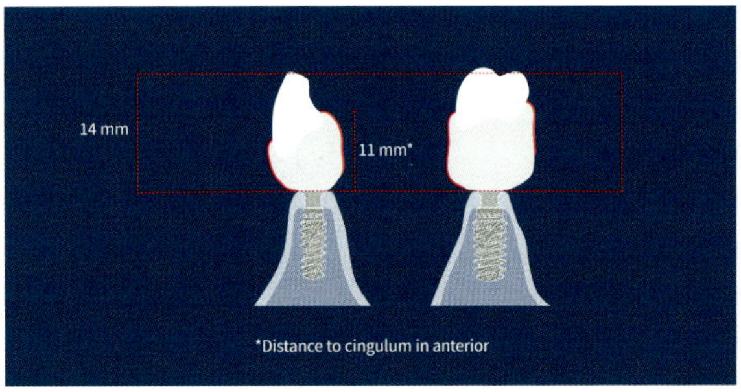

Fig 68. Minimum interocclusal space requirement: Hybrid (monolithic zirconia).

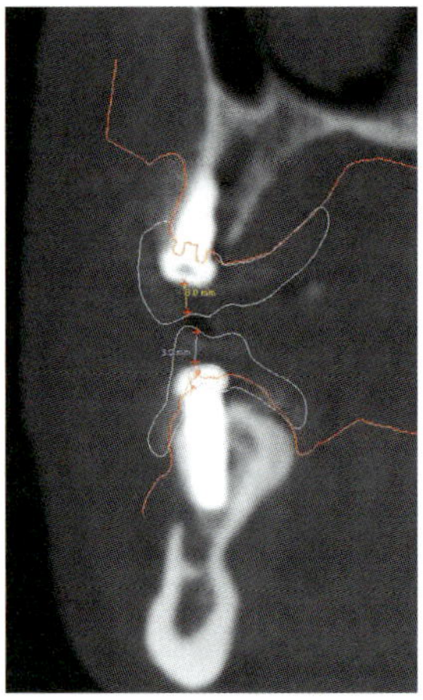

Fig 69. A dual-scan CBCT with an overdenture wax-up (white line) highlighting inadequate interarch space for restoration.

Similar to the prosthetic volume, it is judged according to the ability to create an anatomically and functionally correct restoration which will provide desired esthetics and durability. If this is readily achieved, it is of low risk; if space is compromised but possible to resolve without adjunctive therapy, it is associated with moderate risk. An inadequate space that requires adjunctive therapy to achieve adequate space is a high-risk procedure.

Examples of adjunctive therapy include:

- Orthodontics (intrusion of opposing dentition)
- Restoration of the opposing arch
- Surgical intervention (bone reduction or bone grafting)
- Jaw surgery

Major complications arise in situations where implants have been placed with improper planning for adequate interocclusal space for the planned restoration (Figure 69). In these situations, if no other alternative restorative option exists, the implants will need to be removed and space then created.

3.7.1.3 VOLUME AND CHARACTERISTICS OF THE EDENTULOUS RIDGE

Subject to the extent of dimensional changes following loss of the natural tooth or teeth, the volume and contours of the edentulous ridge may represent a greater or lesser prosthodontic challenge for creation of an ideal restoration anatomy (Figure 70). The assessment focuses on whether prosthetic replacement of soft tissue volume or other adjunctive therapy such as a bone grafting is needed. If there is no need, the situation is deemed low risk. If the volume and characteristics are inadequate and require adjunctive therapy, it is regarded as having high risk.

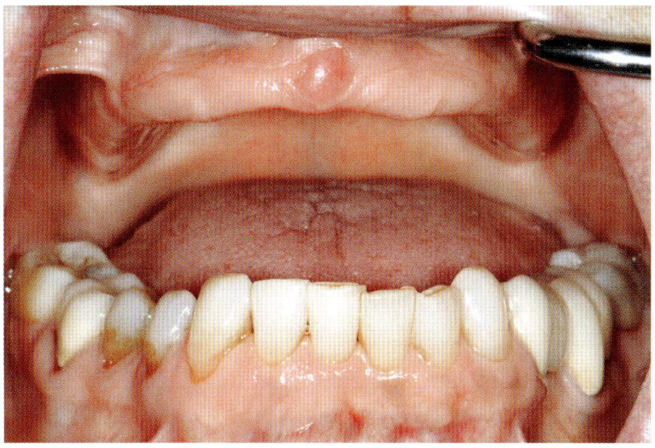

Fig 70. An atrophic maxilla opposing natural dentition, requiring augmentation procedures for an implant-supported restoration.

3.7.2 Occlusal factors

The biophysical response to occlusal force is different for implants and teeth, as teeth are connected to the surrounding alveolar bone via the periodontal ligament. Dental implants, by contrast, are in contact with the bone directly by osseointegration. As a consequence, natural teeth are subject to a mean axial displacement of approximately 25–100 µm, while dental implants get displaced by only 3–5 µm (Kim et al, 2005; Schulte, 1995). This affects capacity for movement and sensory feedback of implants and has been shown to impact risk of—predominantly—hardware complications (Salvi & Brägger, 2009). To adjust and reevaluate the occlusion with implant-supported reconstructions is therefore of fundamental importance, as the absence of the periodontal ligament significantly detracts from their load-sharing ability, occlusal force adaptation, and mechanoperception (Kim et al, 2005). Occlusal considerations are addressed by the ITI in its Academy Learning Module "Occlusion on fixed implant prostheses" (Stilwell, 2015).

ITI Learning Module Occlusion on Fixed Implant Prostheses **by Charlotte Stilwell.**

The characteristics of the patient's occlusal scheme and the extent of involvement of implant prostheses in the scheme affect the degree of difficulty of implant restoration. The presence of occlusal parafunction with greater and unpredictable occlusal forces will further elevate risk. The modifying considerations of three occlusal factors are found in Table 10.

Table 10 Occlusal factors.

Occlusal factors	Risk or degree of difficulty		
	Low	Medium	High
	Site factors		
Occlusal scheme	User-defined occlusal scheme achievable		User-defined occlusal scheme not achievable
Involvement in occlusion	Minimal or no involvement		Implant restoration is involved with guidance
Occlusal parafunction	Absent		Present

3.7.2.1 OCCLUSAL SCHEME

The patient's occlusal scheme, and the extent to which the implant restoration will be involved in this scheme, will affect the degree of difficulty of implant restoration. This may, in turn, influence the likelihood of complications to the definitive restoration.

Patients present with considerable variations in their occlusal schemes, and when determining occlusal stability, the following guidelines can be followed for initial assessment. It must be possible to obtain bilateral, evenly distributed, centered, posterior occlusal contacts in static occlusion and an absence of posterior interferences in dynamic occlusion (lateral and protrusive excursive movements) through anterior guidance. If a slide is present between centric and habitual occlusion, no interferences should be present between the two (Kim et al, 2005; Wismeijer et al, 2012).

Where a user-defined scheme is already present and/or achievable, this is considered of low risk. Where a user-defined scheme is not achievable, it is assessed as being of high risk.

3.7.2.2 INVOLVEMENT IN OCCLUSION

This refers to the degree to which the implant prosthesis is involved in the patient's occlusal scheme. Implant prostheses that are protected in dynamic occlusal excursions by anterior guidance, at the same time as not being part of developing that guidance, present lesser difficulty and are deemed low risk. In contrast, implant prostheses that are part of developing the guidance are considered to carry greater difficulty and are therefore regarded as having high risk.

3.7.2.3 OCCLUSAL PARAFUNCTION

Parafunctional occlusal forces are not proven to present a risk to implant survival, but they are likely to result in more complications for implant prostheses in terms of screw loosening, abutment or screw fracture, and fracture of the veneering material (Salvi & Brägger, 2009). In this context, absence of a parafunctional habit is considered a low-risk situation, whereas presence is elevating difficulty and regarded as high risk. Parafunction as a dental factor is addressed by the ITI in its Academy Learning Module "Patient Dental Factors" (Shahdad, 2015).

ITI Learning Module Patient Dental Factors by Shakeel Shahdad.

3.7.3 Complexity of process

The level of complexity of an implant surgical or restorative treatment may be assessed by considering the number of steps involved in the procedure and the number of areas in which an appropriate outcome must be achieved. As a general principle, the level of complexity rises with an increase in the number of steps involved and the number of objectives that must be achieved to obtain a satisfactory result.

The complexity of the restorative process is influenced by several different factors. They include operator access within the oral cavity, need for additional prosthodontic steps, number of implants, and choice of loading and placement protocols as highlighted in Table 11.

Table 11 Complexity of the process.

Complexity	Risk or degree of difficulty		
	Low	Medium	High
	Site factors		
Access	Adequate		Inadequate
Interim prosthesis	None required	Tooth-supported	Tissue- or interim implant-supported
Implant-supported provisional restoration	None required	Required, reduced esthetic and/ or functional demands	Required, elevated esthetic and/ or functional demands
Number and location of implants	Single	2 (nonsplinted)	> 2 (nonsplinted) or ≥ 2 (splinted)
Loading protocols	Conventional/early		Immediate

3.7.3.1 ACCESS

As for all dental procedures, both the surgical and prosthodontic implant therapy armamentarium requires a certain degree of access to the treatment site. Examples are the ease of access to insert components, make impressions, and undertake future maintenance. The patient's extent of jaw opening and the location and characteristics of the treatment site can all affect the complexity of the treatment. In the context of this factor, adequate access is considered low risk, while inadequate access is high risk.

3.7.3.2 INTERIM PROSTHESIS

Where necessary during the healing phase of implant therapy, the need for interim tooth replacements can add to the difficulty of treatment. A well-designed interim prosthesis should provide esthetic and functional use while protecting the tissues and implants during their healing phase (Markus, 1999). This is often most problematic in the full-arch situation, where an interim denture can place uncontrolled loads on bone grafts and/or healing implants (transmucosal loading), increasing the risk of early failure. In some situations (when anatomy is favorable), consideration should be given to temporary implants being utilized for retention and support of an interim restoration.

In summary, the selection of the type of interim prosthesis should be based on esthetic demands, functional requirements, financial considerations, duration required, and ease of fabrication (Cho et al, 2007).

ITI Treatment Guide Vol. 6 Extended Edentulous Spaces in the Esthetic Zone by Julia-Gabriela Wittneben Matter and Hans-Peter Weber.

3.7.3.3 IMPLANT-SUPPORTED PROVISIONAL RESTORATION

At the time of implant placement or after osseointegration, the fabrication of an implant-supported provisional restoration can aid in developing the peri-implant tissues, testing contours of the definitive restoration and improving patient satisfaction. In 2019, in a study conducted on partially edentulous patients, Furze and coworkers reported a significant difference in esthetic outcomes (modPES) at 36 months when tissues were conditioned with a provisional implant-supported restoration versus no tissue conditioning.

In full-arch situations, a fixed implant-supported provisional restoration can serve several benefits, confirming tooth position, testing esthetics and phonetics, aiding with master cast verification and records, all while improving patient satisfaction. Most importantly, the implant-supported provisional restoration can be utilized as a backup if needed over time.

ITI Learning Module Implant Supported Provisional Restorations by William Christopher Martin.

If an implant-supported provisional restoration is delivered at the time of implant placement (immediate), careful attention should be given to not disturbing the stability of the implant and sutures or to contaminate the submucosal tissue, bone grafts (if present), or implant body (if a horizontal defect is present). These situations are often associated with higher risk or difficulty.

3.7.3.4 NUMBER AND LOCATION OF IMPLANTS

The degree of difficulty and risk of restorative complexity is proportional to the number of implants, their location within the arch, and whether they are splinted or nonsplinted. For example, a single implant with minimal esthetic risk, favorable anatomy, and adequate access for treatment would carry low risk, while multiple implants planned for a splinted restoration in the esthetic zone would carry a higher risk.

3.7.3.5 LOADING PROTOCOLS

When and how implants are loaded by restorations will have an impact on the level of difficulty of the restorative treatment. At the Fourth ITI Consensus Conference, Weber and coworkers (Weber et al, 2009) defined the timing of implant loading relative to its placement. Please refer to Chapter 2.1 to review the details of these definitions. In general, from a prosthodontic perspective, conventional loading (healing time of > 2 months) and early loading (healing time of 1 to 2 months) will likely be more straightforward than loading in which a provisional or definitive restoration is placed within 1 week of implant placement—so-called *immediate loading*. The immediate loading protocol is a more difficult technical procedure, and it requires greater coordination between the surgeon, restorative dentist, and dental laboratory, thus justifying its increased risk.

ITI Learning Module Immediate Restoration and Loading by Diego Bechelli.

Congress Lecture Loading Protocols in the Digital Era – Part I: Single Implants and Extended Edentulous Sites by German Gallucci.

Congress Lecture Loading Protocols in the Digital Era – Part II: Edentulous Jaws – Fixed and Overdenture by German Gallucci.

ITI Treatment Guide Vol. 2 Loading Protocols in Implant Dentistry – Partially Dentate Patients by Jeffrey Ganeles and Dean Morton.

ITI Treatment Guide Vol. 4 Loading Protocols in Implant Dentistry – Edentulous Patients by Daniel Wismeijer, Paolo Casentini, German Gallucci and Matteo Chiapasco.

3.7.4 Complicating factors

No procedure is totally without risk of complicating the treatment outcome or affecting the long-term success and stability of the restoration. A clear understanding of how the restoration design and maintenance following delivery can influence the risk of complications is critical for achieving long-term success. The complicating factors associated with the risk or degree of difficulty of the definitive restoration can be separated into three categories: biologic, mechanical/technical, and maintenance (Table 12).

Table 12 Complicating factors.

Complication factors	Risk or degree of difficulty		
	Low	Medium	High
	Site factors		
Biologic	Screw-retained with appropriate contours and biocompatible materials	Cement-retained single-unit restorations with appropriate contours and biocompatible materials	Cemented multiunit reconstructions or restorations with contours inaccessible for maintenance procedures
Mechanical/technical	Absence of contributing factors	Presence of noncritical contributing factors	Presence of critical contributing factors
Maintenance	Low	Moderate	High

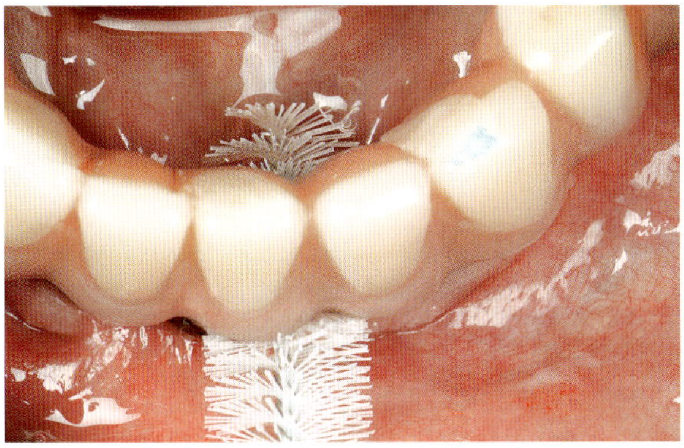

Fig 71. Access for cleaning demonstrated on mandibular hybrid restoration.

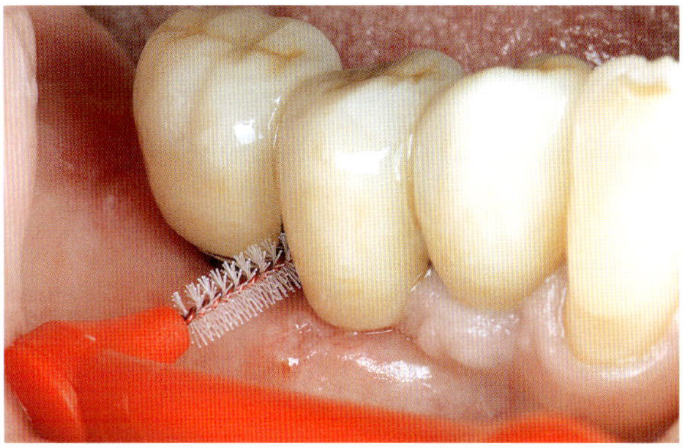

Fig 72. Access for cleaning demonstrated on an implant-supported FDP.

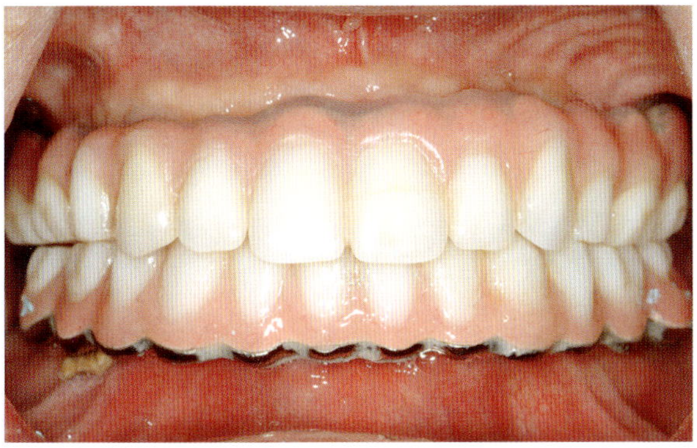

Fig 73. Maxillary and mandibular hybrid restorations demonstrating ridge-lap design.

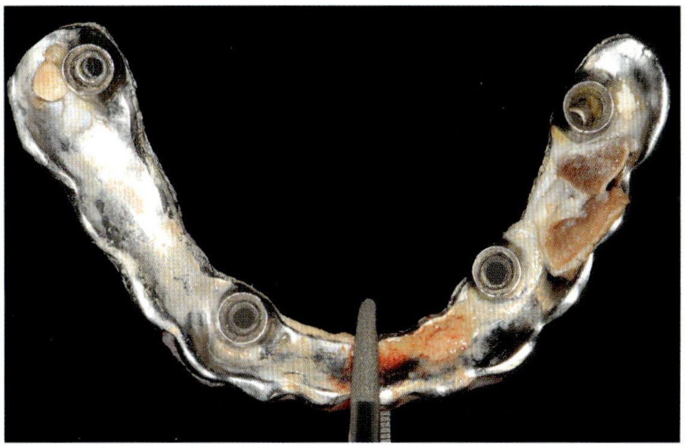

Fig 74. Intaglio view of mandibular hybrid prosthesis with debris from inability to properly clean.

3.7.4.1 BIOLOGIC

Biologic complications influenced by the implant-supported restoration are not unusual. Their risk can be associated with the design of the prosthesis, management of the occlusion, and ability for the patient to access the peri-implant mucosa for cleaning (Figures 71 and 72). Factors that minimize these complications start with meticulous treatment planning, implant selection (surface, shape, size, and connection), and restoration-driven 3D positioning of the implant(s) that allow for optimal restoration design.

High risk for complications is recognized when an implant-supported restoration prevents access for cleaning and does not allow for removal for maintenance procedures (Figures 73 and 74).

Congress Lecture Prosthetic Planning and Design to Prevent Biologic Complications **by Dean Morton.**

Congress Lecture Biologic and Technical Complications in Implant Dentistry **by Lisa J. A. Heitz-Mayfield.**

ITI Treatment Guide Vol. 8 Biological and Hardware Complications in Implant Dentistry **by Urs Brägger and Lisa J. A. Heitz-Mayfield.**

3.7.4.2 MECHANICAL AND TECHNICAL

Mechanical or technical complications occur about twice as frequently as biologic complications. But, when they occur and are not addressed, they can lead to biologic complications (often more severe), potentially compromising the dental implant(s). With this, mechanical and technical risks play a major role in implant dentistry. They may lead to increased rates of repairs and remakes, and to a waste of time and financial resources, and they may even affect the patient's quality of life (Salvi & Brägger, 2009). In 2009, during a systematic review of the literature for the Fourth ITI Consensus Conference, Salvi and Brägger defined mechanical and technical risks as follows:

- *Mechanical risk:* Risk of a complication or failure of a prefabricated component caused by mechanical forces.
- *Technical risk:* Risk of a complication or failure of the laboratory-fabricated suprastructure or its materials.

From their systematic review, they defined 10 contributing factors for mechanical and technical risk:

1. Type of retentive elements supporting overdentures
2. Cantilever extensions on fixed dental prostheses (FDPs)
3. Cemented versus screw-retained FDPs
4. Angled/angulated abutments
5. Bruxism
6. Crown-to-implant ratio
7. Length of the superstructure
8. Prosthetic materials
9. Number of implants supporting an FDP
10. History of mechanical/technical complications

During the diagnostic and planning phase for implant rehabilitation, consideration should be given to these risk factors in an effort to minimize potential complications following delivery.

Congress Lecture Prosthetic Planning and Design to Prevent Technical Complications by Hans-Peter Weber.

Congress Lecture Prosthetic Planning and Design to Prevent Hardware Complications by Hans-Peter Weber.

ITI Treatment Guide Vol. 8 Biological and Hardware Complications in Implant Dentistry by Urs Brägger and Lisa J. A. Heitz-Mayfield.

3.7.4.3 MAINTENANCE

The need for restoration maintenance should be assessed during the planning of an implant rehabilitation and reinforced to the patient during the treatment phase. Several factors play a role on the risk during the maintenance phase, including patient compliance, span of the restoration, occlusal parafunction, retention, prosthesis design, access for care, and the dentist's preferences. These will all have an impact on overall risk assessment. In general, more complex restorations will be associated with higher maintenance needs.

Congress Lecture Hardware Maintenance of Implant-supported Fixed Dental Prostheses by John Hyun Uk Cho.

CHAPTER 4:

How Does the SAC Assessment Tool Derive a Classification?

A. DAWSON, S. KELLER

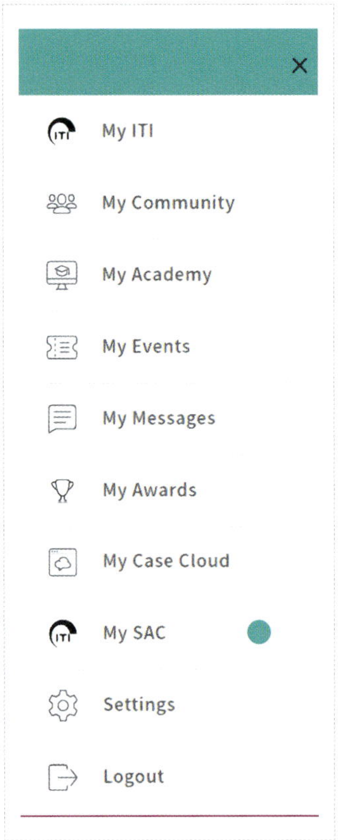

Fig 1. Accessing the SAC Assessment Tool on www.iti.org.

4.1 Introduction

The risk factors identified in Chapter 3 were determined using a consensus approach. The importance of each factor was determined to relate to the impact on the treatment outcome or degree of difficulty that might arise if this risk factor were realized in a case. Thus, some factors were seen to have a higher importance in the determination of risk.

The SAC Assessment Tool was developed based on these identified risk factors. Users are asked to select options for each risk factor (that is relevant to their case type) that most closely relates to their case. The responses to these questions feed into the calculation of the classification determined for that case.

4.2 Definitions

Risk factor: Any characteristic of the patient's presenting history or condition, or of the planned treatment for that patient, that might contribute to the risk of adverse treatment outcomes.

Cluster: A group of thematically similar risk factors.

Group: A selection of clusters making up an assessment (eg, those clusters that contribute to the general risk assessment).

Alert: A risk factor that, when present, would normally block any further treatment. In general, these factors relate to situations that are incompatible with successful implant treatment, or where the risk of suboptimal outcomes would be unacceptable to either the patient or the clinician. Such factors should be resolved, or at least significantly mitigated, prior to commencing implant treatment.

Warning: Risk factors that elevate the SAC level considerably. These factors can have a disproportionate effect on the level of complexity and risk.

4.3 Workflow

The SAC Assessement Tool workflow aims to emulate the normal path of patient assessment and treatment planning. Users start a classification by selecting the "My SAC" option from the dropdown list associated with their iti.org account (Figure 1).

Users are then prompted to start a new classification and then label their assessment. All SAC classification assessments will be saved in the user's profile for future reference, so a unique identifier for the case is recommended. To comply with privacy laws, it is recommended that users **do not** use their patients' names as the label.

The user will then be asked to select the case type (indication) and the treatment region. Finally, they will be asked to select whether they wish to carry out a complete classification (which includes both the surgical and prosthodontic classifications), or one of the partial classification options (surgical classification, prosthodontic classification, or esthetic risk assessment).

Data used to develop a classification are then collected through a series of multiple-choice questions relating to the risk factors considered significant in the presenting case type. An example is shown in Figure 2.

Some questions are common to more than one part of the assessment: The data are collected only once but used to populate the appropriate part of the assessment wherever it is needed.

4.3.1 General risk assessment (GRA)

The processes of anamnesis and clinical assessment will provide much of the information involved in this part of the classification process. Data relating to three major themes (clusters) contribute to this assessment:

- The patient's medical history
- Patient-related factors such as habits and attitudes
- Site-related characteristics, such as the ease of accessing the treatment site

4.3.2 Esthetic risk assessment (ERA)

The case type and treatment site will determine how esthetic risk will be assessed. One of four options will be incorporated into the classification process:

1. The ERA developed by Martin and coworkers (Martin et al, 2017). This is used in most cases in the esthetic zone that involve missing single teeth and short edentulous spans.
2. The Edentulous Esthetic Risk Assessment (EERA) developed to address the assessment of cases involving extended edentulous areas and full-arch replacements.
3. An abbreviated esthetic assessment in cases where there is minimal esthetic impact associated with the case. These issues are addressed in questions in the general, prosthodontic, and surgical risk assessments.
4. No esthetic assessment in cases where there is no perceptible esthetic involvement in the case.

4.3.2.1 ERA

A single cluster of factors contributes to this assessment. Some of these factors are addressed as part of the other risks assessments that make up the SAC classification. Those factors not addressed elsewhere are assessed in the ERA specific cluster.

4.3.2.2 EERA

The EERA aims to measure esthetic risks in cases where there are extended edentulous spaces, or where all teeth are missing. A single cluster of factors contribute this assessment to the overall SAC classification. These factors are discussed in more detail in Chapter 3.4.

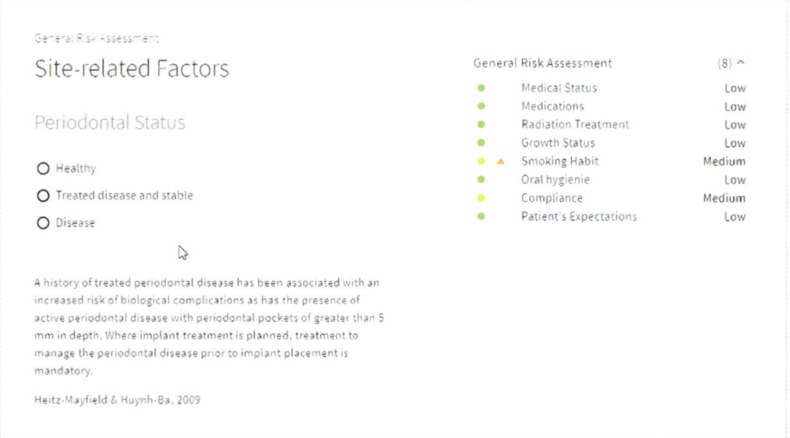

Fig 2. Data are entered by responding to a series of multiple-choice questions. Note that a running tally of selections is also displayed.

4.3.3 Surgical risk assessment (SRA) and surgical classification

Five clusters of risk factors contribute to the SRA:

- The surgical protocol to be used
- Anatomical factors relating to the planned site
- Factors relating to adjacent teeth
- Issues related to the residual bony anatomy in the site after the recent removal of the tooth (if applicable)
- Risks related to the complexity of the surgical procedure

These factors are discussed in detail in Chapter 3.5. The overall calculation of these risk factors determines the surgical classification.

4.3.4 Prosthodontic risk assessment (PRA) and prosthodontic classification

The prosthodontic risk is based on five clusters:

- Restorative factors
- Esthetic factors
- Occlusal factors
- Factors that contribute to the complexity of the restorative process
- Factors that might contribute to the risk of complications

The esthetic cluster contains a subset of the risk factors from the ERA. When a complete ERA is needed, the remaining factors are assessed as part of the esthetic assessment. Edentulous esthetic risk also contributes to the esthetic cluster score (where applicable). A complete discussion of these prosthodontic risk factors can be found in Chapter 3.6.

4.4 Calculating a Classification

Each risk factor can potentially have low, moderate, and high risk values. The characteristics of these levels form the options in the tool's multiple-choice question for the respective risk factor.

4.4.1 Calculation mechanism

A complexity/risk level and an impact level were assigned to each of the available options. The complexity/risk level ranged from Low (1), through Medium (2), to High (3), while the impact levels were designated as Baseline, Elevated, and Severe. Besides the effect on the calculation, impact levels are also used to raise alerts in the application.

For each cluster of risk factors, the weighted mean of the complexity/risk levels was calculated, and the overall risk of the factors determined according to the following risk matrix (Table 1). The weight of the complexity/risk levels was determined during the testing of the algorithm (see Chapter 4.5).

Table 1 The risk matrix used in the calculation of cluster score.

	Complexity/risk level (1)		
Impact level (2)	Low	Medium	High
Baseline	Low	Medium	High
Elevated	Medium	Medium	High
Severe	High	High	High

1) Weighted mean
2) Maximum impact level in the group of risk factors

After the determination of the risk of each cluster, the overall classification for surgical and prosthodontic cases was determined using the risk levels of the groups within the classification. In addition, the results of the GRA were also included in the evaluation of the different case types. During the calibration and consensus phase, it became apparent that the ERA needed to be excluded from the overall determination of the surgical and prosthodontic assessment. The weight of the ERAs was considered too high, and the impact on the overall risk should be considered separately by the clinician.

It can be argued that the risk level of the case should be determined by the highest risk present in the grouped factors. However, to provide consistent results with the earlier tool, each group of factors was treated as having equal weight in the evaluation of the overall SAC classification. The mean risk of the grouped factors was treated as the base risk and elevated to a higher risk level as shown in Table 2.

Table 2 Exceeding the maximum number of groups allowed at a specific level will result in the elevation of the risk to the next level.

	Max. number of groups at medium risk level	**Max. number of groups at high risk level**
Straightforward	2	1
Advanced	NA	2
Complex	NA	NA

4.5 Testing the Algorithm

The SAC Assessment Tool was tested by experienced clinicians who were familiar with the SAC classification concept. Using real cases, these users tested the tool's assessments against their own expectations for the cases being assessed. Alternative calculation methods were provided (although the testers were blinded to the actual methods being offered), and testers were asked to select the method that produced a result that best fitted their expectation. The testers were also asked to select what they thought the prosthodontic and surgical classifications should be for the case. Over a number of iterations, this process fine-tuned the algorithm to ensure that this new tool would provide results that were consistent with earlier methods.

4.6 Presenting the Results

The 2009 version of the SAC Assessment Tool determined a normative classification for a specific case type and highlighted additional modifiers that might contribute to added complexity. It did not, however, classify to the individual case level; that is, award a higher-level classification if these additional modifiers added significant risk. The assessment determined a classification for the case type, and users had to decide if the additional modifiers might be significant. The new tool calculates a SAC classification for the case and incorporates all relevant risk factors into this assessment.

The online tool presents the results of the assessment of the outcomes at the surgical, prosthetic, and esthetic risks

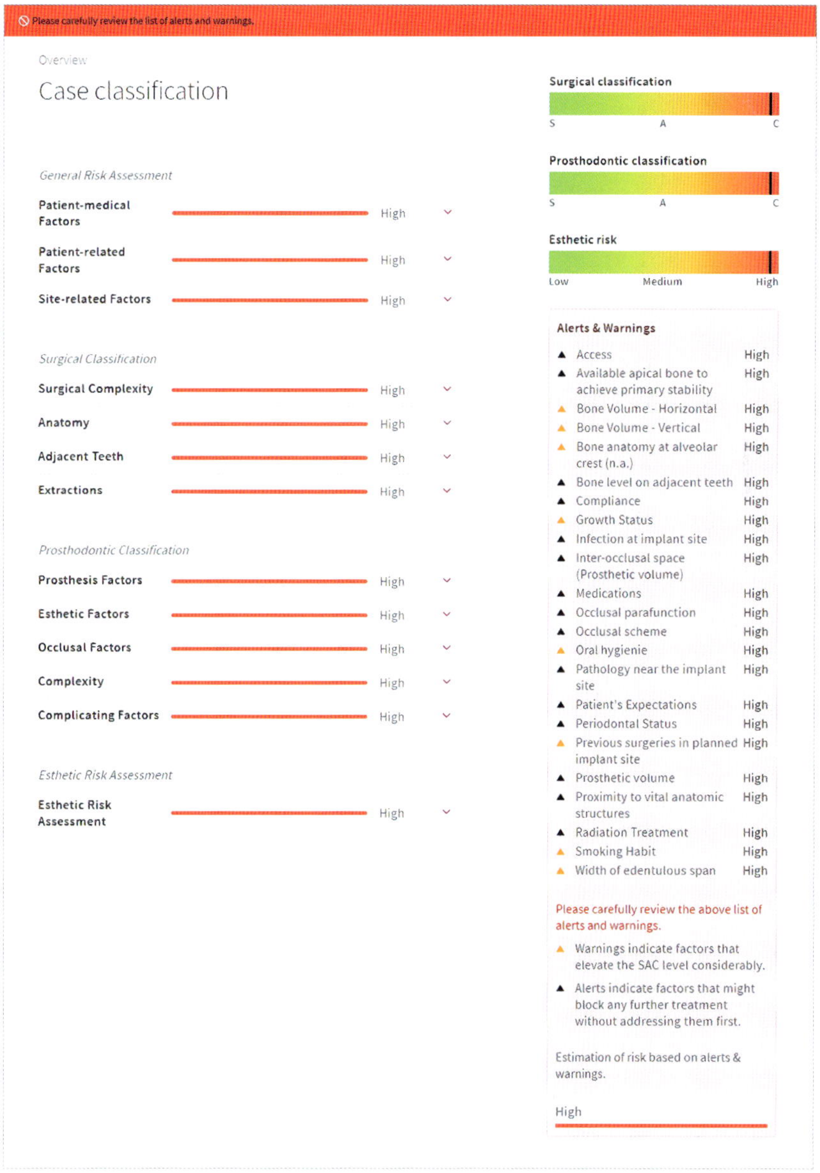

Fig 3. Result screen showing a combined surgical and prosthodontic classification. The estimation of the risk based on impact levels is high.

scores (Figure 3). Users can also assess the input of various risk factors on the assessment by reviewing color-coded responses to each of the clusters and, when expanded, the individual risk factors. The colors green, yellow, and red indicate low, moderate, and high-level responses, respectively. Alerts and warnings are also tabulated on the results screens. Each group of factors can be expanded to display the information collected in that assessment. For example, the ERA for this case can be expanded to display the relevant information (Figure 4).

The online tool will also suggest educational material that might be relevant to the case being assessed. Links to ITI Academy learning items and papers and statements from the ITI Consensus Conferences can be followed to expand on the issues related to the case. Access to some of this material will incur costs for users who are not members of the ITI. ITI Members and Fellows have free access to all material.

The use of the SAC Assessment Tool is probably best demonstrated practically. So please check it out on www.iti.org.

Esthetic Risk Assessment

Esthetic Risk Assessment	Medium
Medical Status	High
▲ Smoking Habit	Medium
Gingival display at full smile	High
Width of edentulous span	Low
Shape of tooth crowns	High
Restorative status of neighboring teeth	High
Gingival Phenotype	Medium
Infection at implant site	Medium
Soft tissue anatomy	High
Bone level on adjacent teeth	Medium
Thickness of buccal wall	Low
Bone anatomy at alveolar crest (n.a.)	Medium
▲ Patient's Expectations	High

Fig 4. Details of the ERA. Black and orange risk icons indicate factors with elevated or severe impact levels.

CHAPTER 5:

Practical Application of the SAC Assessment Tool

W. MARTIN, A. DAWSON, W. D. POLIDO

5.1. Introduction

Every patient's dental situation is a unique circumstance with the treatment approach customized to fit their needs. At the core of the SAC classification is its ability to assist in categorizing the overall treatment risk and difficulty based on the clinical factors presented by the patient prior to the initiation of care. The ability to evaluate the patient from a restorative and surgical perspective aids the clinician and/or treatment team in generating a comprehensive approach to treatment, and in some situations, it assists in identifying the appropriate clinician for providing care. In addition, the patient's SAC classification can be a valuable communication tool between the treatment team and their patient(s) as well as for educational content and events (study clubs, CE courses, webinars, publications, in-person implant meetings, etc).

In an effort to make this classification system streamlined, easily accessible, and utilizable online, the interactive SAC Assessment Tool was created (see Chapter 4). The SAC Assessment Tool allows the user to answer specific questions related to the patient and their planned treatment, after which the overall assessment is generated along with available learning resources in the ITI Online Academy specific to that assessment. In addition, the SAC Assessment Tool was recently redesigned to identify critical and subcritical clinical factors that could negatively influence treatment outcomes and develop algorithms to influence the designation of overall treatment difficulty.

This chapter highlights a variety of clinical scenarios authored by ITI Fellows that utilized the SAC Assessment Tool during the evaluation and planning process, followed by their treatment approach and reflection during follow-up visits.

5.2 Implants for Restoration of Single-Tooth Spaces: Areas of Low Esthetic Risk

5.2.1 Mandibular molar

M. ROCCUZZO

A 40-year-old-man was originally referred by his general dentist for extraction of tooth 47 and placement of two implants in positions 46 and 47. The patient's medical history did not reveal any significant findings, and he was in good general health.

The clinical examination of the right posterior mandible revealed the absence of tooth 46 and a mesiobuccal gingival recession at tooth 47 (Figure 1). A thermal test confirmed that tooth 47 was still vital. The radiograph showed the presence of a significant bone defect, with a slope shape from the distal aspect of tooth 45 to the apex of tooth 47 (Figure 2).

Probing revealed the presence of a 9-mm pocket mesial to tooth 47 (Figure 3). The periapical radiograph confirmed the absence of periapical osteolysis and a normal level of the interproximal bone between teeth 47 and 48 (Figure 4).

The presence of a deep pocket has been associated with increased probability of tooth loss, even in patients attending supportive periodontal therapy (SPT) (Matuliene et al, 2008). Teeth with deep pockets, associated with deep intrabony defects, have been classified as having either a questionable prognosis (ie, need complex treatment) or a hopeless prognosis, and therefore should be extracted as soon as possible (Kwok & Caton, 2007).

In clinical practice, the prognostic system should be based not only on the amount of periodontal supporting apparatus, but also on the evaluation of local and general risk factors, like plaque and infection control, smoking habit, and systemic conditions. Clinicians should be cautious before declaring a tooth "hopeless," as it has been demonstrated that even teeth with severe loss of periodontal support, like attachment loss to the apex, can be retained and kept healthy with appropriate periodontal therapy and strict SPT (Cortellini et al, 2011). Furthermore, patients with a history

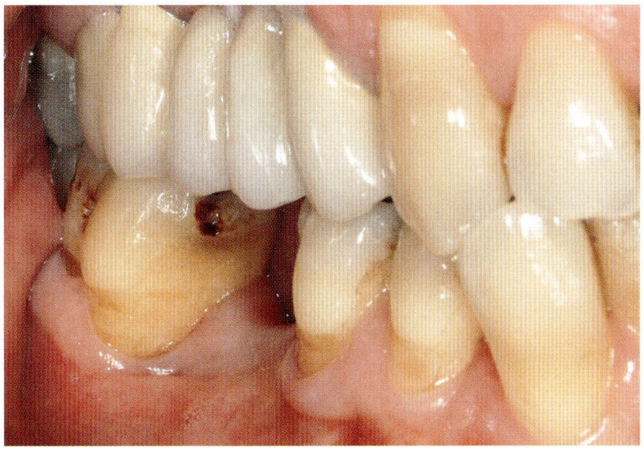

Fig 1. Pretreatment lateral view. Missing tooth 46 and gingival recession on tooth 47.

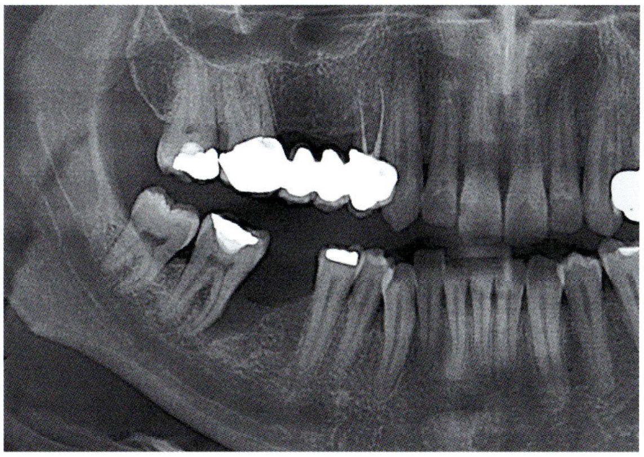

Fig 2. Panoramic radiograph demonstrated the presence of a deep vertical periodontal defect mesially to tooth 47.

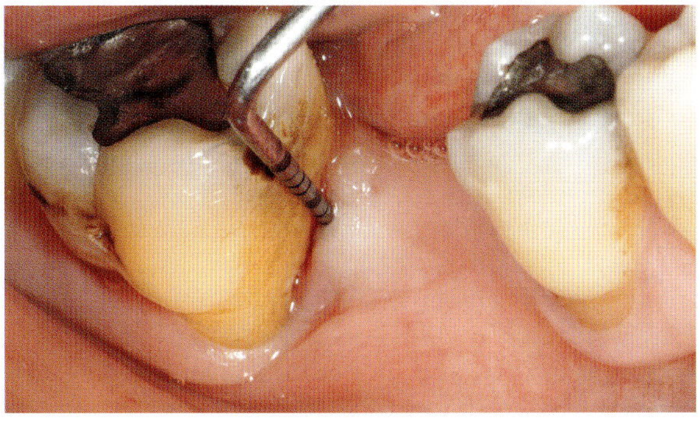

Fig 3. Probing revealed the presence of a 9-mm pocket mesial to tooth 47.

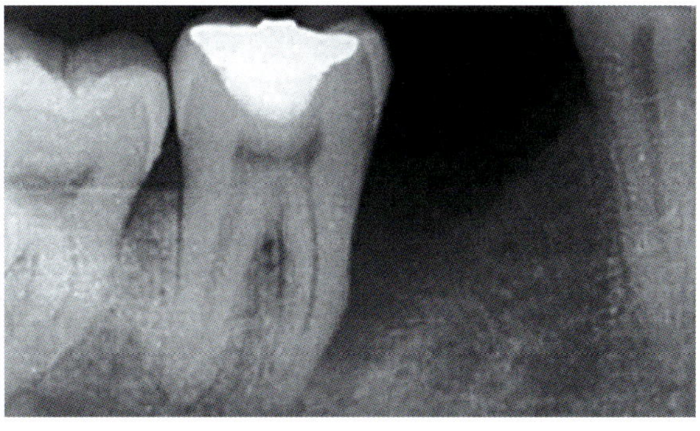

Fig 4. Periapical radiograph revealed an intrabony defect reaching the apex of the mesial root of tooth 47.

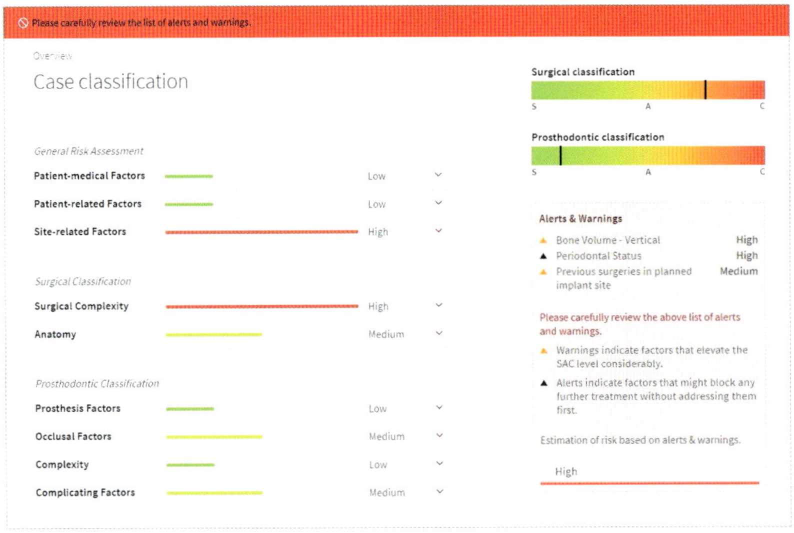

Fig 5. Overall treatment classification: Surgical classification = complex; Prosthodontic classification = straightforward.

of periodontitis should be informed that they are at higher risk of peri-implant disease and may need further therapy to limit the nature and extent of biologic complications over time (Roccuzzo et al, 2012; Roccuzzo et al, 2014).

Based on these considerations, two therapeutic options were presented to the patient:

1. Extraction of tooth 47, guided bone regeneration (GBR), and placement of two implants.

Treatment surgical risk = Advanced

2. Implant placement in site 46 in combination with guided tissue regeneration (GTR) on 47.

Treatment surgical risk = Complex (Figure 5)

The patient was therefore informed about the pros and the cons of both procedures and gave his informed consent for the second treatment.

Surgery was performed after the assurance of good motivation and compliance from the patient (full-mouth plaque score < 20%; full-mouth bleeding score < 20%). The clinical procedure for periodontal and peri-implant bone regeneration was based on following: (1) increase in flap/wound stability, (2) improvement of primary closure of the wound, and (3) minimization of intraoperative and postoperative patient morbidity.

After flap elevation, the granulation tissue was removed from the defect using curettes followed by ultrasonic instrumentation. The root surface was thoroughly scaled and conditioned with 24% ethylenediaminetetraacetic acid (EDTA) gel (PrefGel, Straumann) for 2 minutes to remove any smear layer. The site was then copiously rinsed with sterile saline solution (Figure 6).

One Tissue Level Implant (Standard Plus, Ø 4.8 mm wide neck, SLActive 10 mm, Straumann) was positioned at site 46 according to the International Team for Implantology (ITI) principles: "The apicocoronal positioning of the implant shoulder follows the philosophy as shallow as possible; as deep as necessary" (Buser et al, 2004). This meant a placement of 1 mm below the cementoenamel junction (CEJ) of the adjacent teeth. Ideal positioning created a dehiscence-type bone defect on the buccal and distal aspects of the implant. After placement of the implant, amelogenin (Emdogain, Straumann) was applied on the previously dried surface of the root (Figure 7). Autogenous bone was placed in contact with the implant surface, followed by a thick layer of deproteinized bovine bone mineral (DBBM; Bio-Oss, Geistlich) to completely fill the defects and rebuild an ideal crest profile (Figure 8).

A resorbable collagen membrane (Bio-Gide, Geistlich) was trimmed, punched with a Ø 5.0 mm biopsy punch, and adapted around the collar of the implant to stabilize the graft (Figure 9).

A 2-mm healing cap was used to stabilize the membrane and to facilitate the close adaptation of the flap in the interproximal area (Figure 10).

Modified vertical mattress Vicryl (Johnson & Johnson) sutures were used to seal the flap around the implant for nonsubmerged healing and were kept in place for 2 weeks (Figure 11).

Six weeks after surgery, the patient was instructed to resume regular and normal plaque control (Figure 12).

Three months after surgery, the mucosa appeared healthy and free from inflammation, around both the implant and the adjacent teeth (Figure 13). The radiograph demonstrated complete bone fill (Figure 14), and a solid abutment was in-

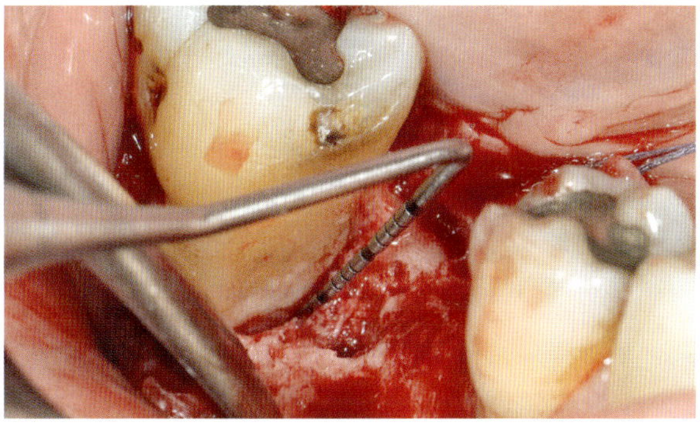

Fig 6. A full-thickness flap was raised to expose the defect and to thoroughly scale and root plane the root surface.

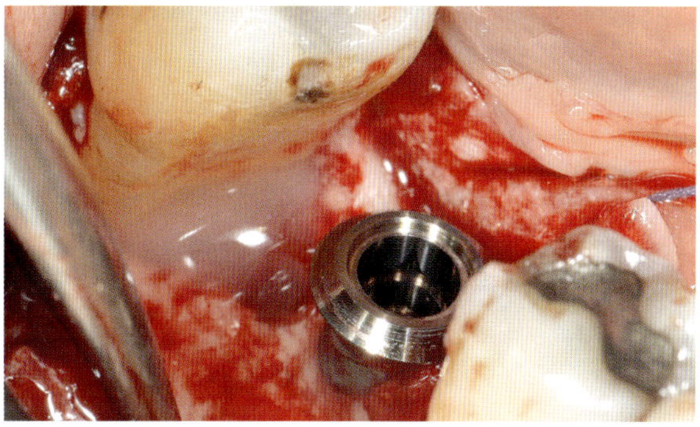

Fig 7. After implant placement, Amelogenin (Emdogain, Straumann) was applied on the root to stimulate periodontal regeneration.

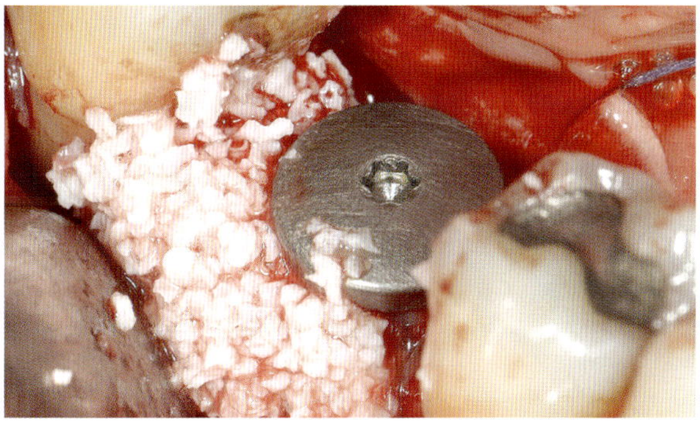

Fig 8. Autogenous bone and deproteinized bovine bone mineral (DBBM; Bio-Oss, Geistlich) were used to fill the defects and rebuild an ideal crest profile.

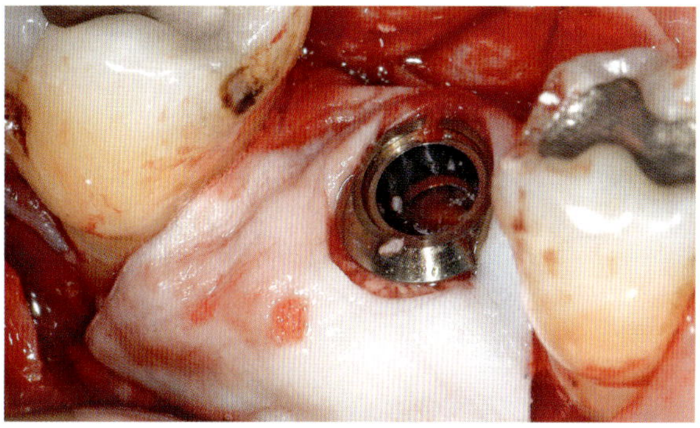

Fig 9. A collagen membrane (Bio-Gide, Geistlich) was trimmed, punched, and adapted around the collar of the implant.

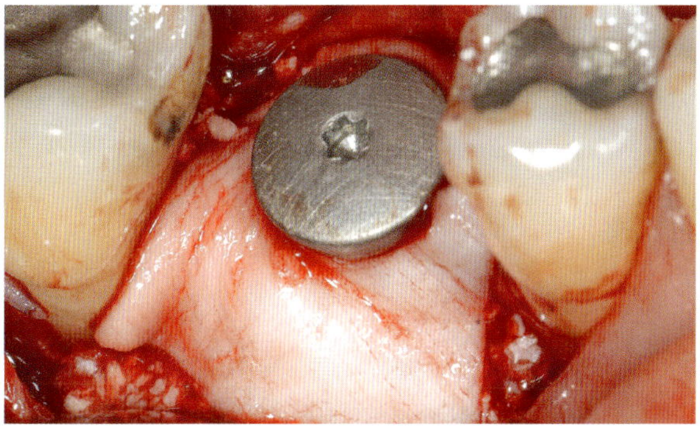

Fig 10. The collagen membrane was stabilized by a 2-mm healing cap.

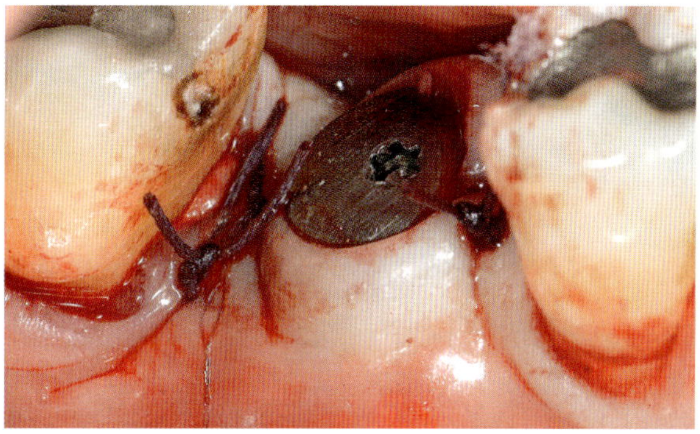

Fig 11. The flap was secured with modified vertical mattress sutures.

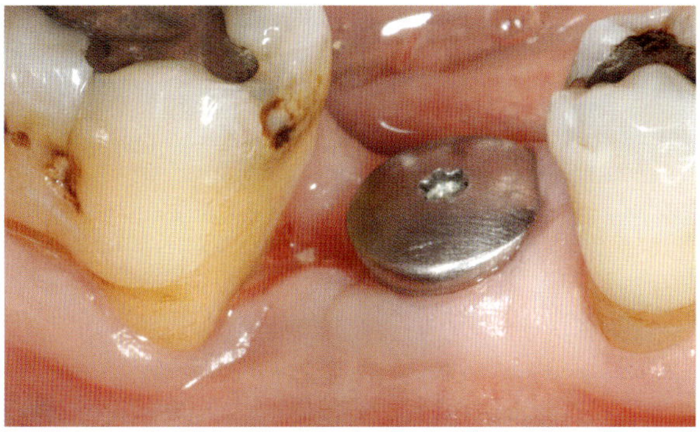

Fig 12. Clinical view 6 weeks after surgery.

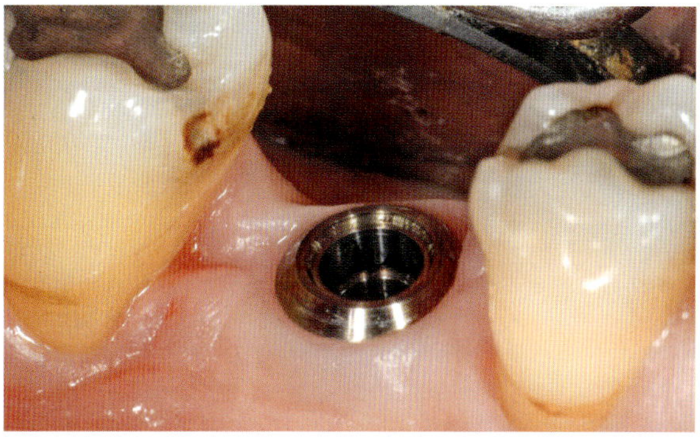

Fig 13. Clinical view 3 months after surgery.

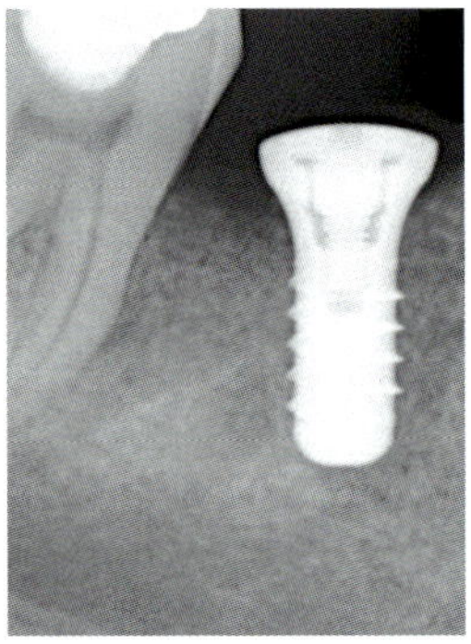

Fig 14. The periapical radiograph confirmed the correct implant position and the complete fill of the bony defect.

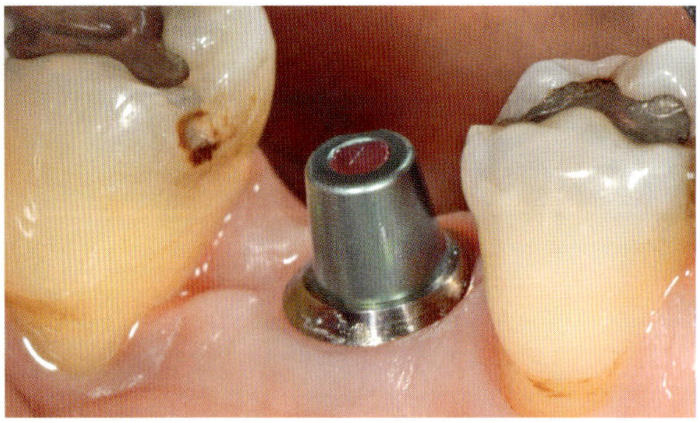

Fig 15. Inserted solid abutment, height of 4mm, 3 months after the implant placement. The implant shoulder is located 1mm below the cementoenamel junction (CEJ) of the adjacent teeth.

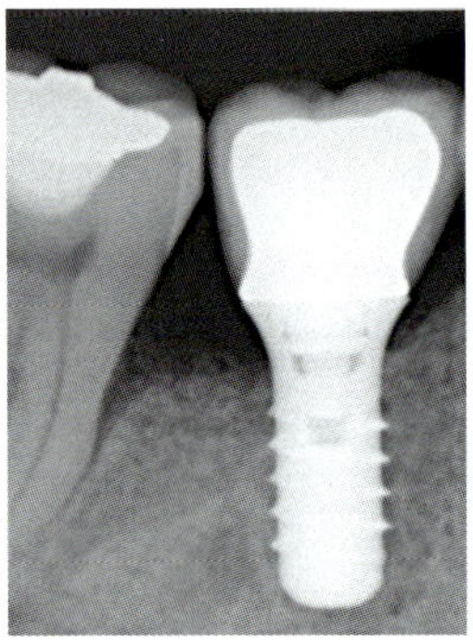

Fig 16. Post-cementation periapical radiograph.

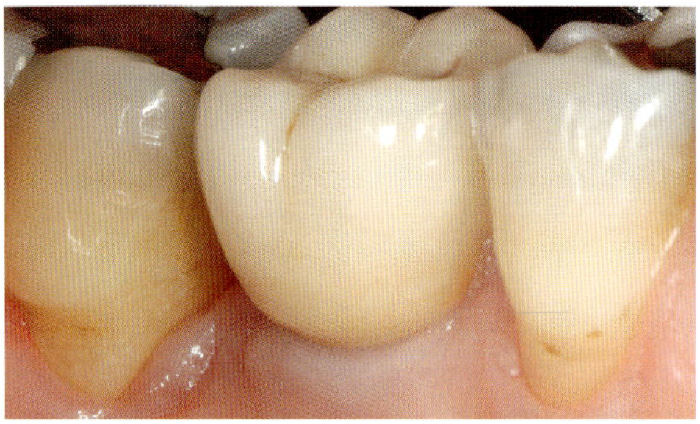

Fig 17. The definitive metal-ceramic crown in situ. The peri-implant tissues are healthy.

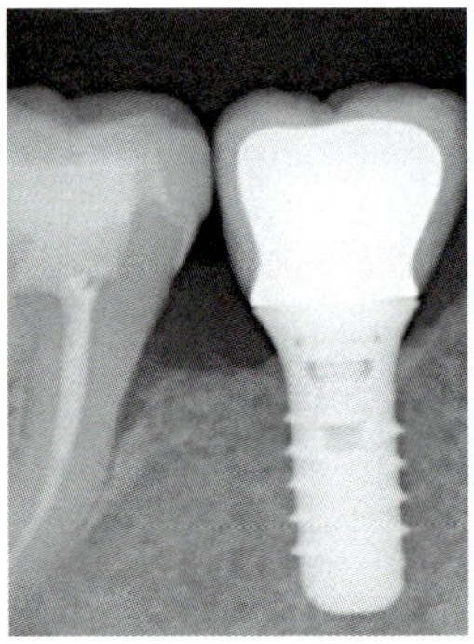

Fig 18. Periapical radiograph 5 years after the implant placement. The peri-implant bone levels are stable.

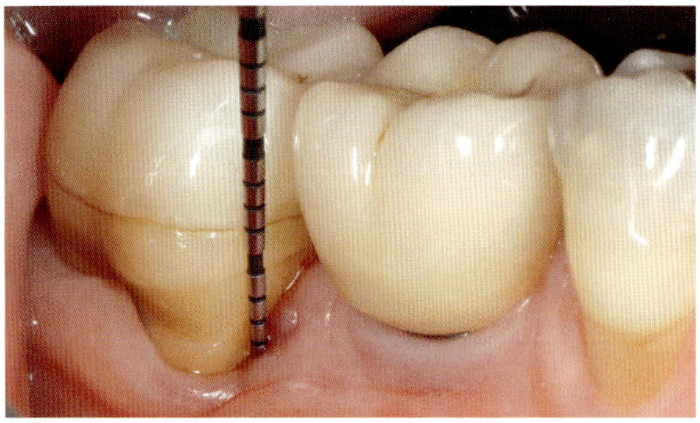

Fig 19. Clinical view 5 years after the surgical treatment reveals minimal probing depth and minimal gingival recession.

serted into the implant and tightened to 35 Ncm in order to proceed with the provisional restoration (Figure 15).

Two months after the cementation of the provisional crown, a metal-ceramic crown was completed and cemented. After the cementation of the definitive crown, cement remnants were thoroughly removed. Gap-free seating of the definitive crown on the implant shoulder was confirmed on the postcementation periapical radiograph (Figure 16). The radiograph confirmed stable peri-implant bone levels (Figure 17).

The patient was sent back to his general dentist, who provided prosthetic reconstructive treatment of tooth 47 and an individualized supportive periodontal therapy plan. The last clinical picture, taken more than 5 years after the surgery, revealed stable soft tissue contours, no signs of inflammation and physiologic probing depth. The radiograph revealed good and stable interproximal bone fill (Figures 18 and 19).

Treatment team:
Surgery and prosthetics: Dr. Mario Roccuzzo
Laboratory: Francesco Cataldi, MDT

5.2.2 Mandibular molar

L. GONZAGA

A 31-year-old woman presented to our clinic to seek replacement of a missing mandibular first molar (tooth 36). She reported that the tooth was extracted approximately 12 months ago after a failed root canal treatment. No bone grafting was performed at the time of extraction, and post-extraction healing was uneventful (Figure 1). The patient desired to have the missing tooth replaced by an implant-supported crown in an effort to prevent involvement of the adjacent teeth or the need for a removable prosthesis.

A review of her past medical history highlighted no contributing factors that would prevent routine surgical and restorative treatment. She reported no allergies and no medications other than birth control. She also denied the use of tobacco in any form. The clinical examination of the edentulous space showed complete healing from the tooth extraction with minimal buccal concavity, an adequate amount of keratinized mucosa (4 mm), and ideal prosthetic volume for a molar tooth replacement (mesial/distal space = 10 mm; interocclusal space = 7 mm). On a favorable note, the opposing tooth maintained its occlusal plane due to a slight distal contact with tooth 37. A diagnostic tool (Diagnostic T, Straumann) was used to confirm that the patient could open, allowing the access needed for the template, handpiece, and twist drills (Figure 2). A mandibular CBCT with the planned restoration and proposed implant position highlights the available bone volume and distance to the inferior alveolar nerve (IAN) canal (Figure 3). Note: A digital tooth arrangement is necessary to allow for detailed examination of available bone and anatomy from a "crown-down" planning process.

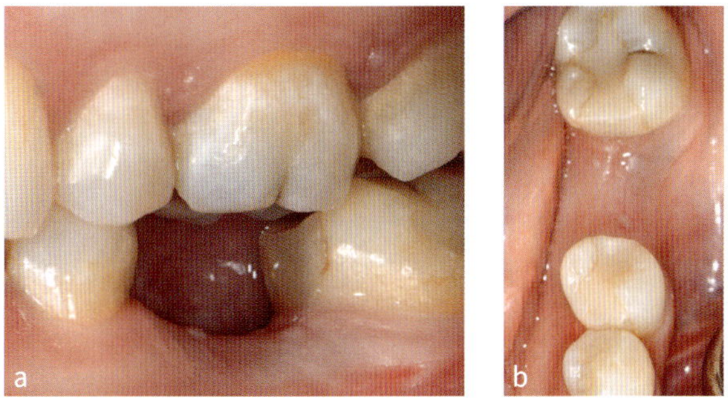

Fig 1 a-b. Lateral and occlusal views of site 36.

The treatment risk was assessed utilizing the SAC Assessment Tool (Figure 4). When evaluating the esthetic risk, the patient was graded as a low risk because the edentulous space was not visible at full smile and the patient had realistic expectations. Surgical risk factors of consideration were the proximity with the IAN and the minor horizontal tissue deficiency at the alveolar crest. The CBCT planning confirmed the ability to place a 4.8-mm-diameter implant inside the bony envelope with simultaneous correction of the minor buccal deficit. The prosthetic risk factors in this rehabilitation are low due to the available prosthetic volume, absence of parafunctional habits, and need for a provisional restoration during the osseointegration phase.

TREATMENT PLANNING

Utilizing the information from the clinical and radiographic examination aligned with the evidence in the literature and digital planning, the patient was presented with a plan for implant placement with simultaneous soft tissue augmentation of the buccal defect followed by an early loading protocol. The treatment planning was performed digitally utilizing surface scans merged with CBCT information (3Shape Implant Studio®). A surgical guide was designed in the same software and then fabricated utilizing 3D printing technology.

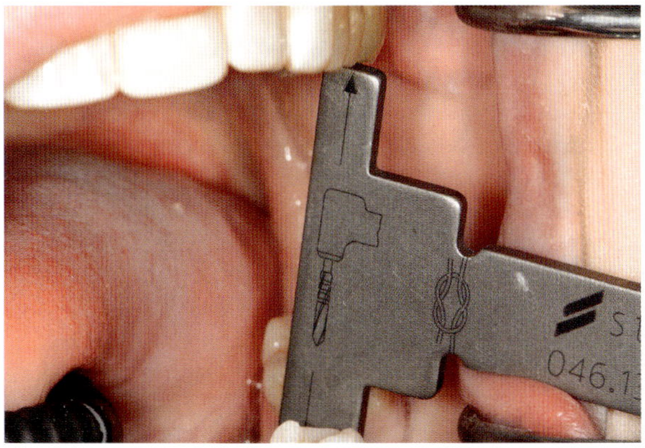

Fig 2. Positioning the Diagnostic T to evaluate maximum mouth opening for implant instrumentation.

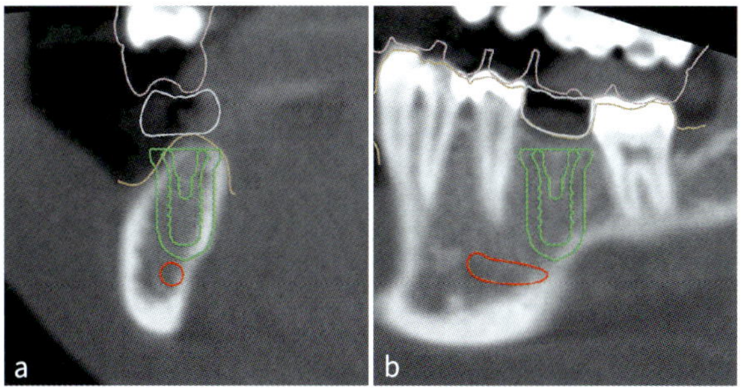

Fig 3 a-b. Cross-sectional and tangential views highlighting the planned restoration and proposed implant position with predetermined safety zone and its relationship to bone volume and IAN position.

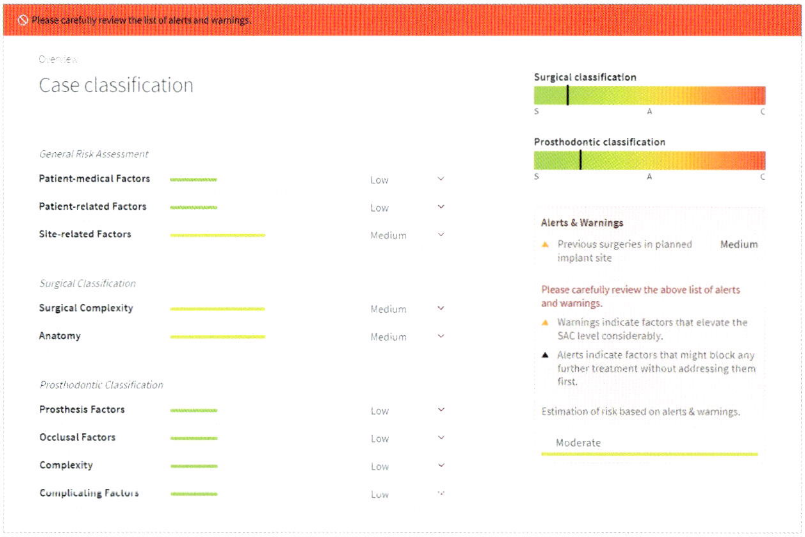

Fig 4. Overall treatment classification: Surgical classification = straightforward; Prosthodontic classification = straightforward.

SURGERY

At the time of surgery, anesthesia was accomplished with inferior alveolar and lingual nerve blocks using lidocaine 2% with epinephrine 1:100,000. A crestal incision was made extending into the sulcus of the adjacent teeth, allowing for minimal tissue reflection. The surgical template was positioned and confirmed seated. Incremental osteotomy preparation was performed through the surgical template with copious irrigation (normal saline [0.9% NaCl]) according to the manufacturer's instructions (Figure 5). The final osteotomy preparation was for a 4.8-mm-diameter wide-neck implant (Straumann) (Figure 6). Following placement of the dental implant, a soft tissue substitute (Fibro-Gide, Geistlich) was used to address the minor buccal defect (Figure 7). A transmucosal healing cap was placed, and the site was sutured with 5-0 nylon sutures following a semisubmerged approach (Figure 8).

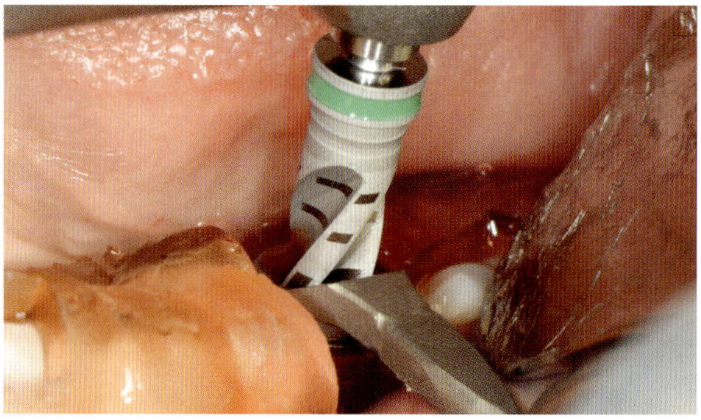

Fig 5. Preparation of the osteotomy though a surgical template.

RESTORATIVE

After 8 weeks of uneventful healing, the healing cap was removed and osseointegration was confirmed with clinical and radiographic examination. Implant stability was confirmed with resonance frequency analysis (Osstell). For definitive crown fabrication, a recording of the implant position (with a scan body) and perimucosal tissue was made through an intraoral scanning process (Trios, 3-Shape) (Figure 9). The plan for the definitive restoration was a screw-retained prosthesis utilizing a titanium base abutment (Variobase, Straumann) with a bonded (extraorally) full-contour zirconium dioxide monolithic crown.

At delivery, interproximal contacts, full restoration seating, and occlusion was confirmed both clinically and radiographically (Figure 10). The abutment screw was tightened to 35 Ncm (according to manufacturer's specifications) and the access channel filled with PTFE tape (Teflon, Chemours) and sealed with light-cured composite resin (Figure 11). Occlusion was confirmed. The patient was scheduled for recall and continued maintenance with the hygienist every 6 months.

REFLECTION

While a straightforward approach, upon reflection there are some surgical and restorative considerations that can be explored based upon my treatment approach. The use of the 3D stable collagen matrix is fairly new, and more long-term results are needed for such an indication. Another approach that could have been used to address a minor buccal defect would be the contour graft utilizing a slow-resorbing bone substitute material. When considering trends in implant dentistry, another restorative option would have been scanning the patient at the time of implant placement, allowing for delivery of the definitive restoration, risking confirmation osseointegration prior to loading.

Treatment team:
Surgery and prosthetics: Dr. Luiz Gonzaga
Laboratory: Glynn Watts, Advantage Dental Design

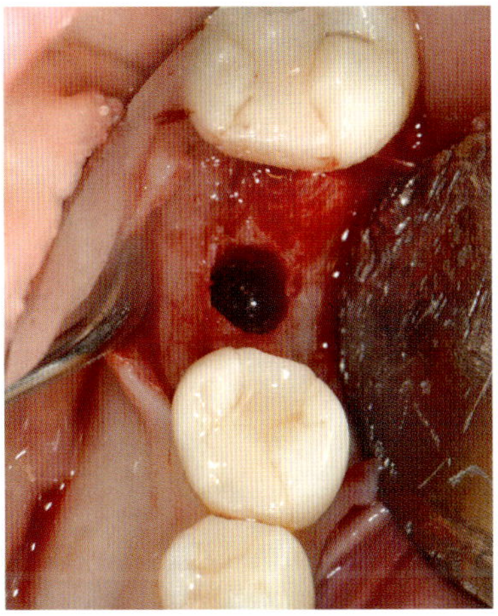

Fig 6. Final osteotomy at site 36.

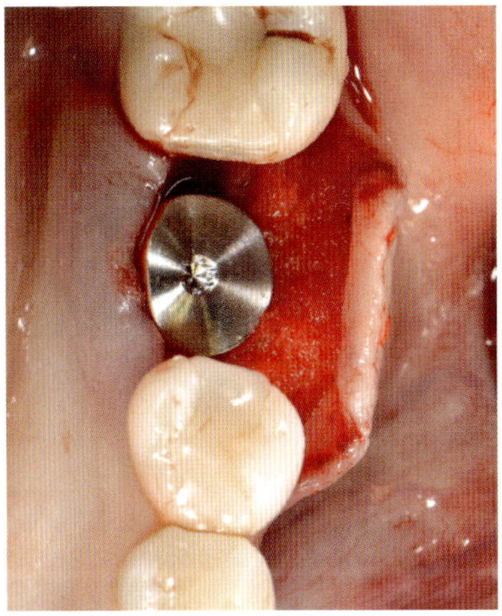

Fig 7. Placement of collagen matrix in buccal defect.

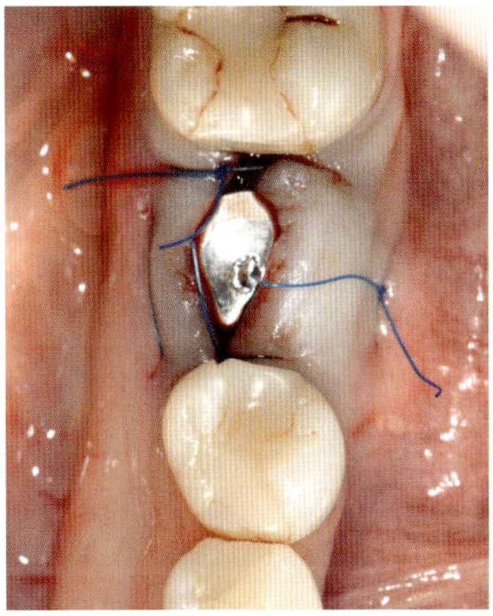

Fig 8. Final implant position with semisubmerged healing approach.

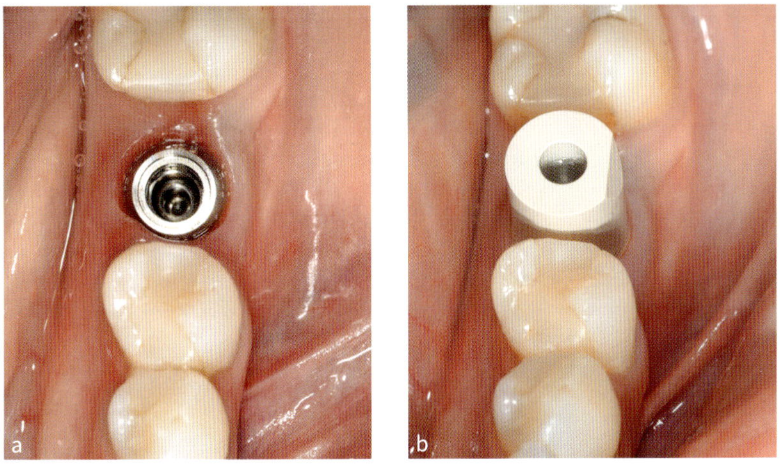

Fig 9 a-b. An occlusal view of the dental implant and scan body.

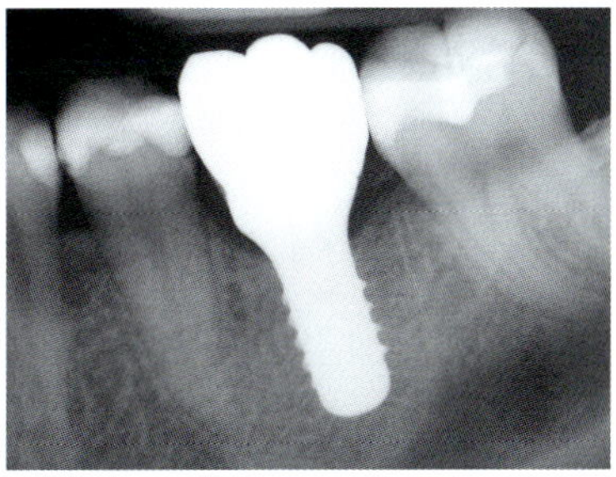

Fig 10. Periapical radiograph of restoration seated on implant.

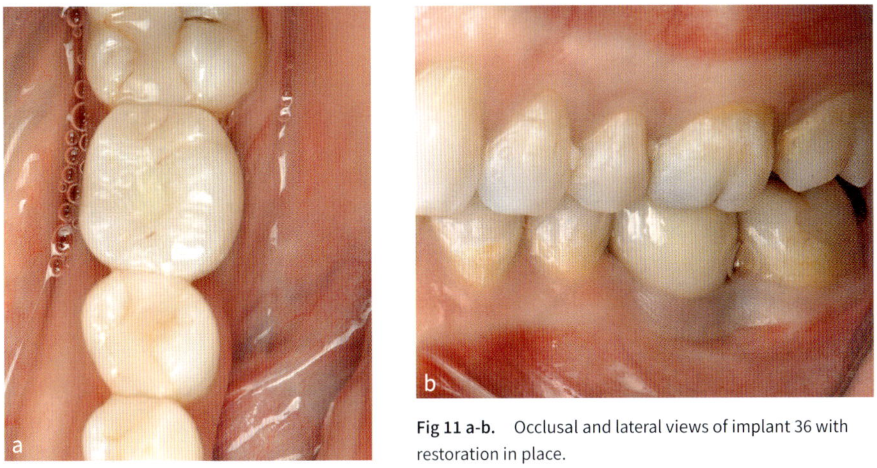

Fig 11 a-b. Occlusal and lateral views of implant 36 with restoration in place.

5.3 Implants for Restoration of Single-Tooth Spaces: Areas of High Esthetic Risk

5.3.1 Maxillary central incisor

L. GONZAGA, W. MARTIN

A 60-year-old woman presented to our clinic to address a nonrestorable central incisor (tooth 11) and explore available treatment options (Figure 1). She was seen previously by an endodontist who diagnosed the tooth as having a vertical root fracture. This tooth had a long history of dental procedures to address function and esthetics involving two root canal treatments in addition to an apical surgery. According to the patient, a fistula was once present facial to the tooth, but is no longer present. At this visit, she expressed an interest to explore options to replace the tooth with an implant-supported crown in an effort to prevent involvement of the adjacent teeth or the need for a removable prosthesis.

A review of her past medical history revealed no contributing factors that would prevent routine surgical and restorative treatment. She reported no allergies nor medications other than multivitamins and supplements. She also denied the use of tobacco in any form. Clinical examination of tooth 11 highlighted a porcelain-fused-to-metal (PFM) crown with minimal mobility. A periodontal probing exam was performed showing normal (1 to 3 mm) depths other than a 6-mm probing at midfacial. The tooth was asymptomatic with no evidence of an acute infection. A localized CBCT scan was taken which allowed the central incisor's root to be viewed in relation to the axial thickness of the maxilla, highlighting missing bone in the facial aspect and a chronic periapical lesion (Figure 2).

The treatment risk was assessed utilizing the SAC Assessment Tool highlighting key esthetic, surgical, and prosthetic risk factors resulting in an overall treatment risk (Figure 3). When evaluating the esthetic risk, the patient presented with high gingival display at full smile, adequate prosthetic space for restoration. The tissue phenotype was high scalloped thin, and the soft tissues were intact. A review of the CBCT highlighted a facial plate < 1 mm, with adjacent tooth interproximal bone heights of 5.5 mm to the interproximal contact points. This patient presented with realistic treatment expectations. Surgical risk factors of consideration were the need for bone augmentation (socket or horizontal) after extraction of tooth 11. The area of treatment being located in a region of esthetic importance and the potential for poor primary stability of the implant at the time of tooth extraction were additional considerations. The prosthetic risk factors in this rehabilitation are favorable due to the available prosthetic volume and absence of parafunctional habits. The

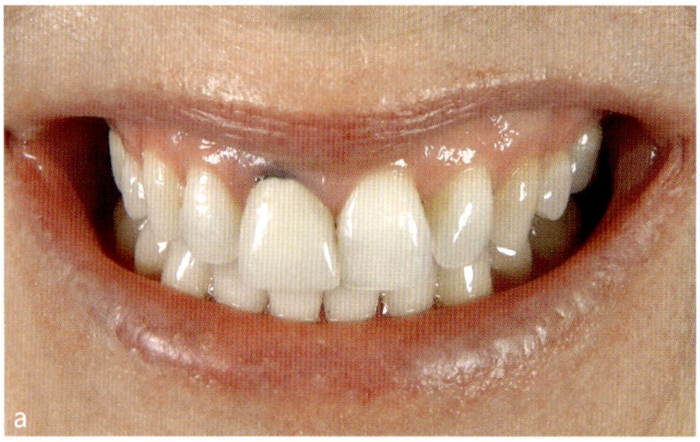

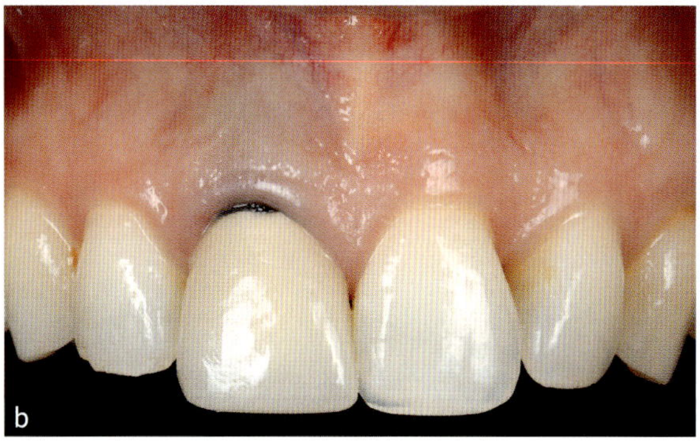

Fig 1 a-b. Full smile and an open-retracted view of the right central incisor (tooth 11).

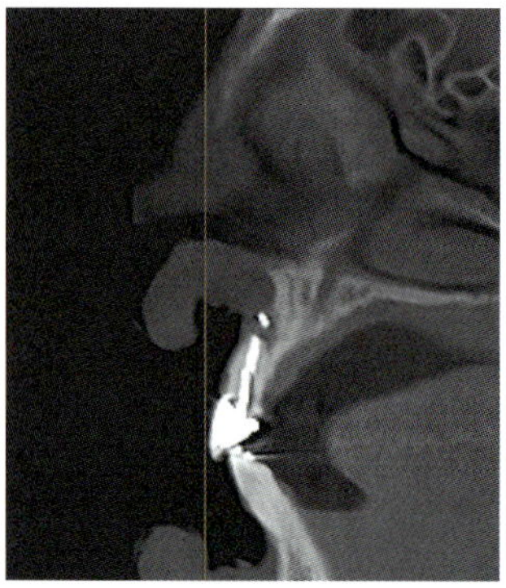

Fig 2. Localized CBCT of maxilla with isolation of tooth 11.

Fig 3. Overall treatment classification: Esthetic risk = high; Surgical classification = advanced to complex; Prosthodontic classification = advanced

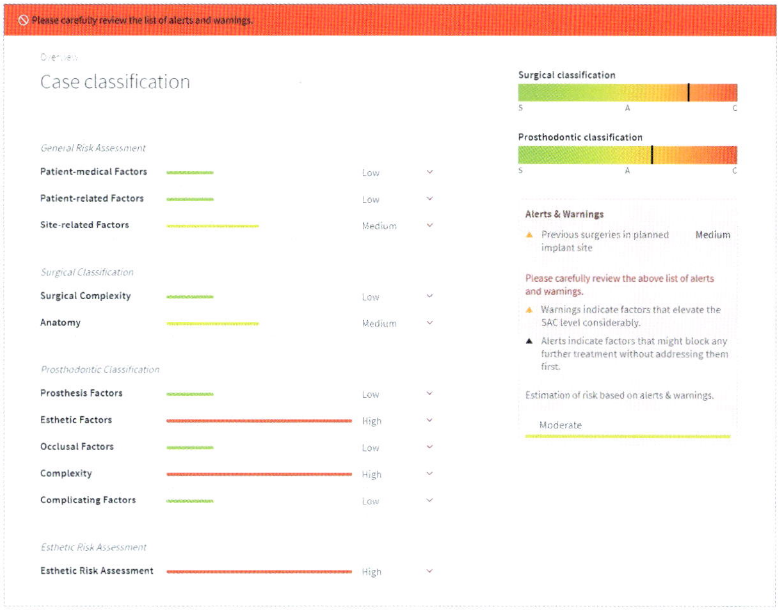

main prosthetic risk was related to the removable provisional restoration during the postextraction healing phase. Treatment alternatives involving dental implant therapy were discussed with the patient (timing of implant placement and load, need for grafting, restoration type, and treatment time).

TREATMENT PLANNING

Utilizing the information from the clinical and radiographic examination aligned with the evidence in the literature, it was determined that we would proceed with the extraction of tooth 11 and perform a ridge preservation graft.

SURGERY

At the time of surgery, anesthesia was accomplished with nerve blocks using lidocaine 2% with epinephrine 1:100,000. The surgical approach involved a minimally invasive technique with no flap elevation during the extraction of tooth 11 (Figure 4). The apical lesion was removed with hand curettes, and the socket was cleaned with a carbide round bur used in reverse (Figure 5). The socket was augmented with allograft corticocancellous chips and a collagen membrane (Figure 6). A vacuum-formed Essix retainer with an acrylic resin duplicate of the patient's crown was used as a provisional restoration. Attention was given to the intaglio contours of the restoration so as not to apply excessive pressure to the site.

Use this QR code to view a highlight video of the extraction and subsequent ridge preservation.

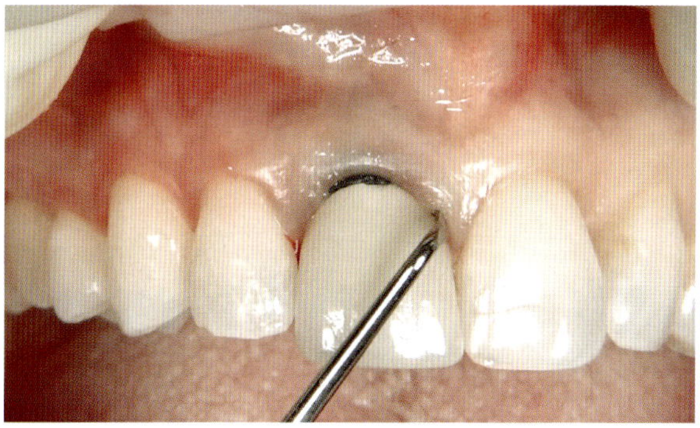

Fig 4. A periotome used during the extraction of tooth 11.

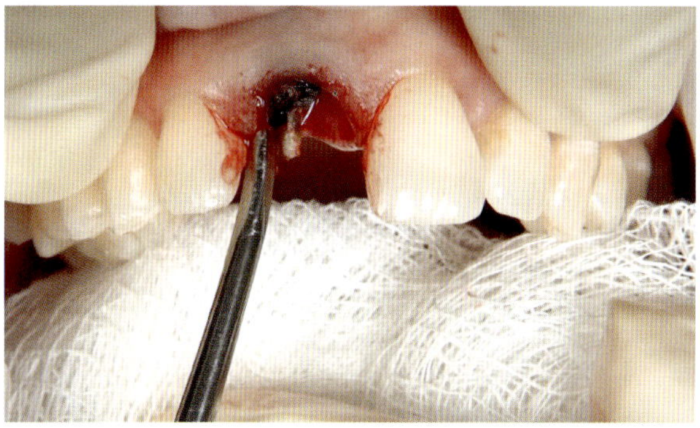

Fig 5. Curette used for removal of apical granuloma.

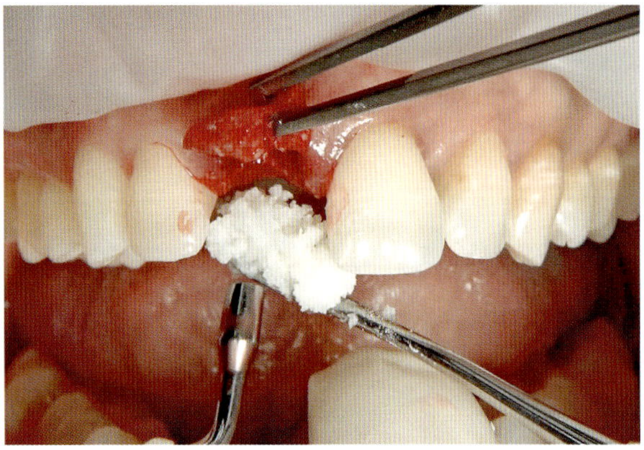

Fig 6. Placement of the allograft corticocancellous chips into the socket.

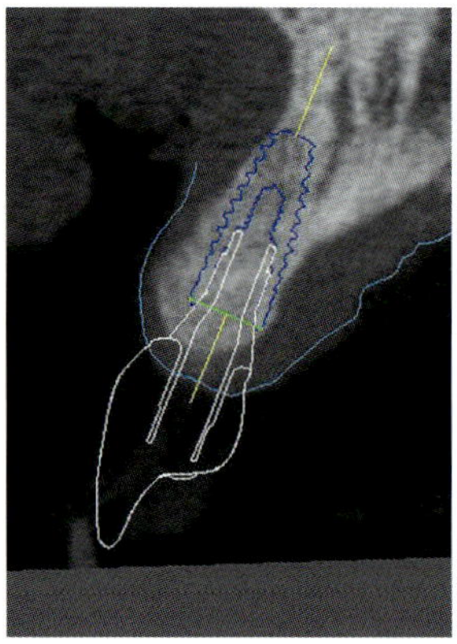

Fig 7. Restoration-driven digital treatment planning for implant and restoration of site 11.

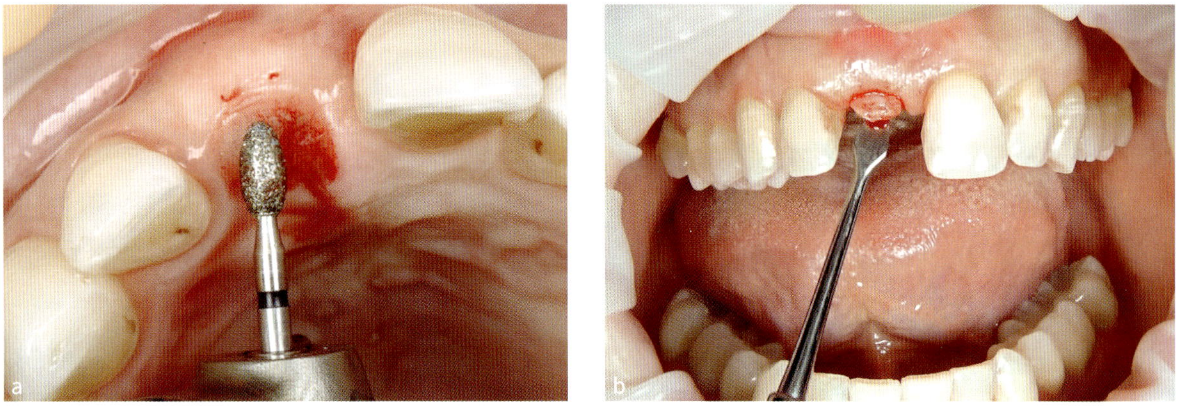

Fig 8 a-b. Modified role technique utilized for access to place implant at site 11.

After 6 months of healing from the extraction and graft, treatment planning was performed utilizing intraoral surface scans (Trios) merged with CBCT information (coDiagnostiX, Straumann) (Figure 7). A surgical guide was designed and then fabricated utilizing 3D SLA printing technology. At surgery, a modified role technique was used to create a mini-flap while simultaneously increasing the thickness of the facial tissue (Abrams, 1980) (Figure 8). A fully guided approach in the preparation and placement of a tapered implant (Bone Level Tapered Ø 4.1 mm × 10 mm, Straumann) was performed according to the manufacturer's recommendations. Confirmation of adequate primary stability was assessed clinically and with the Beacon (Osstell) with implant stability quotient (ISQ) values of 79/79. It was determined that an immediate screw-retained provisional restoration could be placed with careful adjustment to prevent occlusal contacts in maximum intercuspation and during excursive movements (Figure 9).

Use this QR code to view a highlight video of implant placement and loading.

RESTORATIVE

After 8 weeks of uneventful healing, the provisional restoration was removed and osseointegration was confirmed through clinical examination, a second ISQ measurement, and radiographic evaluation. The final impression of the implant position and transition zone was made utilizing a customized impression post as described by Patras and Martin in 2016 (Figure 10). The definitive restoration was planned as a screw-retained all-ceramic restoration bonded to a titanium base abutment (Variobase RC) (Figure 11). The lithium disilicate crown was cemented extraorally to the titanium base with multilink implant resin cement (Ivoclar Vivadent). Interproximal contacts and proper transition zone tissue support

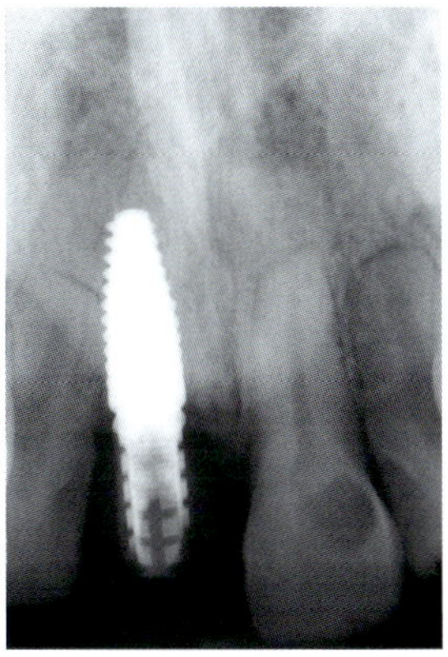

Fig 9. Postsurgical periapical radiograph at site 11.

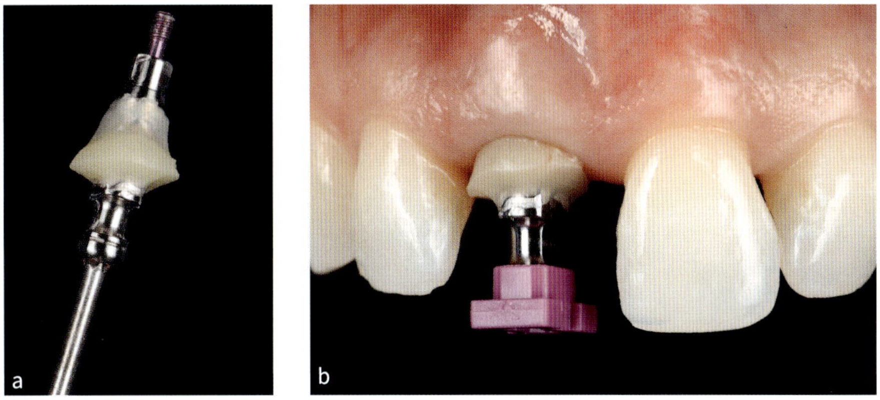

Fig 10 a-b. Customized impression post extra- and intraorally.

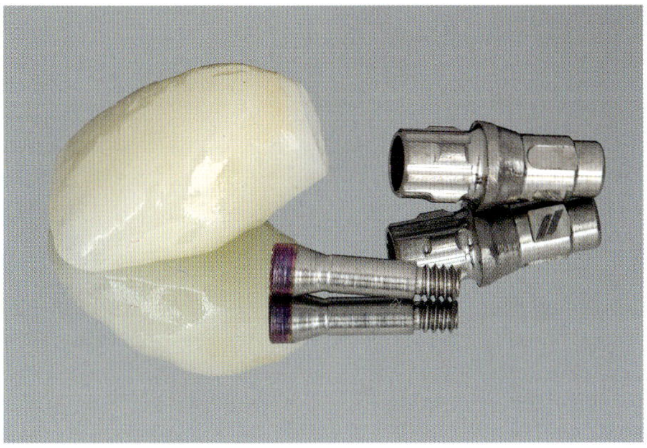

Fig 11. Lithium disilicate crown and titanium base.

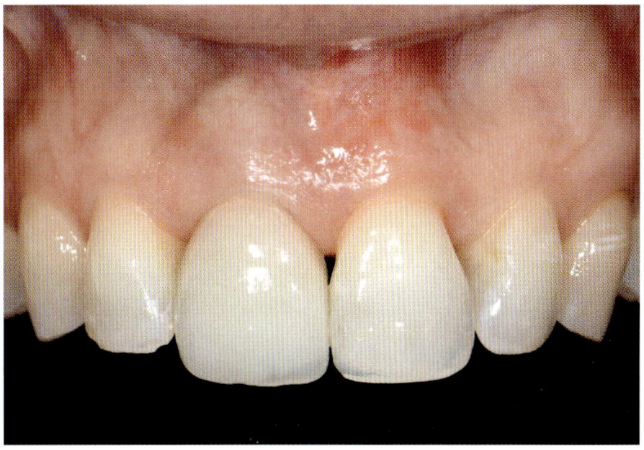

Fig 12. At delivery of implant crown 11.

were confirmed followed by radiographic confirmation of the abutment/implant seating. The abutment screw was tightened to 35 Ncm (according to the manufacturer's specifications) and the access hole sealed with PTFE tape (Teflon) and light-cured composite resin (Figure 12). A direct composite-resin restoration was added to the distal aspect of tooth 21 to improve the emergence profile and symmetry of the central incisors. Occlusion was confirmed, and the patient was scheduled for a 12-week recall visit.

At the 12-week follow-up visit, the patient was instructed to continue maintenance care with hygiene visits every 6 months. Figure 13 highlights a 2-year follow-up evaluation showing good hard and soft tissue esthetics as well as a periapical radiograph highlighting good interproximal bone support.

REFLECTION ON THE TREATMENT APPROACH AND OUTCOME

This treatment approach had a total treatment time of 9 months. We chose a conservative approach due to the evaluated pretreatment esthetic risk. Another sound treatment option would have involved a routine extraction followed by a type 2 implant placement with simultaneous graft. Our concern with this approach is that we felt that, due to the hard tissue defect, we would not be able to place the implant in an ideal position with primary stability, eventually ending up with a formal graft, which would have increased the number of surgical interventions. Also, in review of our treatment approach with regard to implant selection, we could have proceeded with a 3.3-mm body, allowing for more native bone surrounding the implant. But, due to the size of the implant we would have had to place it slightly deeper to allow for a proper emergence profile into a standard central incisor contour. There are obvious pros and cons to each approach.

Treatment team:
Surgery: Dr. Luiz Gonzaga
Prosthetics: Dr. William C. Martin
Laboratory: Glynn Watts, Advantage Dental Design

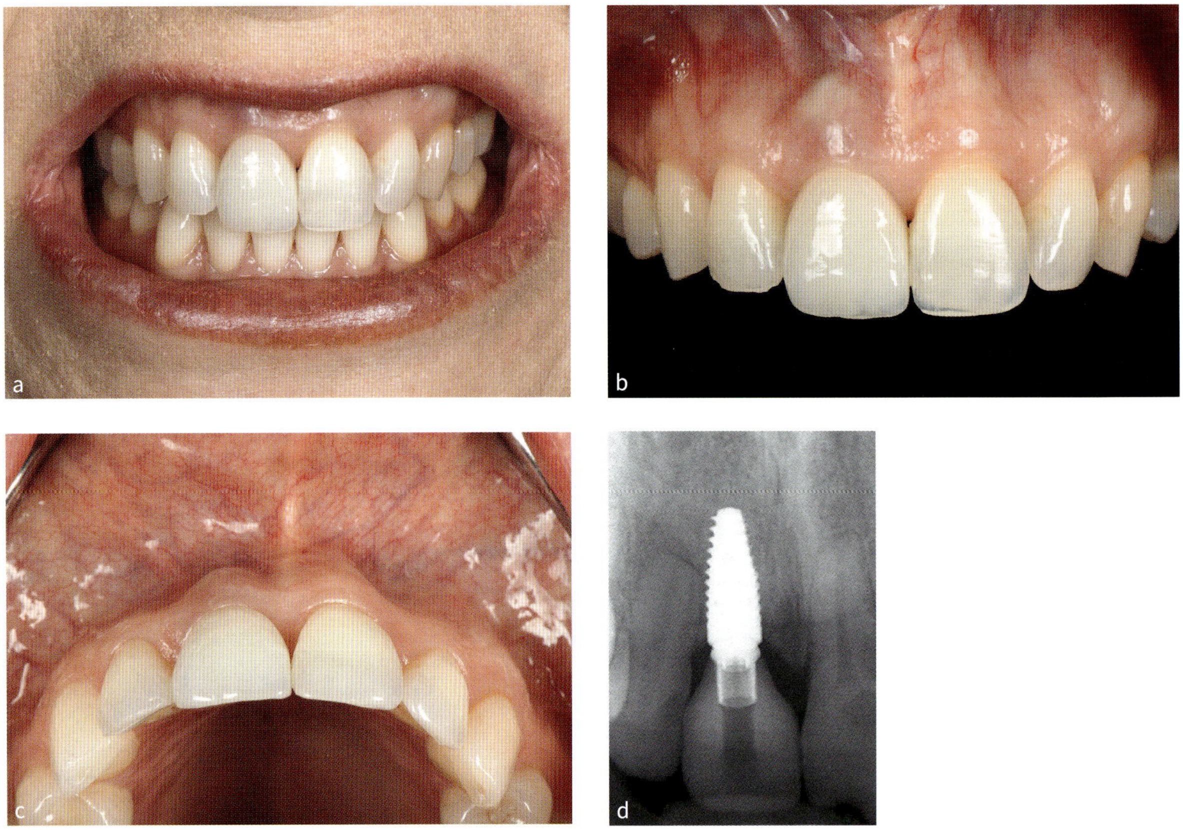

Fig 13 a-d. Two-year follow-up of implant crown 11.

5.3.2 Maxillary lateral incisor

A. TREVIÑO SANTOS

A healthy 29-year-old man had agenesis of the maxillary right lateral incisor and was wearing a removable prosthesis (Figure 1). Tooth agenesis is the most clearly recognized developmental dental anomaly in humans and can be challenging to manage clinically. Maxillary lateral incisor agenesis affects approximately 2% of the population. Bilateral cases are more common than unilateral cases, and women have a slightly higher prevalence than men. This is a condition that involves dental asymmetries and compromised facial esthetics, particularly the smile. His chief complaint was the lack of comfort and esthetic issues.

A review of his past medical history highlighted no contributing factors that would prevent routine surgical and restorative treatment. Clinical examination of the region of site 12 regarding the esthetic risk assessment presents healthy soft tissue, anatomy defects with a thin facial bone wall phenotype, and horizontal bone deficiency at alveolar crest (Figures 2 and 3).

TREATMENT PLANNING

The CBCT scan showed a reduced bone availability in the mesiodistal and orofacial dimensions in region 12 (Figures 4 and 5). For this reason, a Straumann 2.9-mm small-diameter implant was chosen. This option resolves the need to obtain an esthetic solution in narrow gaps, optimize the specific anatomical situation, achieve primary stability, reduce GBR procedures, and simplify the implant placement (Figure 6).

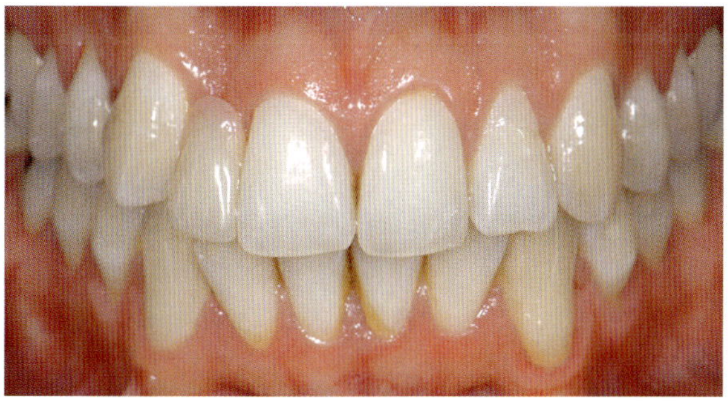

Fig 1. Frontal view with removable prosthesis at site 12.

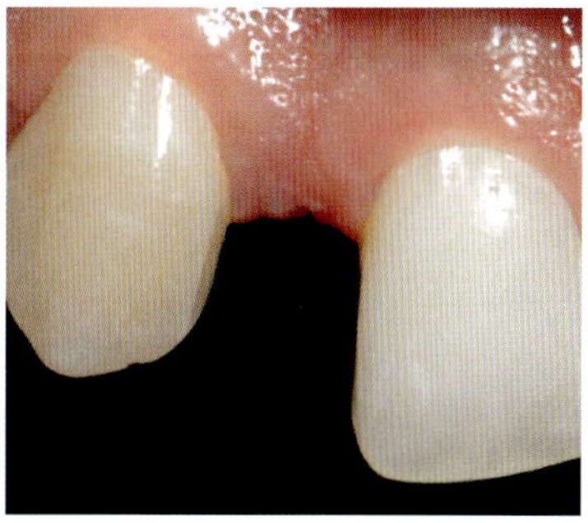

Fig 2. Frontal view, agenesis of tooth 12 with mesiodistal space 4.2 mm.

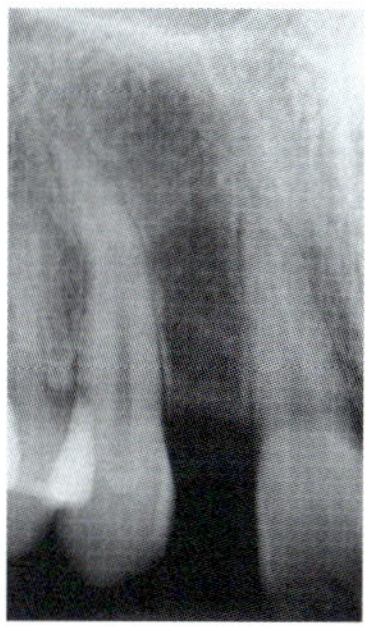

Fig 3. Initial radiograph.

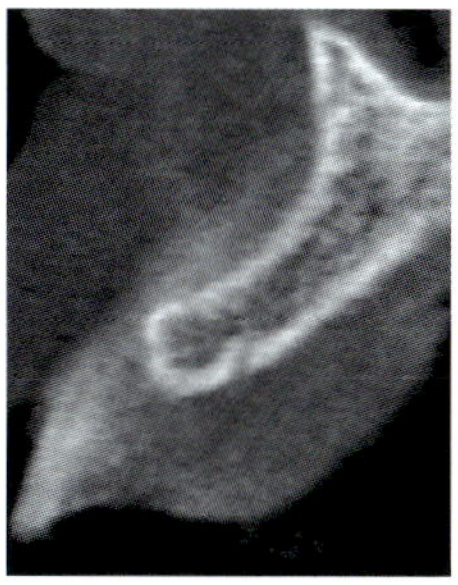

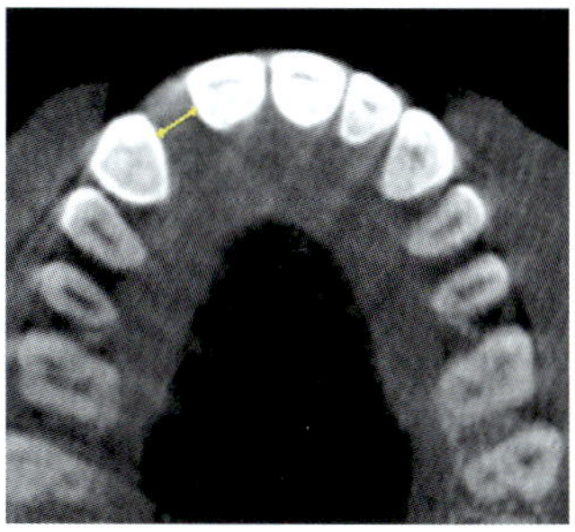

Figs 4, 5. Initial CBCT of region 12 (orofacial and mesiodistal).

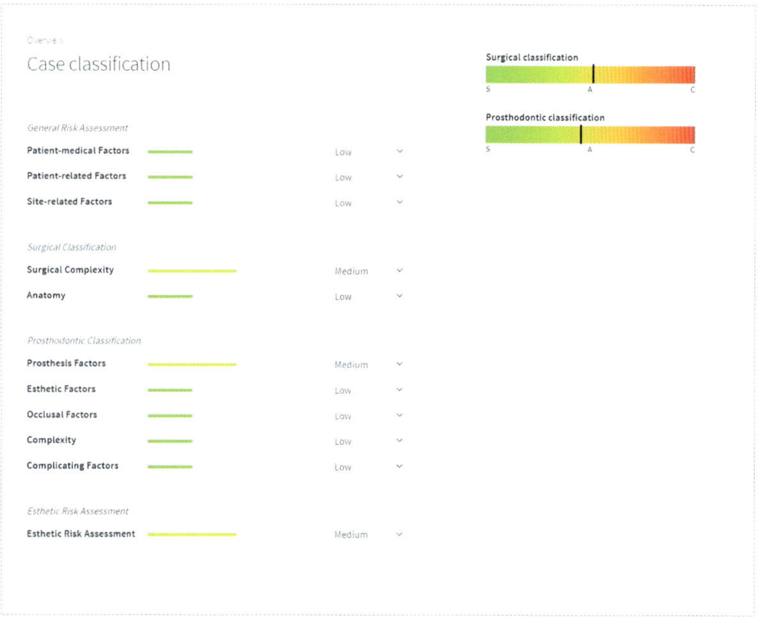

Fig 6. Overall treatment classification: Esthetic risk = medium; Surgical classification = advanced; Prosthodontic classification = advanced.

SURGICAL PROCEDURE

To avoid scar formation in the esthetic zone, a marginal incision was made with a releasing incision distally to reflect a mucoperiosteum flap (Figure 7a). The implant bed preparation was made following the Straumann 2.9-mm workflow, needle drill (Figure 7b), pilot drill (Figure 7c), position indicator (Figure 7d), profile drill (Figure 7e), and implant placement with an ideal implant orientation. Due to the oval shape of the prosthetic components, the correct implant orientation needs to be ensured by verifying that the markings on the transfer piece are oriented exactly in the bucco-oral direction (Figure 7f).

The facial bone was intact (Figure 8a), but GBR was needed for long-term prognosis of the implant. A xenograft was added on the facial wall and covered with a double layer of collagen membrane to avoid gingival recession (Figure 8b). Esthetic results are crucially determined by successful soft tissue management, and an oval healing abutment was placed to enable soft tissue sculpting during the mucosal healing (Figure 8c). The implant was left to heal for 3 months before loading with a provisional restoration.

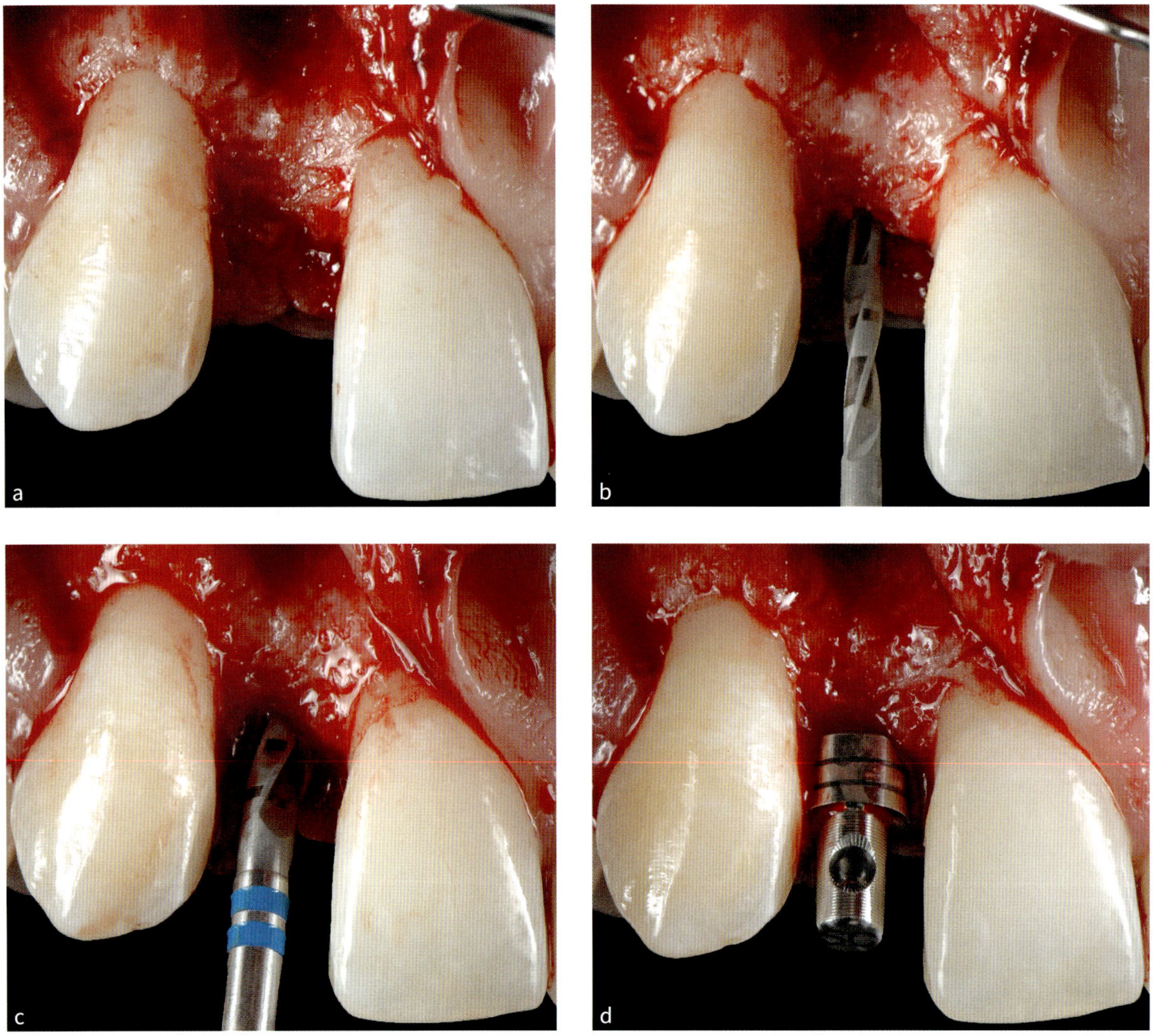

Fig 7 a-d. This implant with a reduced diameter has all the necessary characteristics to solve problems of spaces, narrow interdental ridges, or reduced bone availability thanks to its apically conical and cutting body, with excellent mechanical resistance due to the Roxolid (Straumann) material and the extensive healing potential of the SLActive surface. (Bone Level Tapered [BLT] Ø 2.9 × 10-mm Small CrossFit implant).

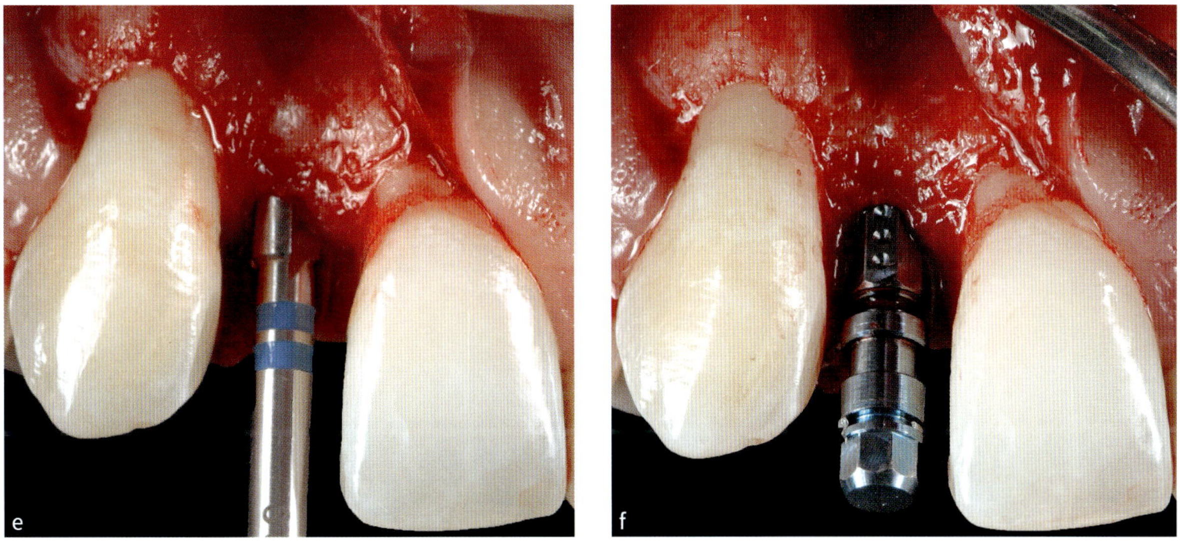

Fig 7 e-f. This implant with a reduced diameter has all the necessary characteristics to solve problems of spaces, narrow interdental ridges, or reduced bone availability thanks to its apically conical and cutting body, with excellent mechanical resistance due to the Roxolid (Straumann) material and the extensive healing potential of the SLActive surface. (Bone Level Tapered [BLT] Ø 2.9 × 10–mm Small CrossFit implant).

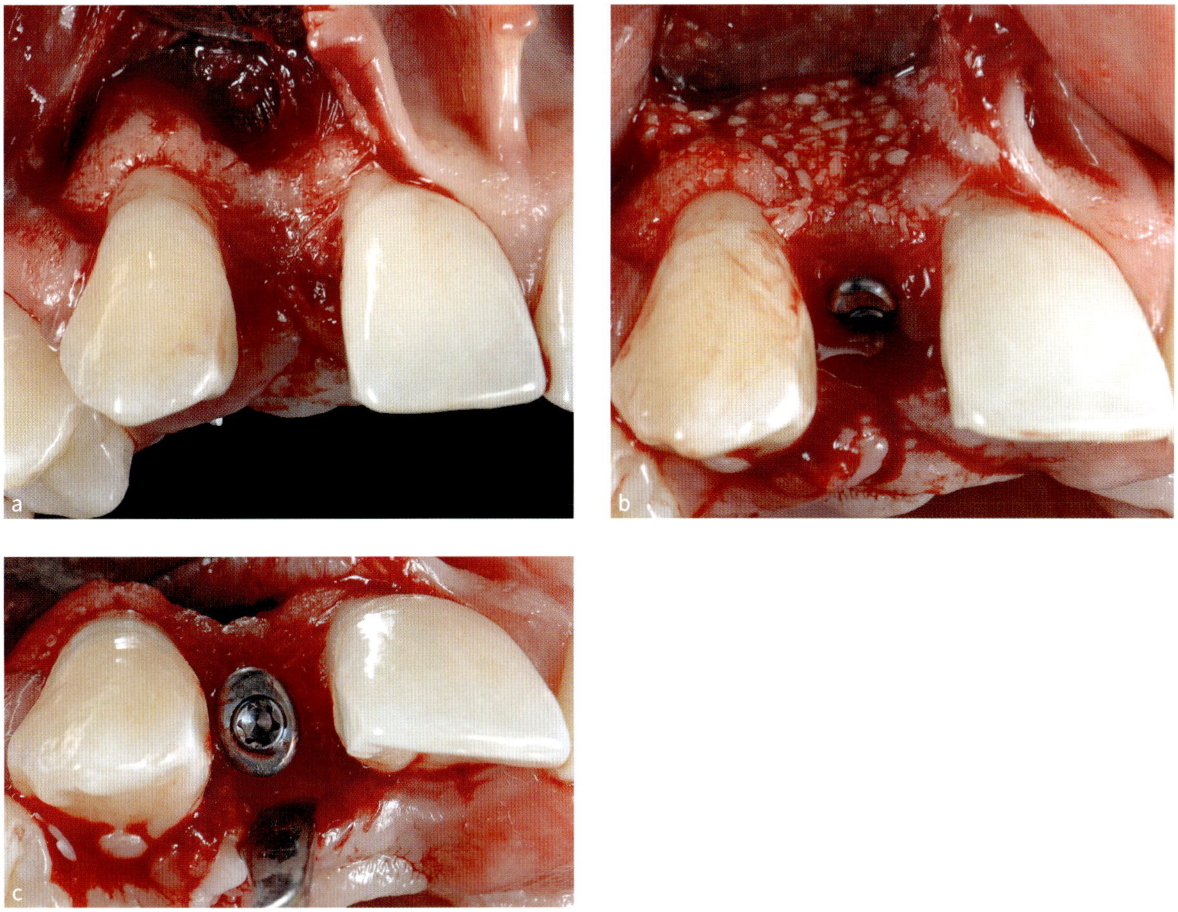

Fig 8 a-c. The BLT Ø 2.9 implant is indicated for narrow interproximal spaces and deficient bone ridges. In the palatine vestibule direction, it was necessary to perform a bone augmentation with xenograft and a double layer of resorbable collagen membrane. A 2.0-mm-long healing screw was placed in the implant. The flap was repositioned, and the wound was closed with tension-free sutures.

PROSTHETIC PROCEDURE

After 3 months, a provisional prosthesis was placed with an oval temporary abutment, placing the longer platform dimension parallel to the buccopalatal direction to achieve an esthetic emergence profile during the transmucosal healing of the soft tissue (Figure 9).

A customized impression technique was utilized with polyvinyl siloxane to copy the emergence profile of the provisional restoration, and the shade of the future restoration was determined (Figure 10).

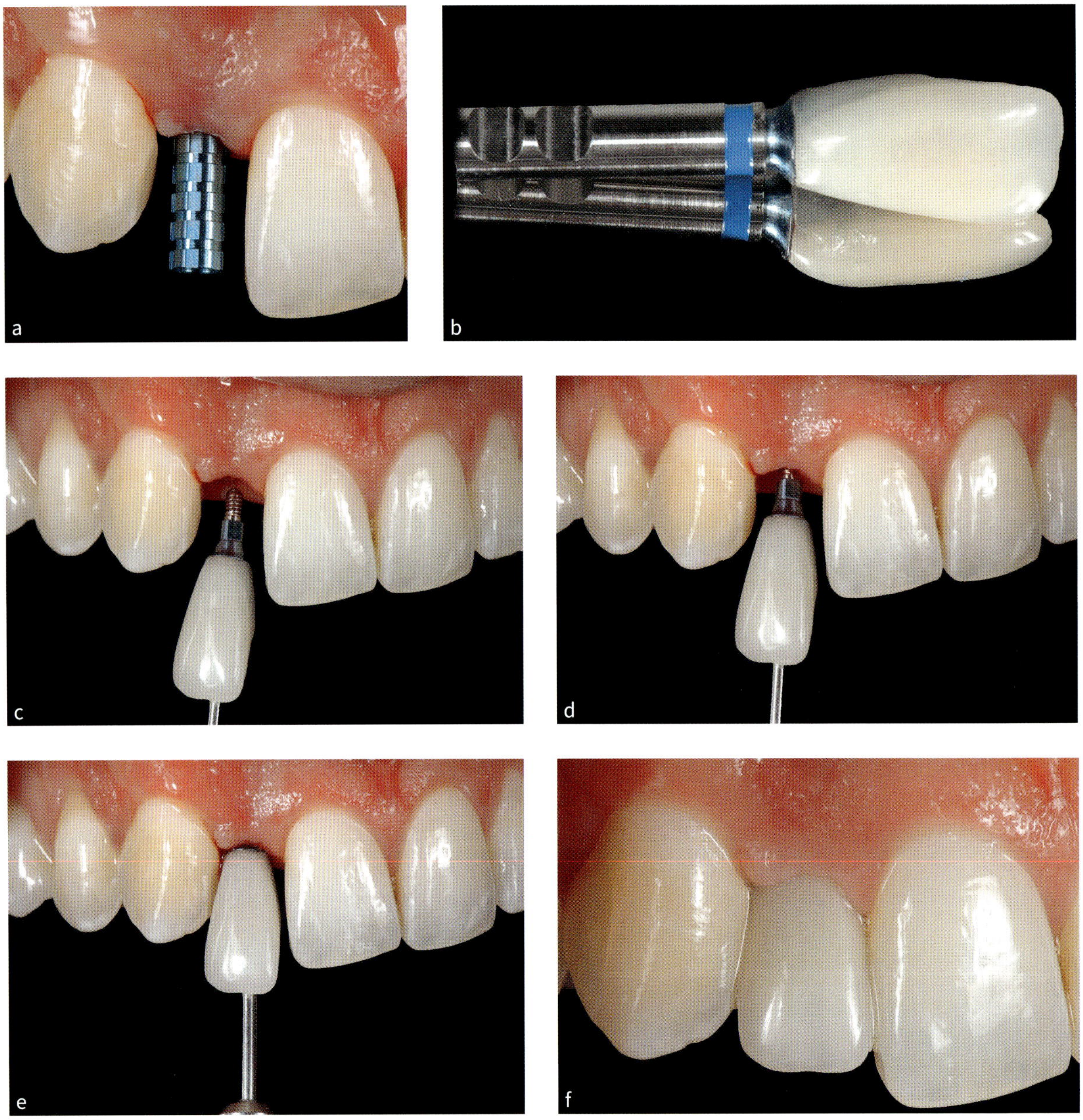

Fig 9 a-f. We know that implants in the anterior region represent a great challenge. Obtaining esthetic results is crucially determined by the successful management of soft tissues; for this, the new prosthetic components of the BLT Ø 2.9-mm implant has a unique oval design and consistent emergence profile to address esthetic challenges. This makes it easy for the clinician to have enough space for the surrounding soft tissue to achieve satisfactory esthetic results.

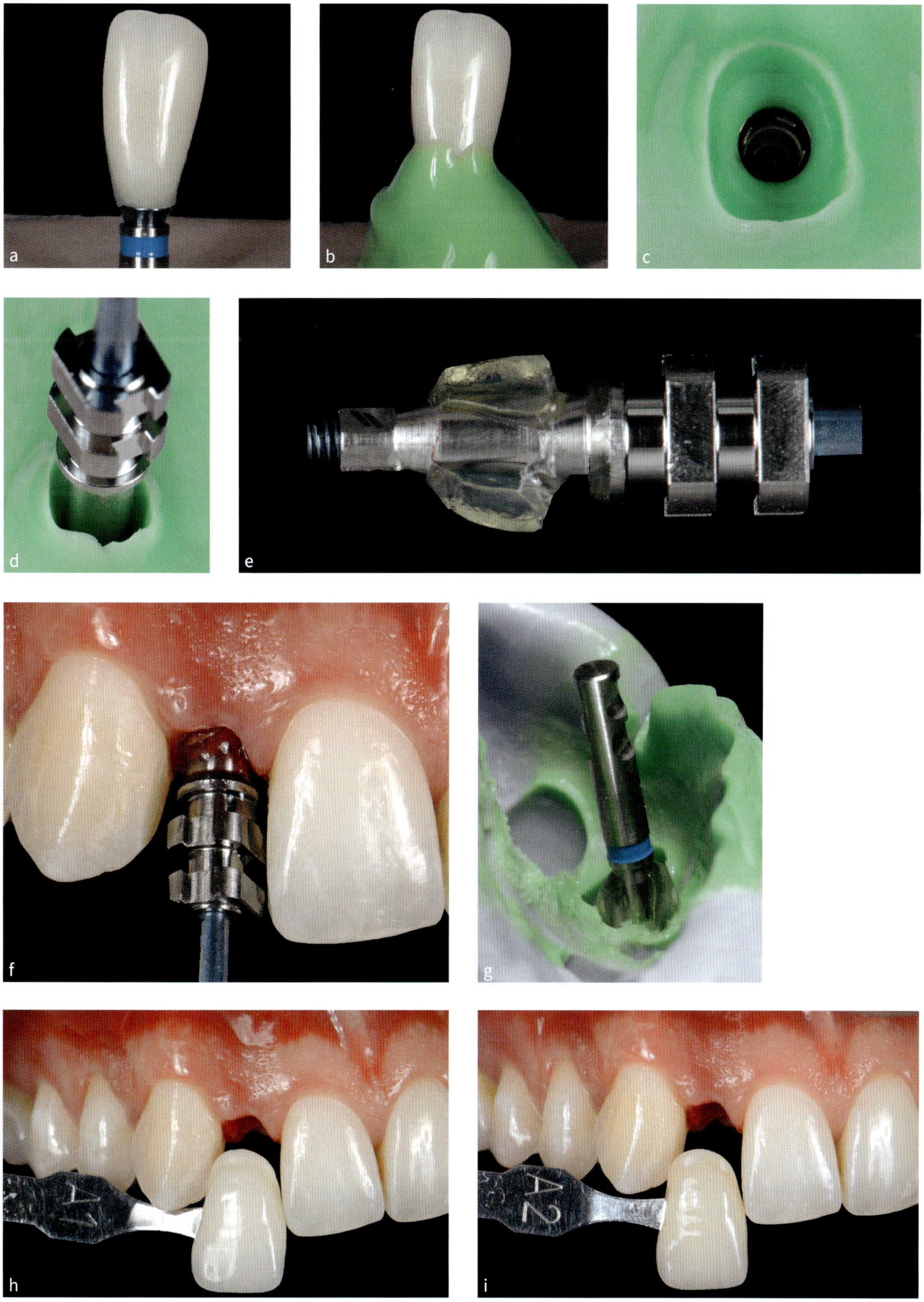

Fig 10 a-i. Replica of the provisional prosthesis, oval design of the connection and the emergence profile, customized impression post, impression taking, analog transfer, and shade selection.

The definitve zirconia crown was fabricated and cemented extraorally onto a ti-base abutment (Small CrossFit [SC] Variobase) (Figure 11).

The SC Variobase offers restoration options with maximum design freedom, thanks to the patented engaging mechanism with four cams allowing exact seating and rotational lock of the crown having a bonding surface without sand-blasting. This allows us to save valuable time by reducing the processing steps (Figure 12).

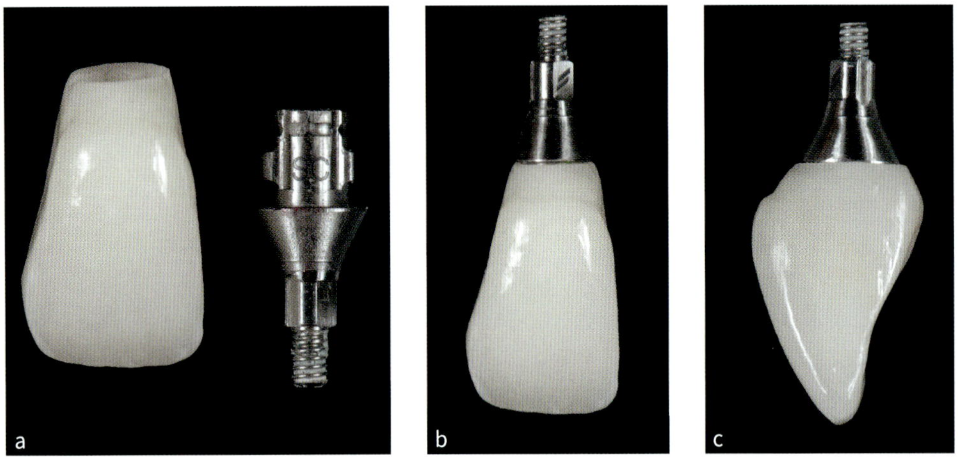

Fig 11 a-c. The Small CrossFit Variobase abutment has a cylindric platform shape from a vestibular perspective, but it has an oval platform shape from a mesial and distal perspective for a better adaptation in tight interdental spaces.

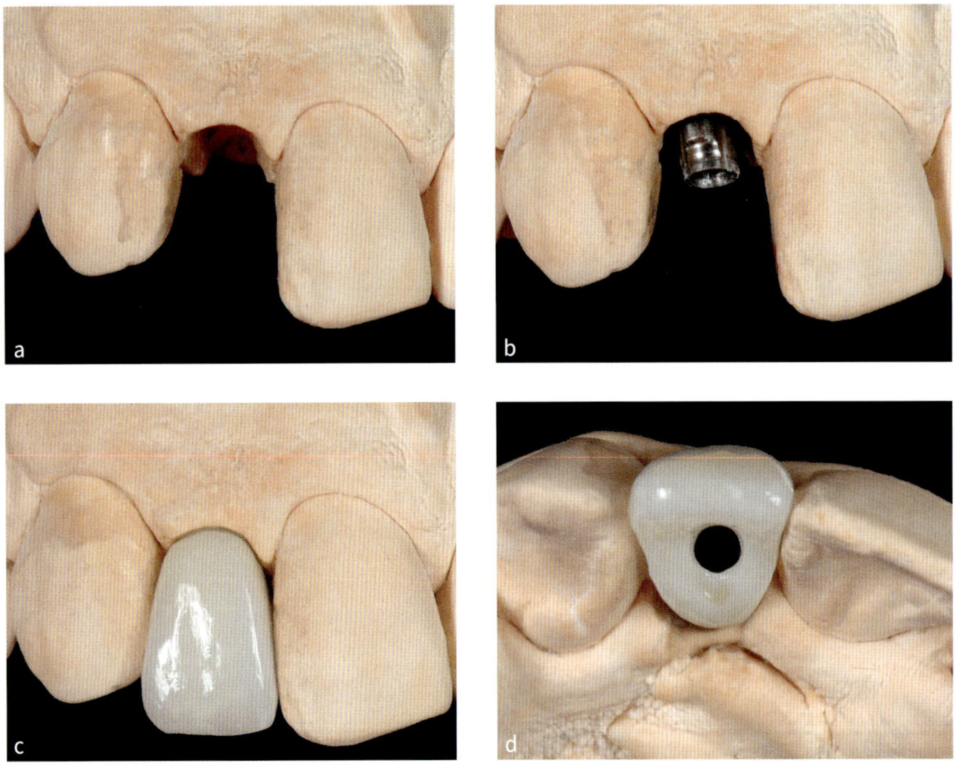

Fig 12a-d. Frontal and occlusal view of the master cast. A cement-screw-retained restoration was manufactured in the laboratory, taking care that the access hole was free of cement.

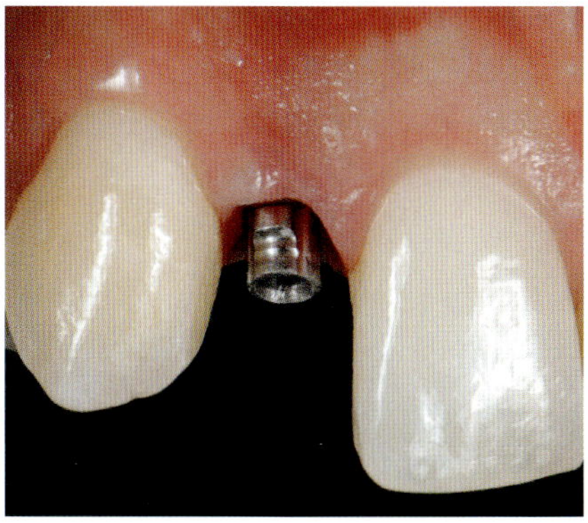

Fig 13. Frontal view of the SC Variobase abutment.

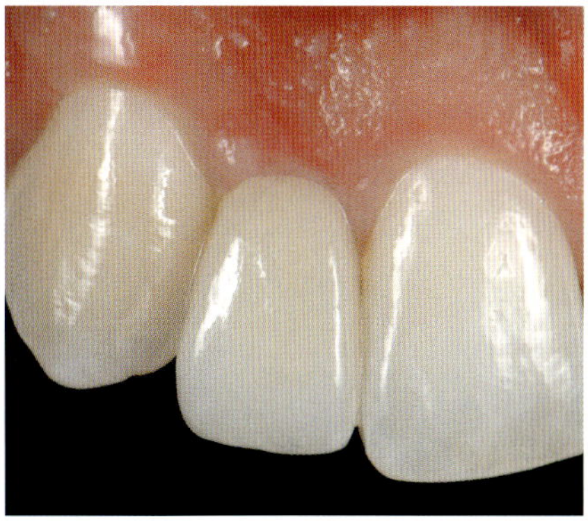

Fig 14. Frontal view of definitive zirconium dioxide screw-retained restoration.

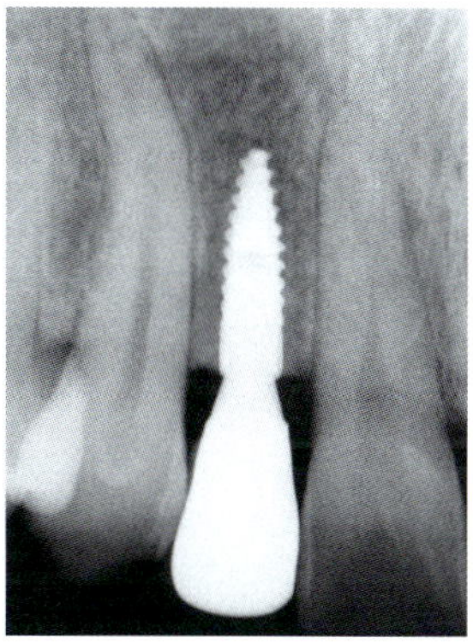

Fig 15. Follow-up periapical radiograph.

A cement-screw-retained restoration was placed (Figures 13 and 14).

Figure 15 shows 6-month radiographic follow-up.

CONCLUSIONS

The comparison in the tension of the passive fit between screwed versus cemented structures shows us that the allowed gap must be between 50 and 150 mm to avoid micromovements.

The better passive adjustment of the structures, the greater reduction in stress that is transferred to the peri-implant tissue.

The microtension values reported in the literature for structures of a single premachined (screwed) piece present an average of 2,517 mε (measure of tension), while the cement-screwed prostheses present an average of 844 mε. The conclusion follows that cement-screwed prostheses generate much less stress on the implants than single-piece screw-retained prostheses.

Treatment team:
Surgery: Alejandro Treviño & Brenda Papadopulos
Prosthetics: Alejandro Treviño Santos
Laboratory: Thomas Graber, Estudio de Porcelana Suizo

5.4 Implants in Extraction Sockets: Single Rooted Teeth

5.4.1 Maxillary central incisor

W. MARTIN, L. GONZAGA

A 60-year-old woman presented to our clinic to address a nonrestorable central incisor and evaluation for treatment options. She was seen previously by an endodontist, who diagnosed the tooth as having a vertical root fracture. This tooth had a past history of endodontic treatment with a direct composite resin restoration that fractured during function (Figure 1). The patient wished to explore options to replace the tooth with an implant-supported crown in an effort to prevent involvement of the adjacent teeth or need for a removable prosthesis.

A review of her past medical history highlighted no contributing factors that would prevent routine surgical and restorative treatment. She reported no allergies and no medications. She also denied the use of tobacco in any form but admitted the use of tetrahydrocannabinol products. Clinical examination of tooth 11 highlighted the clinical crown fracture with mesiopalatal extension of the fracture subgingivally toward the location of the vertical root fracture. The tooth is asymptomatic with no mobility, and there was no evidence of an acute or chronic infection. A localized CBCT highlights the position of interproximal bone on the adjacent teeth, thickness of facial bone, as well as the orientation of the root in relation to the axial thickness of the maxilla (Figure 2).

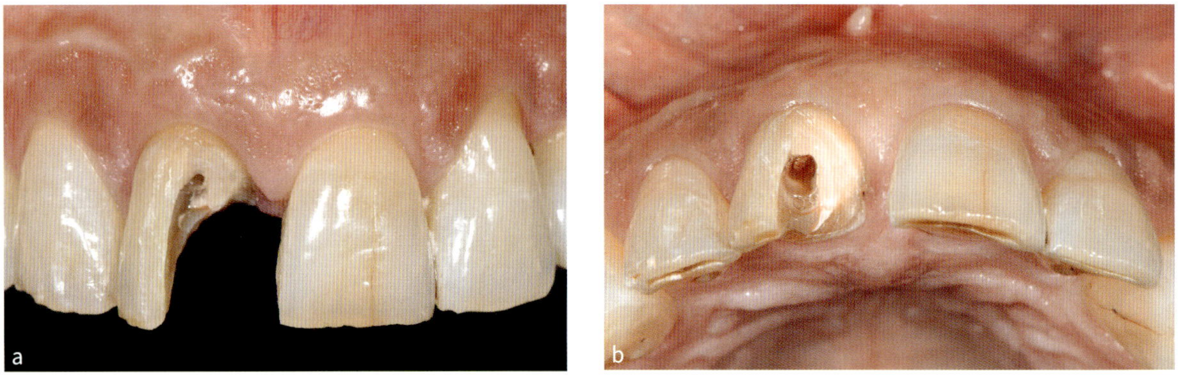

Fig 1 a-b. Frontal and occlusal views of tooth 11.

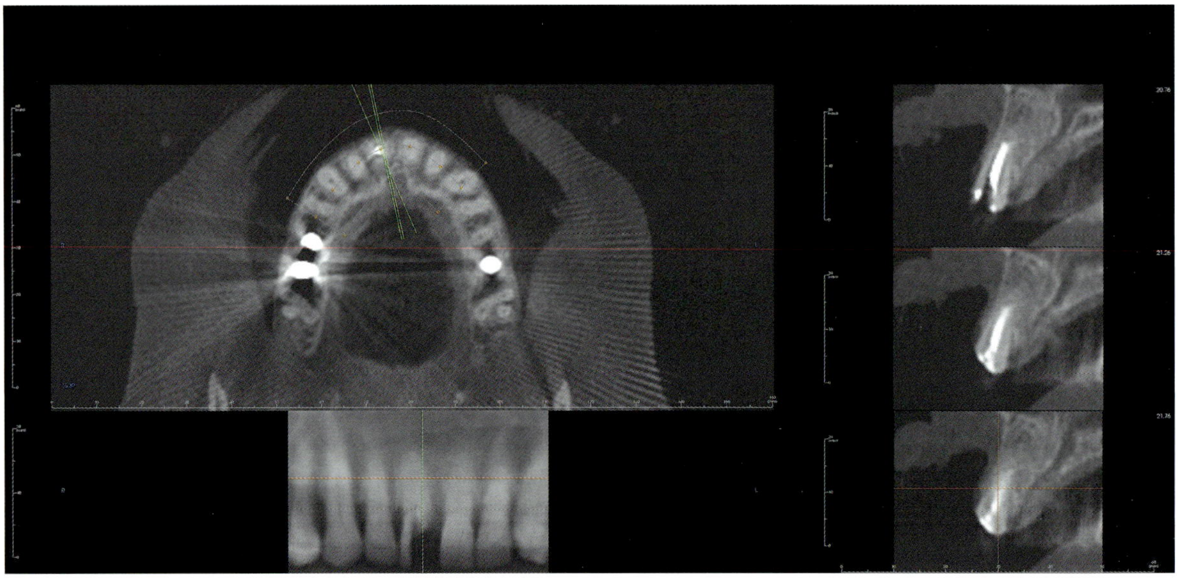

Fig 2. Axial and coronal views of CBCT, sagittal view focused on tooth 11. Note upper lip retraction, allowing assessment of soft tissue thickness.

Fig 3. Overall treatment classification: Esthetic risk = medium; Surgical classification = complex; Prosthodontic classification = advanced.

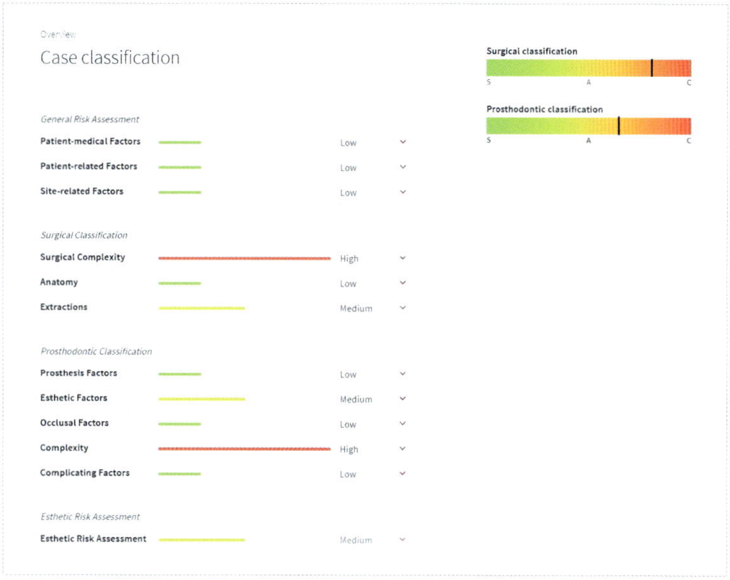

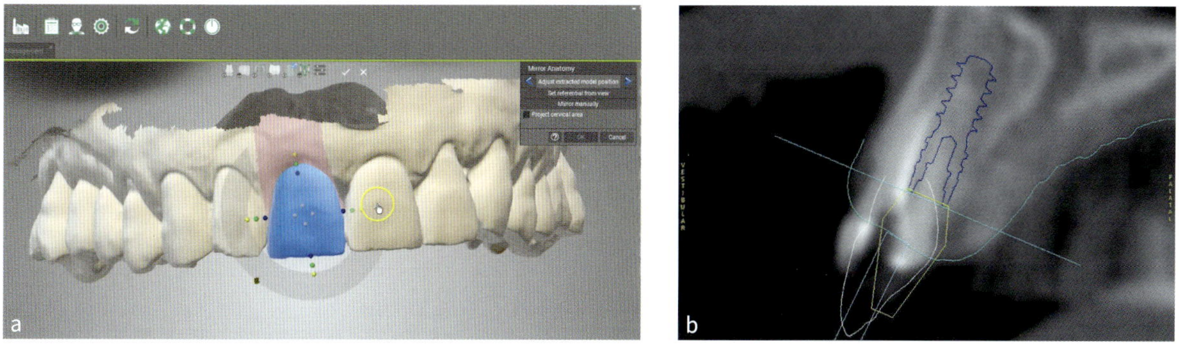

Fig 4 a-b. Digital tooth arrangement of tooth 11 and planning for immediate implant placement.

The treatment risk was assessed utilizing the SAC Assessment Tool highlighting key esthetic, surgical, and prosthetic risk factors resulting in an overall treatment risk (Figure 3). When evaluating the esthetic risk, the patient presented with medium gingival display at full smile and adequate prosthetic space for restoration. The tissue phenotype was medium-scalloped/medium-thick, and the soft tissues were intact. A review of the CBCT highlighted a thin facial plate (< 1 mm), with adjacent tooth interproximal bone heights of 5.5 mm to the interproximal contact points. This patient had realistic treatment expectations. Surgical risk factors of consideration were the need for bone augmentation (socket or horizontal), the area of treatment being located in a region of esthetic importance, and the potential desire to place the implant at the time of tooth extraction. The prosthetic risk factors in this rehabilitation are favorable due to the available prosthetic volume and absence of parafunctional habits. The main prosthetic risk was related to the desire for immediate restoration. Treatment alternatives involving dental implant therapy were discussed with the patient (timing of implant placement and load, need for grafting, restoration type, and treatment time).

TREATMENT PLANNING

Utilizing the information from the clinical and radiographic examination aligned with the evidence in the literature, an immediate implant placement approach was selected with the option for either the delivery of a provisional restoration or a custom healing abutment (based upon implant stability testing) at the time of surgery. This case is classified as Type 1A according to Gallucci et al. 2018.

Treatment planning was performed digitally utilizing surface scans merged with CBCT information (Synergy pathway with coDiagnostiX Dental Wings Care Visual). Prior to template design and fabrication, a digital tooth arrangement was completed and imported into the implant planning software, allowing for a restoration-driven implant positioning (Figure 4). A surgical guide was then fabricated utilizing 3D printing technology, and the provisional restoration and customized healing abutment were milled from a polymethyl methacrylate (PMMA) block. Both are designed to fit a titanium-base prefabricated abutment (Variobase).

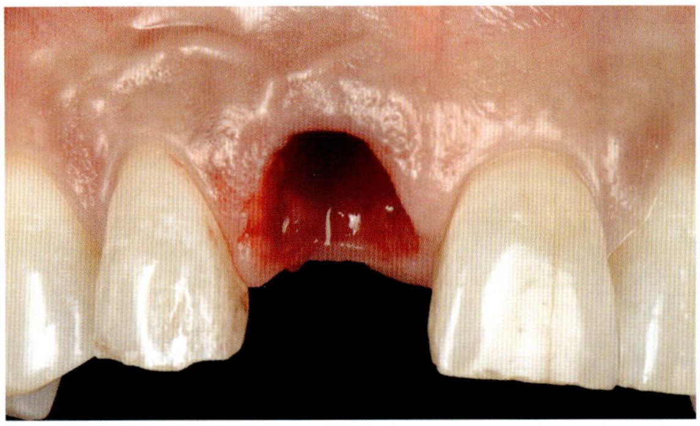

Fig 5. Postextraction socket of tooth 11.

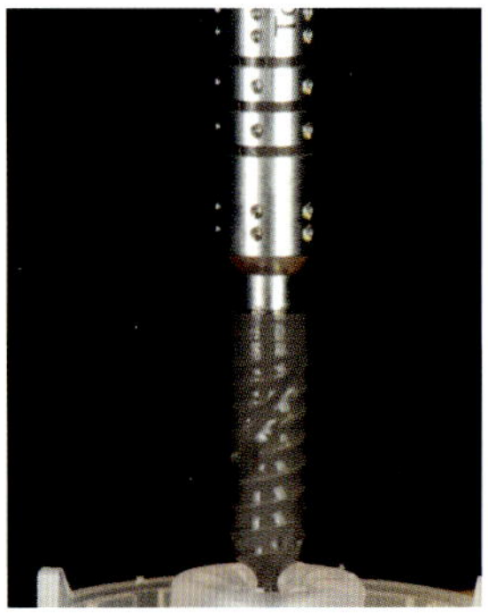

Fig 6. Straumann BLX implant with a guided mount.

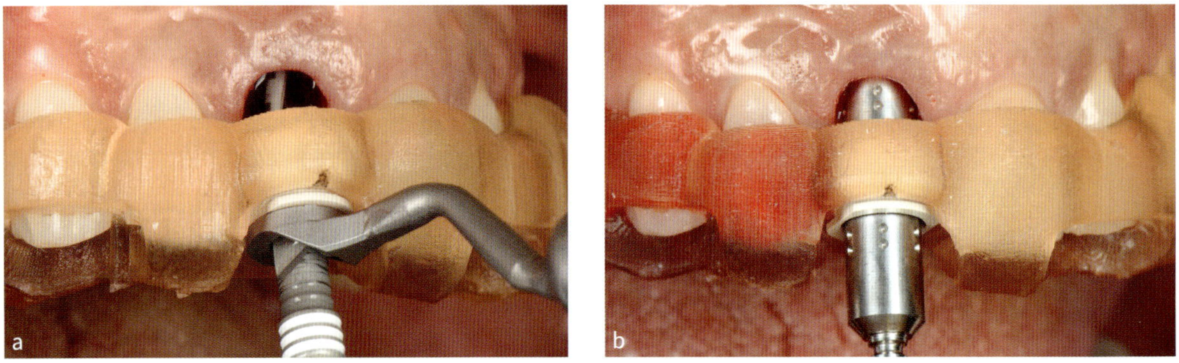

Fig 7 a-b. Preparation of the implant osteotomy through the fully guided template, followed by implant positioning using indicators on template and implant mount.

SURGERY

At the time of surgery, anesthesia was accomplished with nerve blocks using lidocaine 2% with epinephrine 1:100,000 and complemented with bupivacaine 0.5% with epinephrine 1:200,000. Nerve blocks were used to minimize local infiltration that could lead to tissue displacement and possible incomplete seating of the surgical template. Tooth 11 was extracted, minimizing trauma through the use of periotomes approaching from the mesial, distal, and palatal aspects. Evaluation of the socket walls was performed postextraction, and full seating of the surgical template confirmed. All walls were intact, and the fit of the guide could be confirmed (Figure 5).

An implant with aggressive macro design was chosen to maximize primary stability and allow for the potential for immediate restoration (BLX 3.75 mm × 12 mm SLActive implant, Straumann) (Figure 6). The osteotomy was performed per the soft bone protocol recommended by the implant manufacturer. Sequential preparation of the osteotomy was performed under copious irrigation at recommended speeds, continually confirming full seating of the template and guided components (handles and twist drills) (Figure 7a). The guided implant mount had engraved indicators to allow for accurate final positioning of the dental implant in four directions (mesiodistal, orofacial, apicocoronal, and internal connection timing) when used through the sleeve template (Figure 7b).

After the implant was placed and its final position confirmed, the guide was removed and the primary stability evaluated to determine if immediate loading was possible. The two methods utilized to determine implant stability were (1) resonance frequency analysis (RFA) with an ISQ of 72 (Osstell Beacon) and (2) the final insertion torque of 45 Ncm (Figure 8).

Use this QR code to view a highlight video of the surgery and immediate loading.

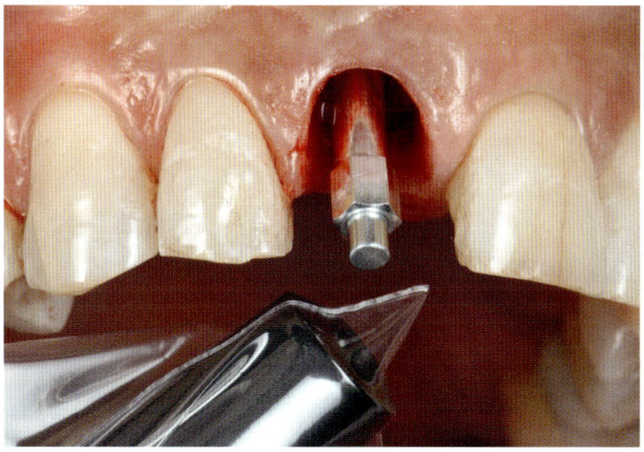

Fig 8. RFA performed on implant 11.

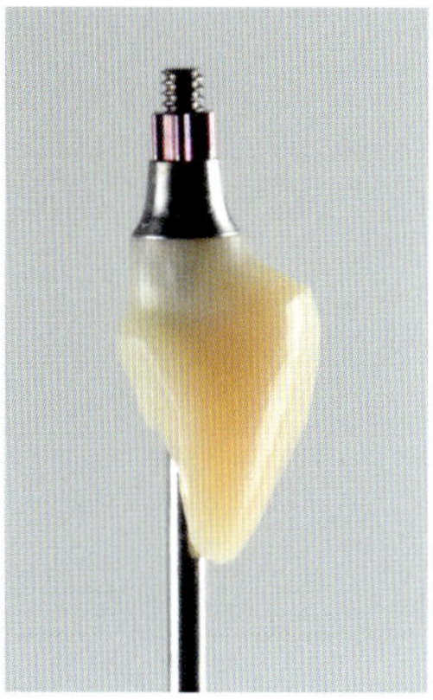

Fig 9. PMMA provisional on Variobase RB abutment.

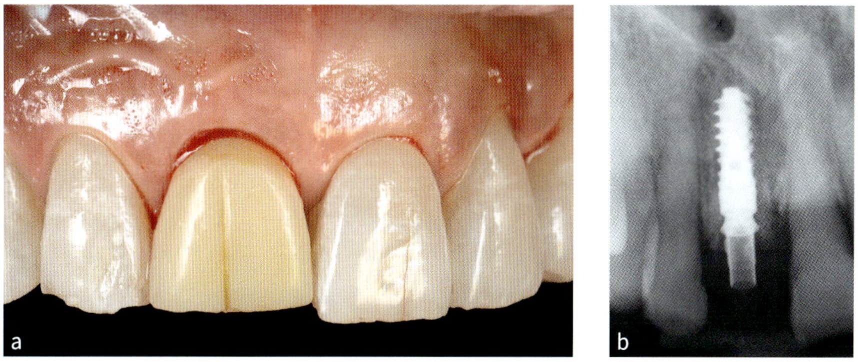

Fig 10 a-b. Facial view of the immediate provisional restoration 11 and periapical radiograph.

IMMEDIATE PROVISIONAL

After confirmation of implant stability, the prefabricated abutment (Variobase RB) was placed onto the implant with finger tightening. The PMMA milled crown was placed onto the abutment for confirmation of correct timing, 3D position, interproximal contacts, and complete setting. Once full seating of the provisional restoration onto the abutment was confirmed, the two were connected together extraorally with flowable composite resin (Figure 9).

Prior to placing the provisional restoration onto the implant, the horizontal defect dimension (HDD) was grafted with a xenograft bone substitute material (Bio-Oss) utilizing the dual-zone technique (Chu et al, 2012). Once the screw-retained provisional was placed and tightened to 15 Ncm, a periapical radiographic confirmation was taken, followed by occlusal adjustments, to avoid contacts in all excursive movements. The screw access was then closed with PTFE tape (Teflon) and temporary composite material (Telio, Ivoclar Vivadent) (Figure 10). The patient was prescribed 500 mg amoxicillin every 8 hours for 7 days, 600 mg ibuprofen every 8 hours for 3 days, and chlorhexidine gluconate 0.12% mouthwash 2 times a day for 15 days.

PROSTHETICS

Ten weeks after implant placement, the provisional restoration was removed and implant stability was tested using RFA (ISQ 78). A digital impression of the implant and provisional contours were made utilizing an intraoral scanner (Trios) (Figure 11).

In the process of fabricating the definitive restoration, it was decided to utilize an angulated solution abutment (AS Variobase RB) to allow for an increased thickness of material in the incisal third of the restoration, thus providing improved esthetics. The material selected for the crown was zirconium dioxide with a facial cutback for layering porcelain (Figure 12). The patient was seen for delivery of the definitive restoration. Upon removal of the provisional restoration, tissues were irrigated and the restoration fit confirmed, followed by abutment screw tightening to 35 Ncm. The access hole was sealed with Teflon

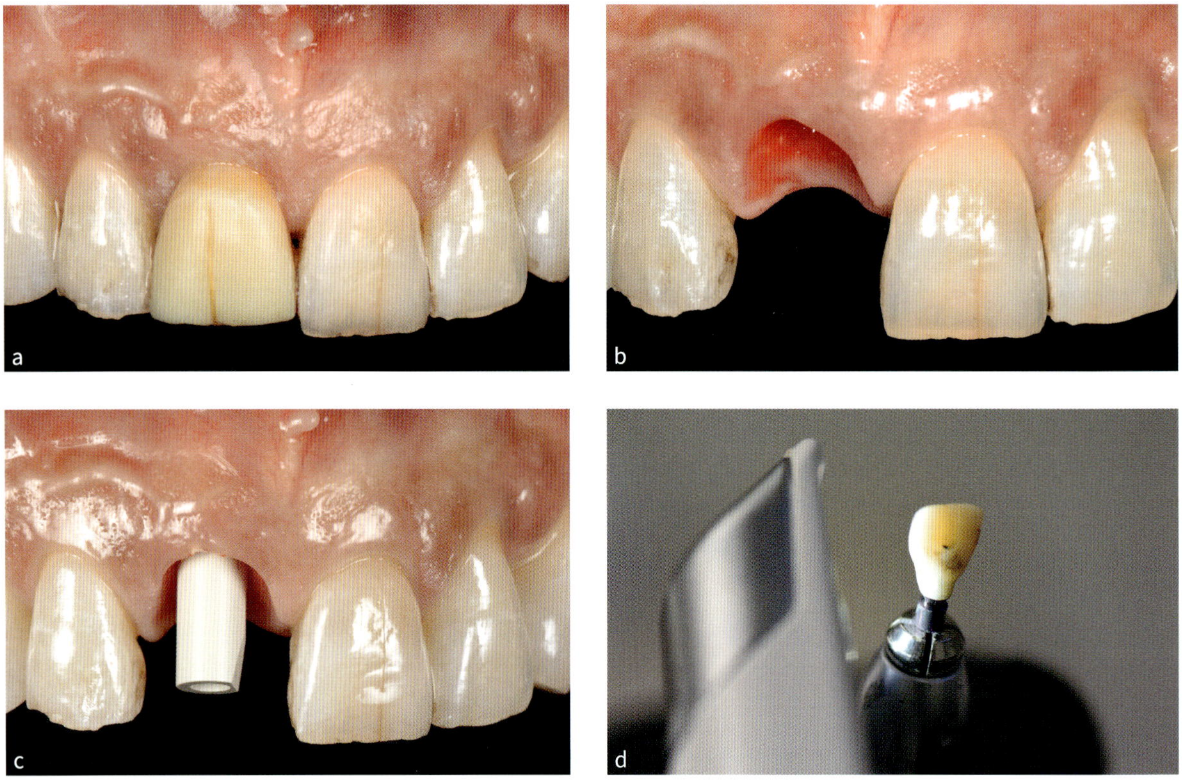

Fig 11 a-d. Implant 11 at 10 weeks healing, transition zone, scan body on implant 11, and chairside scanning of the provisional restoration utilizing an intra-oral scanner.

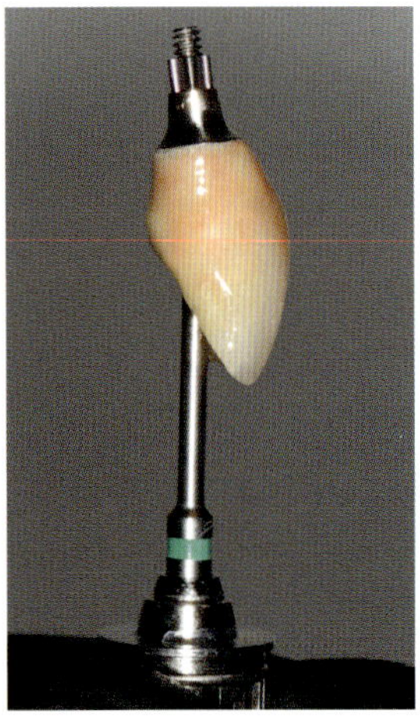

Fig 12. Definitive screw-retained restoration.

and composite resin. Occlusion was adjusted as needed and polished.

The patient was seen for a 12-month clinical and radiographic follow-up visit to confirm mucosal tissue contours, implant health, esthetics, and occlusion (Figure 13).

REFLECTION ON THE TREATMENT APPROACH AND OUTCOME

Based upon the clinical evaluation, this patient was a good candidate for an immediate placement and immediate loading scenario. In hindsight, the placement of a connective tissue graft at the time of surgery to thicken the soft tissue would be seriously considered if done again. The digital workflow with an intraoral scanner made the treatment approach streamlined and allowed for a faster construction and delivery of the immediate provisional. While new digital

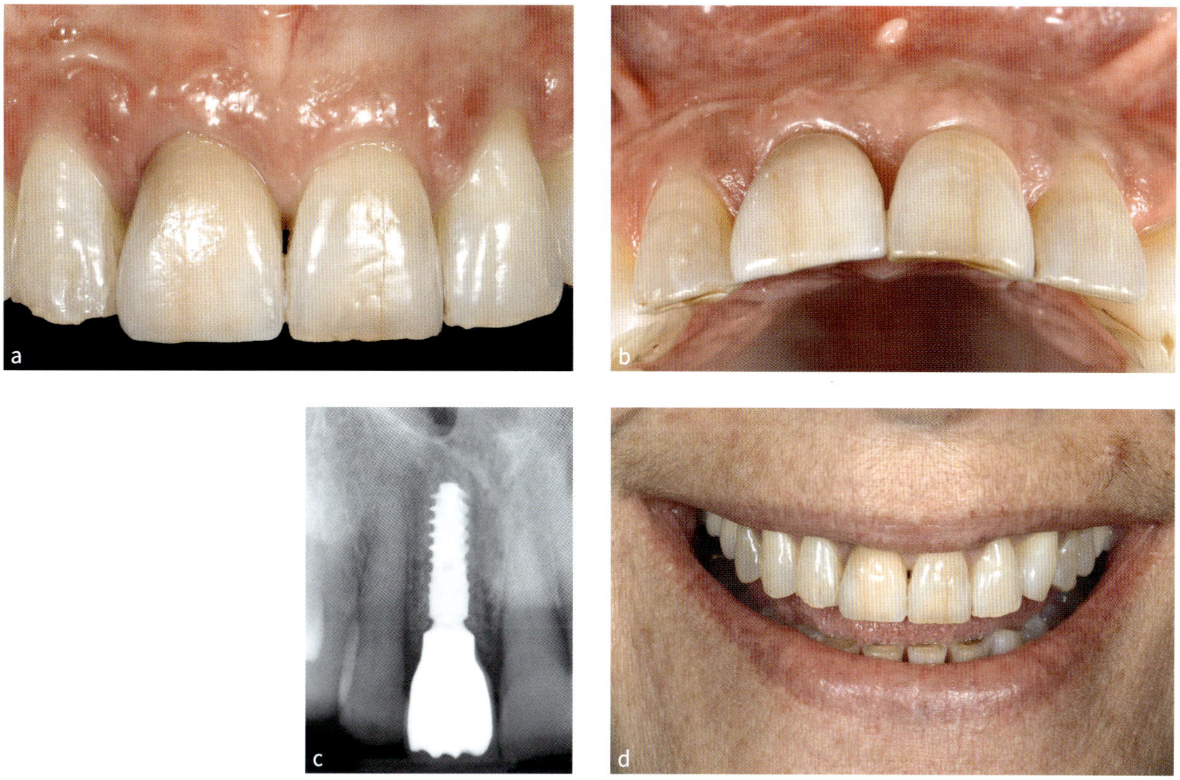

Fig 13a-d. Buccal and occlusal views, periapical radiograph, and smile of implant restoration at site 11 at 12 months.

technology was utilized, some esthetic limitations existed with the color and translucency of the PMMA milled block. This patient was tolerant of the shade of the interim restoration, but in a patient with higher esthetic demands, a cutback or refabrication with conventional PMMA or Bis-GMA material would have been required. Utilizing a Variobase AS abutment in the definitive restoration made a big difference in the esthetic outcome, allowing our laboratory technician to maximize layers in the porcelain to match the adjacent teeth.

Treatment team:
Surgery: Dr. Luiz Gonzaga
Prosthetics: Dr. William C. Martin
Laboratory: Alexander Wuensche, Zahntechnique Inc.

5.4.2 Maxillary premolar

L. GONZAGA

A 58-year-old man presented to our clinic to seek replacement of a fractured, nonrestorable maxillary premolar (tooth 15). His past medical history reported no contraindications to routine dental and surgical procedures. He reported as a nonsmoker, occasional alcohol drinker, no known allergies, and was currently taking the following medications: ramipril 2.5 mg, simvastatin 20 mg and a daily aspirin (81 mg). The clinical and radiographic examination revealed that tooth 15 had extensive caries and was deemed nonrestorable, and tooth 16 had a restoration needing replacement (Figure 1). The patient desired to have the failing tooth replaced by an implant-supported crown in an effort to prevent involvement of the adjacent teeth or the need of a fixed partial denture.

The extraoral clinical examination showed no significant findings, and the tooth was not visible during full smile. Examination of the hard and soft tissues around tooth 15 revealed acceptable amount of keratinized mucosa (3 mm) with ideal prosthetic volume for a premolar tooth replacement (mesial/distal space = 7 mm; interocclusal space = 7 mm). The adjacent tooth (no. 16) needed a full-coverage restoration to replace the failed amalgam restoration and fractured cusp. The plan was to treat tooth 16 after implant placement to avoid a misfit of the surgical guide. A maxillary CBCT with the planned restoration and proposed implant position highlights the available bone volume and distance to the maxillary sinus (Figure 2).

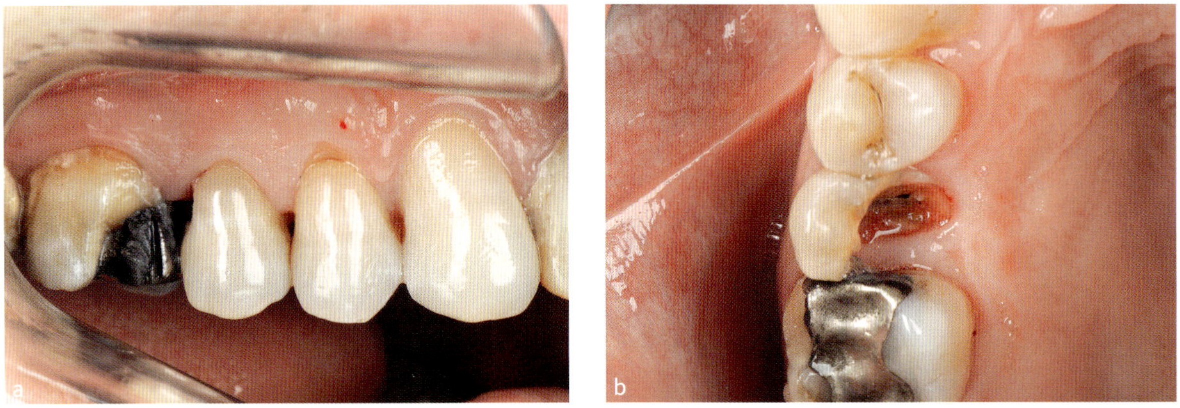

Fig 1 a-b. Lateral and occlusal views of tooth 15.

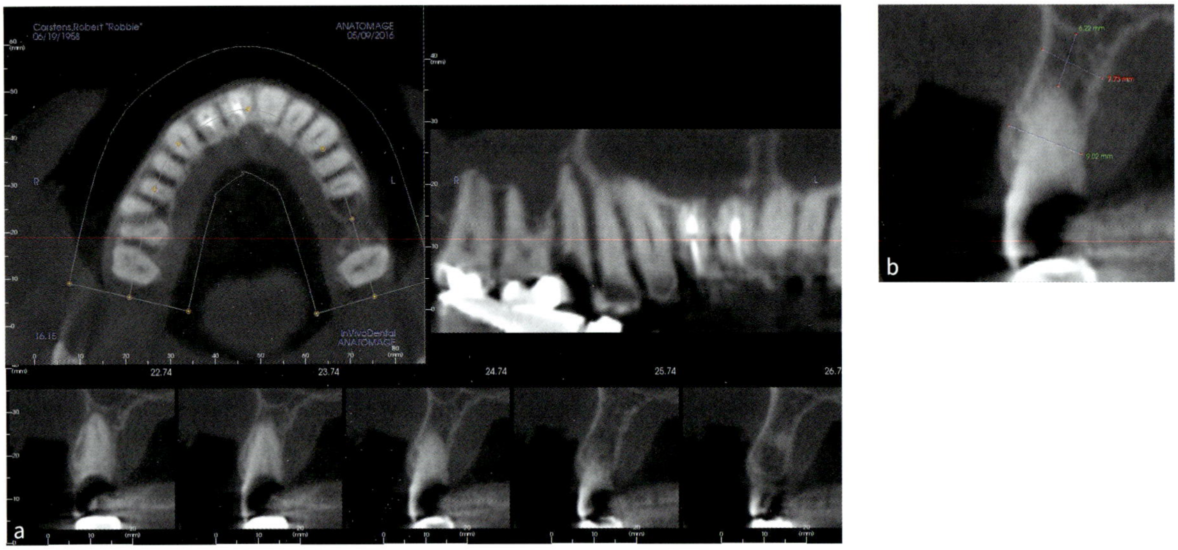

Fig 2 a-b. Panoramic and cross-sectional views highlighting the adjacent bone, including the buccopalatal dimension and the bone volume apical to the socket potentially allowing for good primary stability.

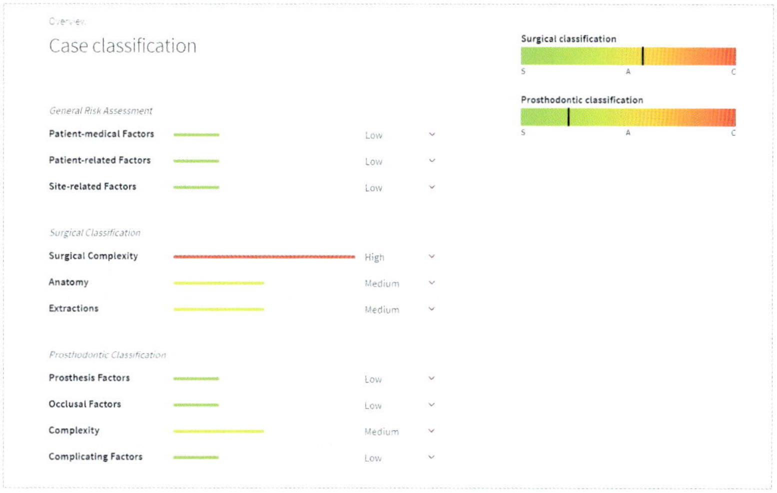

Fig 3. Overall treatment classification: Surgical classification = advanced; Prosthodontic classification = straightforward.

The treatment risk was assessed utilizing the SAC Assessment Tool (Figure 3). When evaluating the esthetic risk, the patient was graded as a low risk because the edentulous space was not visible at full smile and the patient had realistic expectations. Surgical risk factors of consideration were the proximity with the sinus and adjacent roots and need to address the horizontal gap in case of immediate implant placement. The CBCT planning confirmed the ability to place a 4.1-mm-diameter tapered implant inside the bony envelope with simultaneous correction of the minor buccal deficit. The prosthetic risk factors in this rehabilitation were straightforward due to the low esthetic risk, conventional loading, and favorable prosthetic factors.

TREATMENT PLANNING

Utilizing the information from the clinical and radiographic examination aligned with the evidence in the literature and digital planning, the patient was presented with a plan for an immediate implant placement with simultaneous bone augmentation of the buccal defect followed by an conventional loading protocol (type 1C, Gallucci and coworkers 2018). The treatment planning was performed digitally utilizing surface scans merged with CBCT information (coDiagnostiX). A surgical guide was designed and then fabricated utilizing 3D SLA printing technology.

SURGERY

At the time of surgery, anesthesia was accomplished with nerve blocks using lidocaine 2% with epinephrine 1:100,000. The surgical approach involved a minimally traumatic technique with periotomes to extract tooth 15. The socket was debrided with curettage and saline solution irrigation. The surgical guide was positioned and confirmed to be fully seated. Incremental osteotomy preparation with copious normal saline irrigation was performed according to the manufacturer's instructions. The final osteotomy preparation was for a 4.1-mm Regular CrossFit (RC) BLT implant. After the placement of the implant, a 0.5-mm closure screw was inserted into the implant, and the buccal defect was filled with corticocancellous allograft mix (LifeNet Health) and a collagen sponge was stabilized over the socket with a 5-0 resorbable suture (figure-8 suture design) (Figure 4).

RESTORATIVE

After 10 weeks of uneventful healing, an uncovering procedure was performed through a simple crestal incision (Figure 5). Confirmation of osseointegration was done through clinical examination including a torque test and resonance frequency analysis (Osstell Beacon). A polyvinyl siloxane impression of the implant position was made for the indirect fabrication

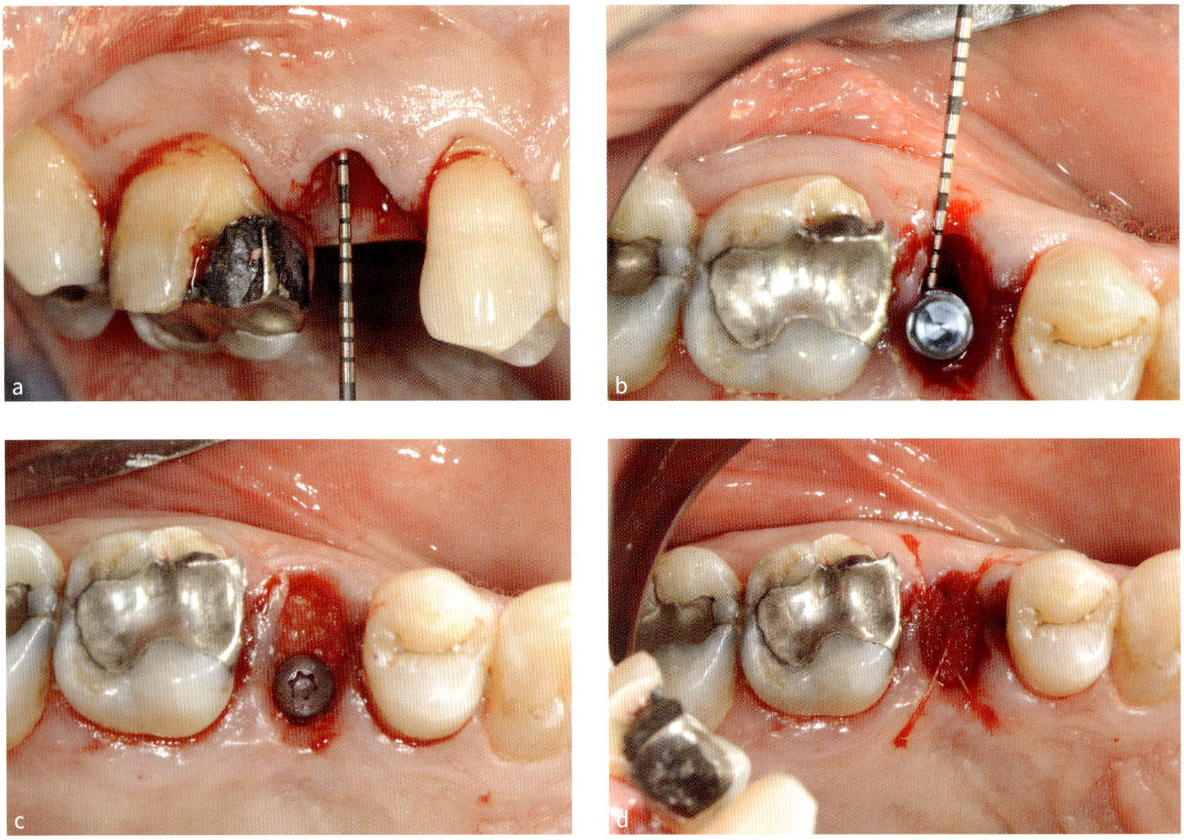

Fig 4 a-d. Clinical series highlighting surgical steps: postextraction evaluation, implant in place and assessment of the buccal defect; closure screw placed with grafted buccal defect; collagen sponge with a figure-8 suture design.

of a provisional restoration. The provisional restoration was designed to provide the ideal support and emergence profile through the transition zone, in addition to testing the occlusion and preventing the adjacent teeth from moving in between the impression appointment and the delivery of the definitive restoration.

The definitive restoration was designed as screw-retained, with a castable abutment (RC Bone Level Implant Gold abutment) veneered with feldspathic ceramic. At delivery, ideal interproximal contacts, peri-implant tissue support, and full seating of the restoration was clinically and radiographically confirmed prior to occlusal adjustments. The abutment screw was tightened to 35 Ncm (according to the manufacturer's specifications) and the access channel filled with Teflon (PTFE tape) and sealed with light-cured composite resin (Figure 6). Occlusion was adjusted and polished. The patient was scheduled for recall and continued maintenance with the hygienist every 6 months (Figure 7).

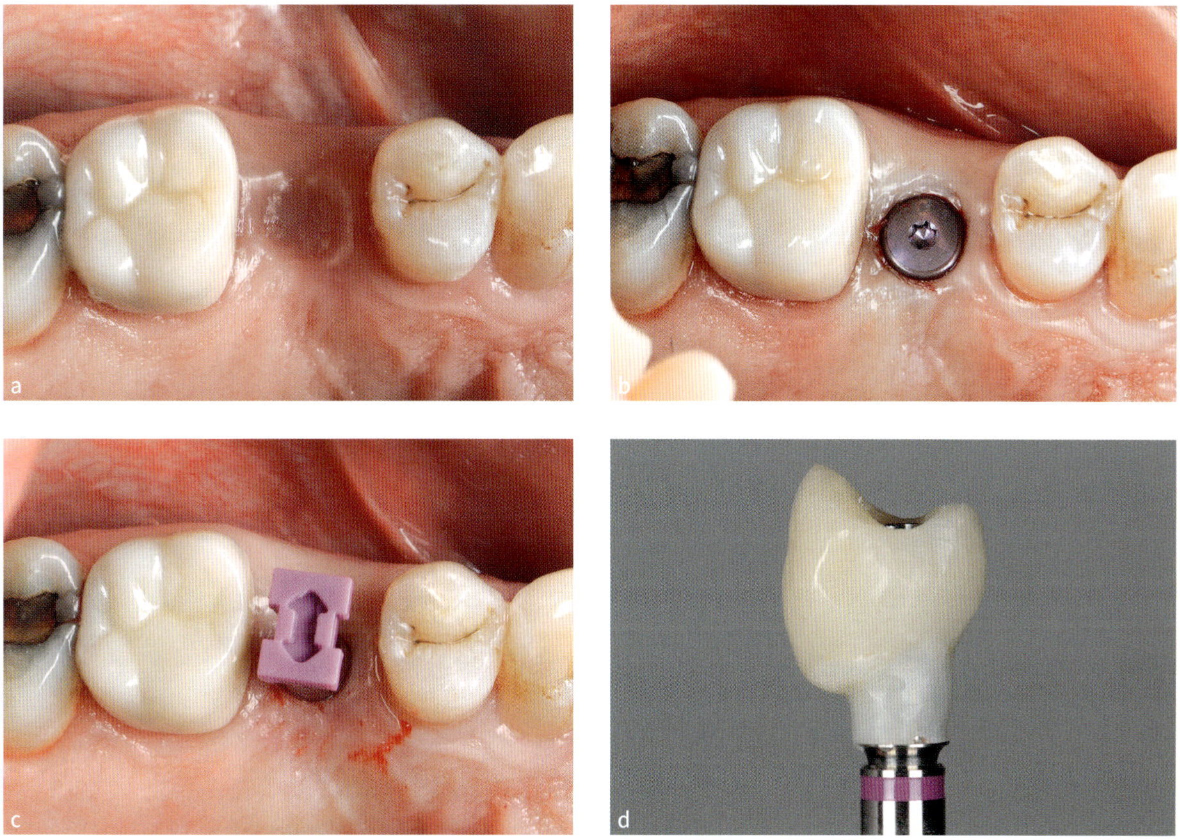

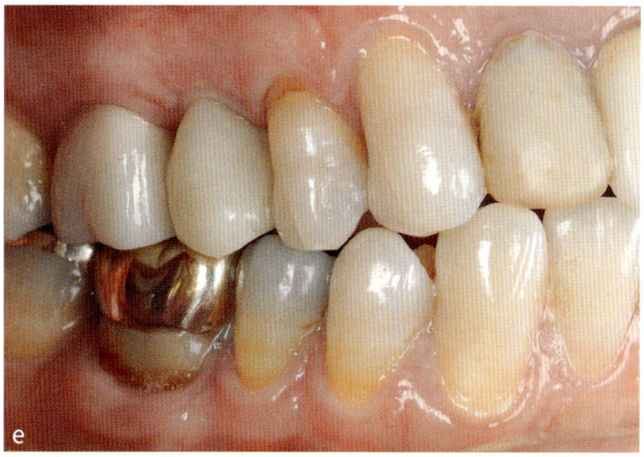

Fig 5 a-e. Clinical series highlighting restorative steps: (a) healing 10 weeks after implant placement, (b) uncovering procedure with healing abutment, (c) closed-tray impression post, (d) screw-retained provisional restoration, and (e) delivery of the provisional restoration at site 15.

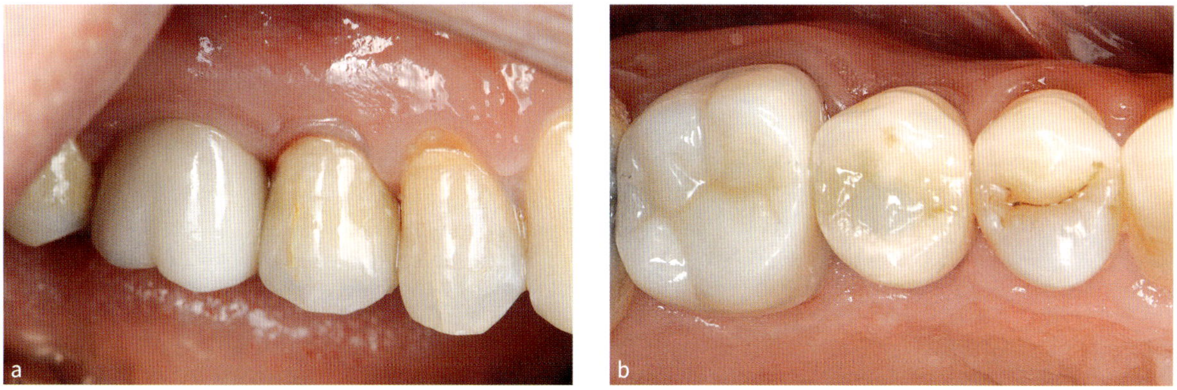

Fig 6 a-b. Lateral and occlusal views of definitive screw-retained restoration at delivery.

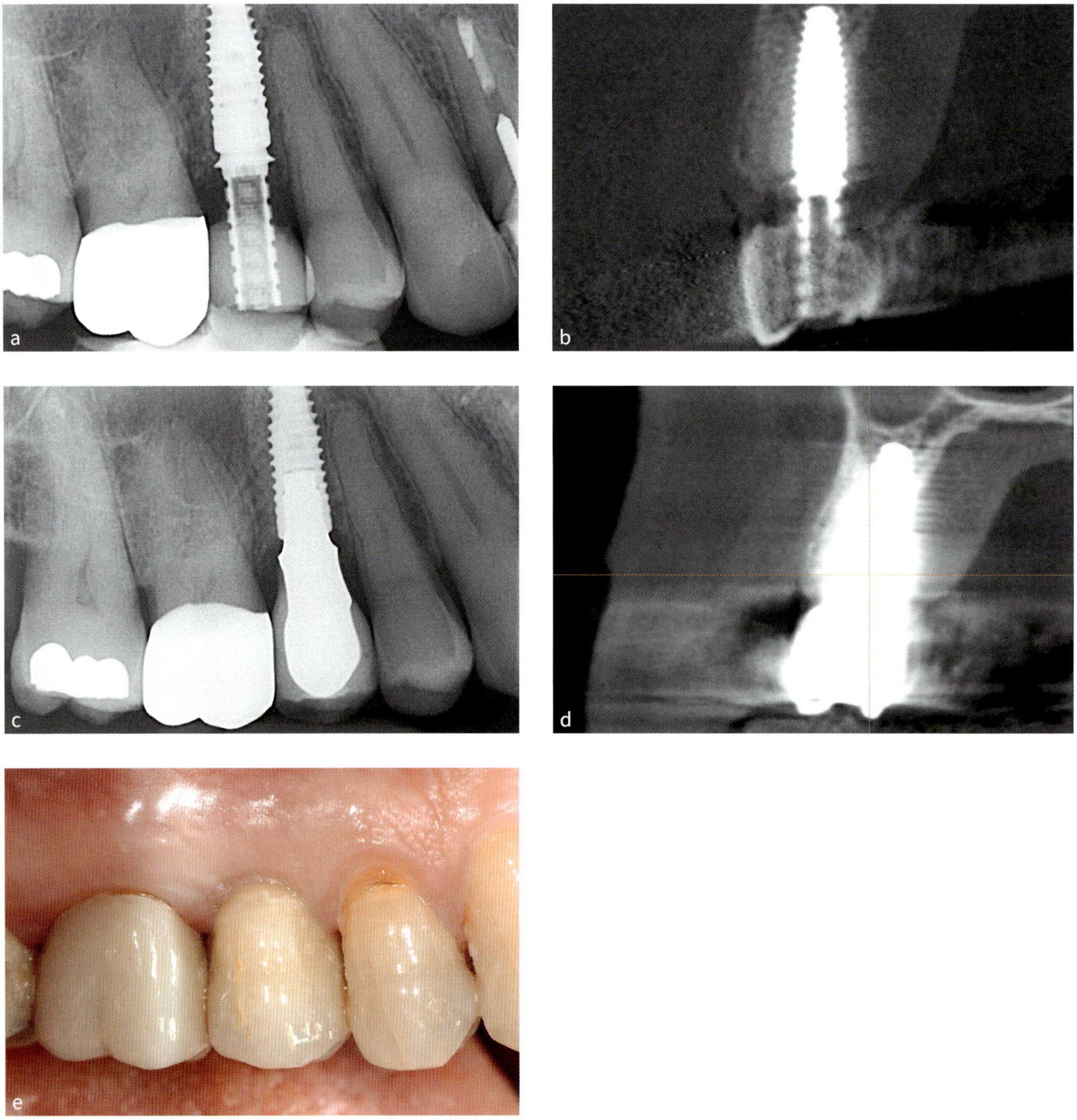

Fig 7 a-e. (a) Periapical radiograph at the time of loading (10 weeks). (b) CBCT at the time of loading (10 weeks). (c) Periapical radiograph at 3 years postdelivery. (d) CBCT at 3 years postdelivery. (e) Lateral view of site 15 at 3 years postdelivery.

REFLECTION

This approach had a positive outcome for the patient and allowed us to decrease the number of interventions since the implant was placed at the time of extraction. In reflection, we could have used a one-stage healing approach utilizing a customized healing abutment providing ideal support for the transition zone. From a restorative perspective, today, this treatment would follow a digital workflow including intraoral scanning, chairside or laboratory milling utilizing a titanium bonding base abutment with an all-ceramic screw-retained restoration.

Treatment team:
Surgery and prosthetics: Dr. Luiz Gonzaga
Laboratory: Glynn Watts, Advantage Dental Design

5.5 Implants in Extraction Sockets: Multirooted Teeth

5.5.1 Maxillary first molar

P. CASENTINI

A 32-year-old man was referred by his dentist to our clinic for treatment of a recently fractured maxillary molar. The tooth had received an endodontic treatment in the past and a direct composite resin restoration. The patient reported a mild discomfort in the area without acute symptoms, and he was interested in replacing the fractured tooth with an implant-supported crown. The patient was not taking any medication, did not smoke, and reported being in good general health.

CLINICAL AND RADIOGRAPHIC EXAMINATION

The intraoral examination showed a visible fracture of tooth 16, crossing the entire surface of the tooth from the mesiobuccal to the midpalatal area. The presence of swelling and an increased probing depth was assessed in the palatal area. In the intraoral periapical radiograph, the fracture was partially visible (Figure 1).

The negative prognosis of the tooth was confirmed, and a CBCT was immediately executed to obtain complete information about the anatomy of the roots and the surrounding bone. The CBCT revealed the presence of divergent roots and an inter-radicular septum with a favorable anatomy in order to place an immediate implant; absence of significant radiolucency was also confirmed (Figure 2).

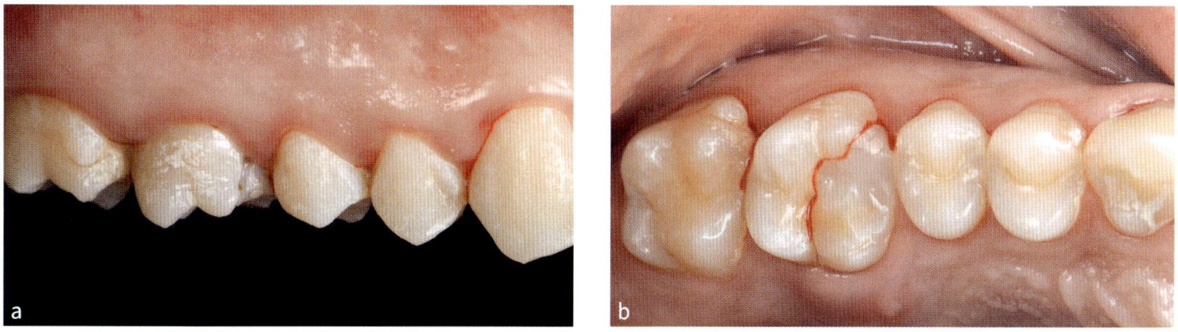

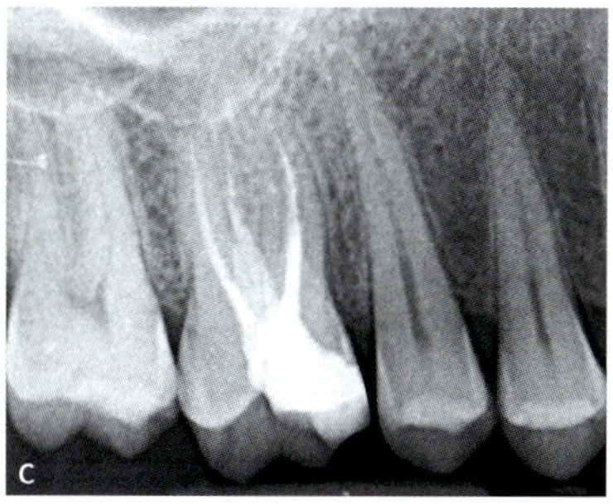

Fig 1 a-c. Buccal, occlusal, and radiographic view of tooth 16.

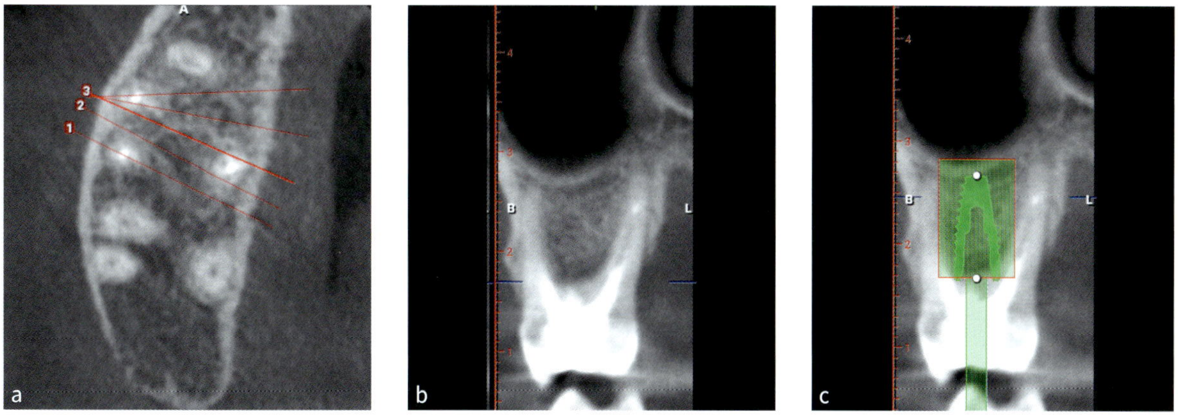

Fig 2 a-c. Localized CBCT of the fractured molar.

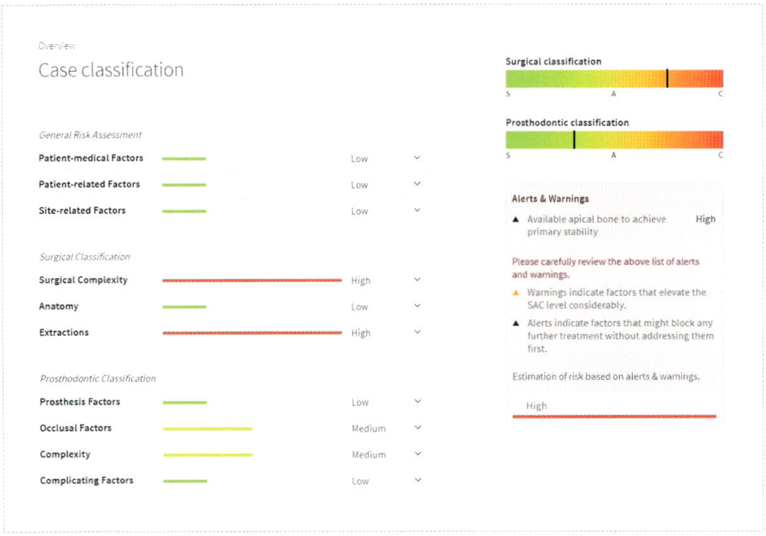

Fig 3. Overall treatment classification: Surgical classification = advanced to complex; Prosthodontic classification = straightforward to advanced.

TREATMENT RISK PROFILE

The treatment risk profile was assessed with the SAC Assessment Tool in order to define specific esthetic, surgical, and prosthetic risk factors (Figure 3). Esthetic risk was judged reduced in this case, since the area of treatment is partially visible when the patient smiles. The patient in any case declared realistic expectations. Main surgical risk factors are represented by the proximity of the sinus floor, the presence of a multirooted tooth that has to be extracted with minimal trauma, the need to achieve primary stability, and a prosthetically driven implant position in a complex anatomical situation. Finally, the need for simultaneous grafting procedures should be considered to manage the residual gap. Prosthetic risk factors for this case are not significant, since restorative space is adequate, occlusion is normal, and immediate loading or temporization are not required.

TREATMENT PLANNING

Based on the clinical and radiological situation, the following treatment plan was proposed:

- Extraction of the fractured maxillary molar
- Immediate implant placement in the area of the interradicular bone septum, combined with a grafting procedure in order to fill the gap between the implant and the socket walls.
- Placement of a custom-made healing abutment to seal the extraction socket and provide immediate soft tissue support.
- Realization and delivery of the definitive implant-supported crown after osseointegration of the implant and healing of the soft tissues.

The patient agreed to the proposed treatment, providing his written informed consent.

SURGICAL TREATMENT

The extraction and implant placement procedure were performed under local anesthesia. A preliminary separation, performed with a carbide bur, allowed the surgeon to remove the crown and achieve accessibility to the roots that were subsequently separated and extracted. Extraction was minimally traumatic, and it was performed by means of thin periotomes and elevators to avoid any damage to the socket walls and to the interradicular bone. After complete extraction of the tooth, integrity of the interradicular septum was confirmed and preparation of the implant bed was performed with a sequence of drills. An implant with an aggressive external design (5 x 10 BLX Wide Base [WB]) was selected to achieve an adequate primary stability, and an hydrophilic implant surface (SLActive) was chosen to shorten the time of osseointegration in a complex anatomical situation. A prosthetically driven implant placement at the center of the socket was achieved (Figure 4).

After implant placement, the gap between the implant and the surrounding socket walls was filled with trimmed fragments of an osteoconductive xenograft represented by DBBM in a collagen matrix (Bio-Oss Collagen). Gentle pressure was applied to the biomaterial in order to obtain perfect adaptation to the defect (Figure 5). The benefit of this material, compared to simple granules of DBBM, is represented by its stability and the tendency to remain in place despite bleeding from the recipient site.

After placement of the graft, a customized healing abutment was used to seal the socket and protect the underlying graft (Figure 6). The custom-made healing screw was obtained, relining a temporary titanium abutment with flowable composite resin. Teflon tape was used to isolate the surgical field from the composite resin. Teflon tape and flowable composite resin were also used to seal the screw access. No sutures were utilized.

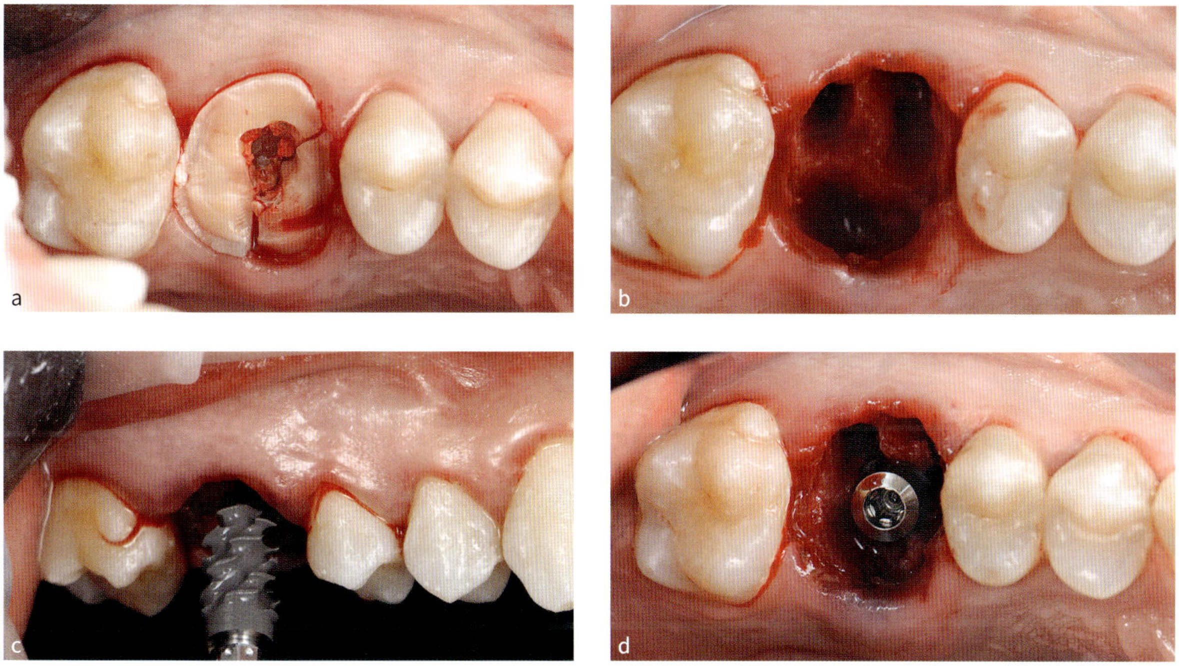

Fig 4 a-d. Occlusal view before and after extraction, and placement of a BLX 5.0 × 10–mm implant.

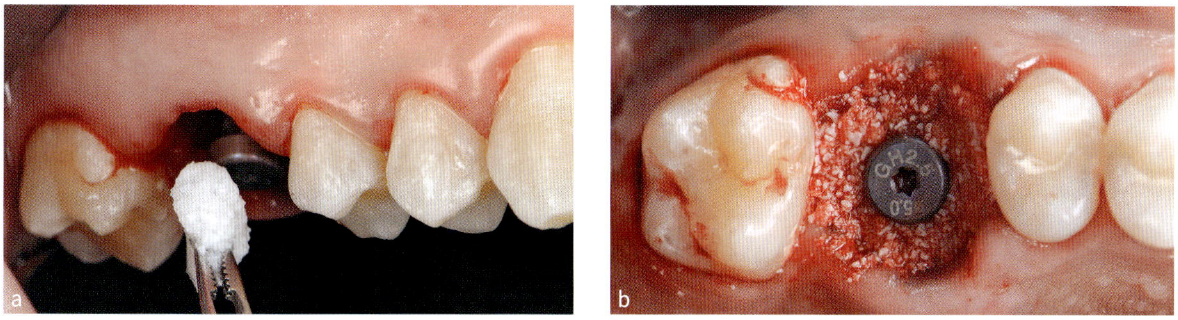

Fig 5 a-b. Placement of a xenograft in order to fill the peri-implant defects.

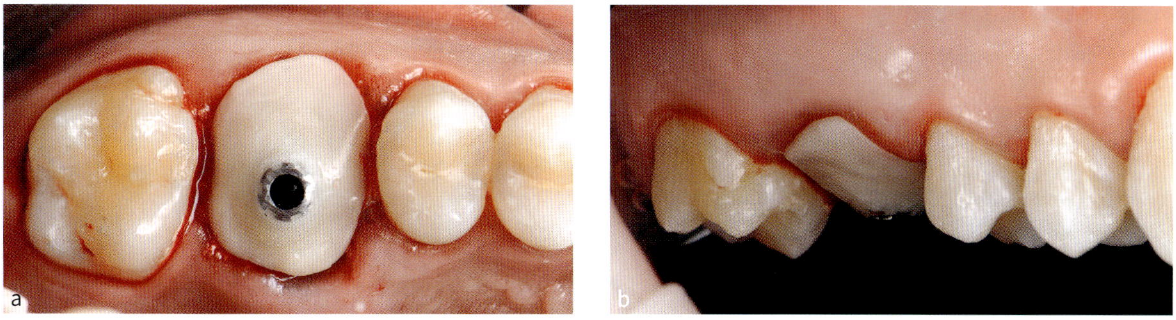

Fig 6 a-b. Occlusal and lateral view of the customized healing screw.

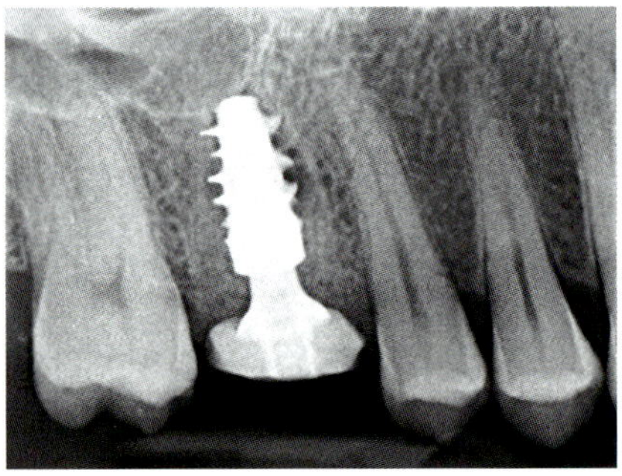

Fig 7. Periapical radiograph after implant placement.

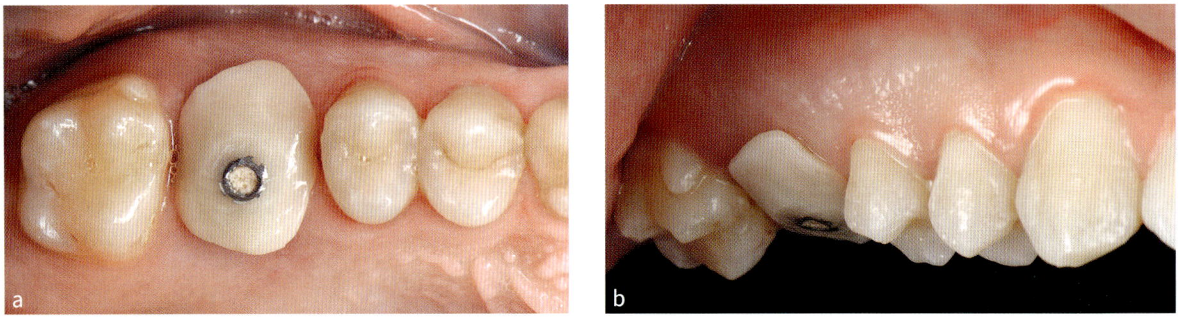

Fig 8 a-b. Occlusal and lateral view after 1 month of healing.

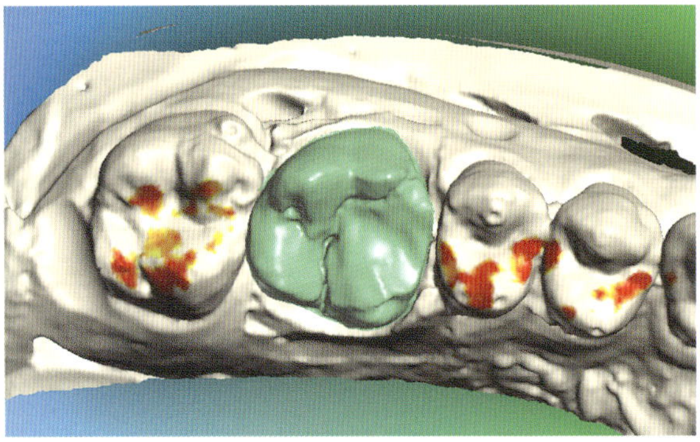

Fig 9. Scan of the original shape of the extracted tooth.

A radiograph confirmed correct placement of the implant underneath the sinus floor and adequate filling of the peri-implant defects (Figure 7).

The postsurgical pharmacologic protocol included antibiotics for 6 days (amoxicillin + clavulanic acid 1 g every 12 hours), chlorhexidine 0.2% mouthrinses for 2 weeks, and ibuprofen 600 mg every 12 hours for pain relief. The patient was advised to avoid brushing the operation site for 2 weeks.

At the 2-week follow-up, no complications were recorded, and the patient did not report significant symptoms. The soft tissues did not reveal any sign of inflammation.

The patient was visited every month (Figure 8), and after 3 months, prosthetic procedures were started.

PROSTHETIC TREATMENT

A preliminary impression before the dental extraction provided a model and a scan of the original volume and shape of the extracted tooth (Figure 9).

The implant position was recorded with a polyether (Impregum, 3M) open-tray impression after connecting metal transfer to the implant. Color information was also transferred to the dental laboratory.

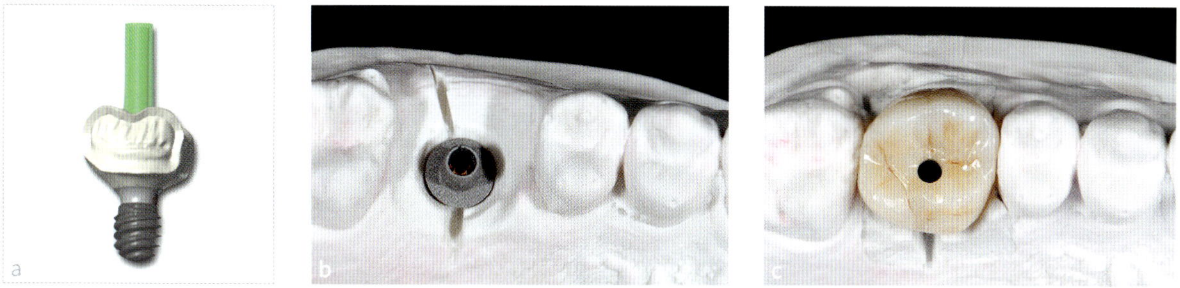

Fig 10 a-c. CAD/CAM design of the crown, selection of the titanium definitive abutment, and occlusal view of the screw-retained crown.

The dental technician, utilizing a CAD/CAM software (CARES, Straumann), selected a titanium abutment (Variobase) and designed the final shape of the screw-retained implant-supported crown (Figure 10). The selected material was zirconium dioxide with a buccal cutback in order to stratify a layer of porcelain.

In the dental laboratory, the titanium abutment was sandblasted and then luted to the zirconia-porcelain crown with an autopolymerizing cement.

DELIVERY OF THE DEFINITIVE RECONSTRUCTION AND FOLLOW-UP

Before delivery of the definitive reconstruction, the internal cavity of the implants was disinfected with a 1% chlorhexidine gel.

After the patient approved the esthetic appearance of the prosthetic reconstruction, the crown was screwed and the screw was activated with a controlled torque of 35 Ncm. A periapical radiograph confirmed precise fit of the crown.

Subsequently, the access hole were sealed with a packed Teflon tape and with a flowable composite. Specific hygienic instructions were provided to the patient, and in particular the use of dental floss was strongly recommended.

The view of the restoration at the 1-year follow-up demonstrates a favorable esthetic integration of the implant-supported crown in the surrounding tissues, and in the smile of the patient (Figure 11). The patient declared himself fully satisfied by the treatment outcome.

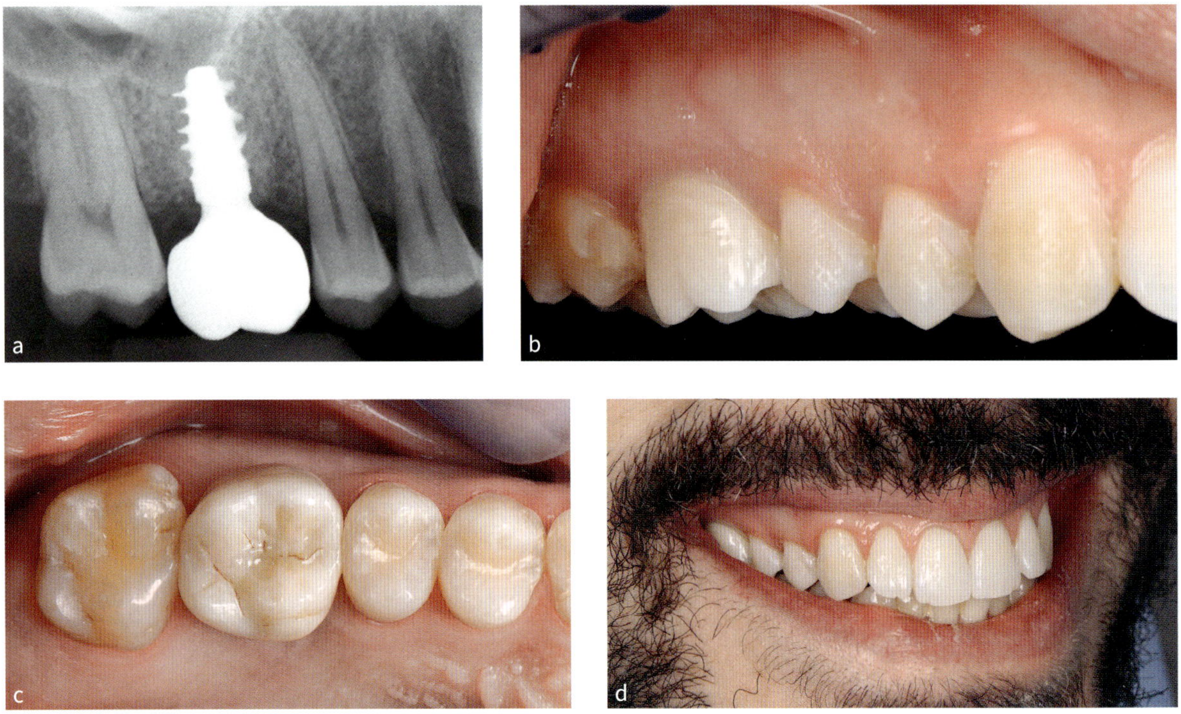

Fig 11 a-d. One-year clinical and radiographic follow-up and extraoral view.

DISCUSSION

Immediate placement of an implant in a post-extraction socket represents an evidence-based procedure, with benefits for the patient in terms of time of treatment and maintenance of the original profile of the tissues. However, placement in a molar site can be critical. The complex anatomy in this area represents a complicating factor, and immediate placement is not always possible. In the presence of a local favorable anatomy, however, immediate implant placement can be considered.

In the presented case, implant placement was combined with a grafting procedure and placement of a customized healing screw.

This approach presents the following benefits:

- The duration of treatment can be reduced.
- The alveolar socket is immediately sealed by the customized healing screw that protects the underlying graft and provides immediate support to the surrounding soft tissues.
- The local soft tissue architecture can be maintained, creating the best conditions for a biomimetic integration of the definitive prosthetic reconstruction.

Finally, the combination of soft tissue contour maintenance and prosthetic reproduction of the original volume and occlusal morphology, captured by scanning a preliminary model, should allow the final aspect of the prosthetic reconstruction to be optimized.

Treatment team:
Surgery and prosthetics: Dr. Paolo Casentini
Dental laboratory procedures: Alessandro Giacometti

5.6 Implants for Restoration of Short Edentulous Spaces: Areas of Low Esthetic Risk

5.6.1 Adjacent maxillary premolars

S. CHEN, A. DICKINSON

INTRODUCTION AND PRELIMINARY ASSESSMENT

A 55-year-old woman was referred to the clinic to manage replacement of the maxillary right second premolar with a dental implant. The tooth had been previously endodontically treated and restored with a post-retained PFM crown. The crown and post structure had dislodged, and the residual tooth structure was deemed to be structurally unsound and insufficient for a similar replacement tooth-supported prosthesis. She had mild asthma, which was being managed with preventers, and osteopenia. She was otherwise healthy and well.

On examination, the following clinical features of the teeth in the maxillary right posterior segment were noted (Figure 1):

- The root of the maxillary right second premolar was in situ. Recurrent caries was noted within the remaining root structure, rendering the tooth nonrestorable.
- The adjacent first premolar was endodontically treated and restored with a PFM crown. Marginal defects on the mesial and distal aspects of the crown were noted. A periapical radiolucency was noted.
- The neighboring first molar was restored with a large amalgam restoration with evidence of marginal leakage. Periodontal probing pockets of 5 mm were noted on the distal aspect with early involvement of the distal furcation.
- The maxillary right second molar was endodontically treated and restored with a post-retained PFM crown. Recurrent caries on the mesial aspect was noted. An 8-mm periodontal pocket was noted on the distal aspect.
- The teeth in the maxillary premolar segment were visible when the patient smiled, but not the gingiva.

Following the clinical and radiographic examination, an initial discussion was held with the patient. The poor restorative prognosis of the maxillary right second premolar was confirmed. In addition, the possibility of recurrent caries affecting the first premolar and the defective amalgam restoration on the first molar were outlined. Furthermore, the second molar had an uncertain restorative, endodontic, and periodontal prognosis. On this basis, the recommendation was made for her to undergo a comprehensive restorative and endodontic assessment prior to finalizing a treatment plan. The patient agreed to a referral to a prosthodontist for further evaluation.

PROSTHODONTIC ASSESSMENT AND TREATMENT OPTIONS

The prosthodontist confirmed the poor prognosis of the second premolar. He recommended an exploratory procedure on the first premolar. The crown was sectioned and removed and the available supporting tooth structure evaluated (Figure 2). Following caries removal, minimal healthy coronal tooth structure remained, insufficient to ensure an adequate ferrule to be prepared. While retention of this tooth with endodontic retreatment and the fabrication of a cast post-retained core and new full coverage crown would be technically possible, the prognosis over a 10-year period was considered as guarded.

Following this procedure, the patient subsequently presented having displaced the crown on the second molar. Clinical assessment confirmed extensive caries around the dental amalgam alloy core and little tooth structure apical to the restorative material. As a consequence, the prognosis with conventional retreatment of the second molar was determined to be poor. The first molar was assessed to have a good prognosis.

It was therefore recommended to the patient that maxillary right first and second premolars and the maxillary right second molar be extracted.

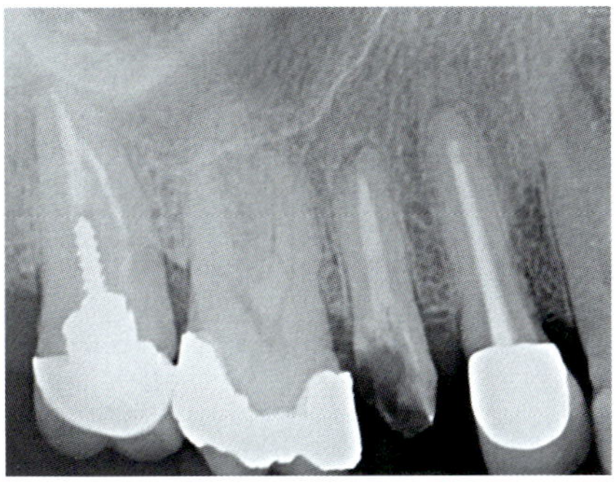

Fig 1. A periapical radiograph of teeth in the maxillary right posterior segment.

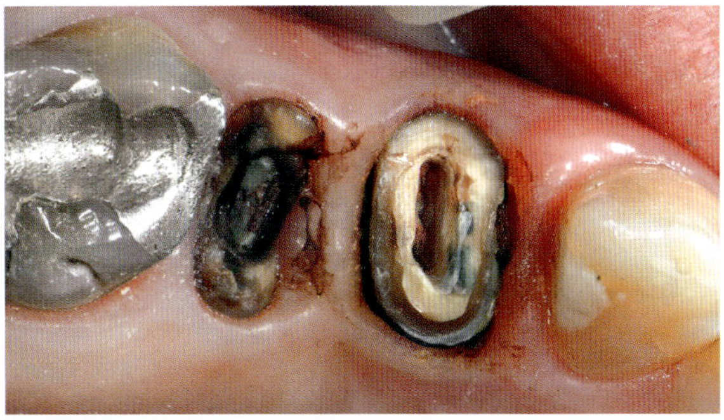

Fig 2. Occlusal view of the roots of the maxillary premolars immediately following the initial explorartory procedure.

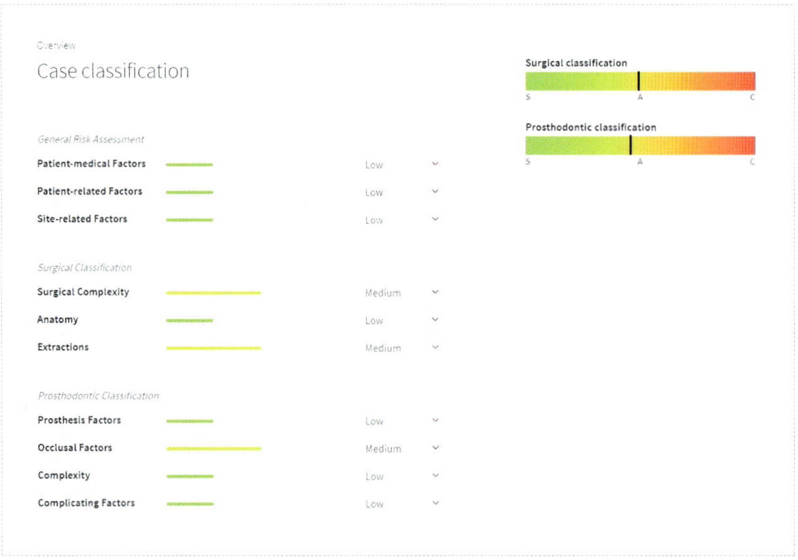

Fig 3. Overall treatment classification: Surgical classification = advanced; Prosthodontic classification = straight-forward to advanced.

Subsequently, the prosthodontics options for replacement of the first and second premolars discussed were:

1. A single implant replacing either the first or second premolar sites for the fabrication of a two-unit cantilevered fixed dental prosthesis (I-cFDP), supported by the single implant
2. Two implants; one placed in each of the first and second premolar sites for two implant retained single crowns (I-SC)

The prosthodontic plan for the first molar was a full-coverage all-ceramic crown.

SURGICAL ASSESSMENT

The patient then returned for a surgical assessment of the site. Clinical and radiographic examination confirmed sufficient bone volume to permit the placement of implants in both premolar sites. The mesiodistal space for both teeth was determined to be 14 mm. This gap would permit the placement of a standard-diameter 4.1-mm implant and a reduced-diameter 3.3-mm implant while maintaining a distance of 3 mm between the shoulders of the implants and at least 1.5 mm between the implants and adjacent teeth. An early implant placement (type 2) was recommended.

Following presentation of the treatment options to the patient, she opted for two implants in the first and second premolar sites so that two individual crowns could be constructed.

SAC ASSESSMENT

The treatment approach recommended to the patient was for an early implant placement protocol following tooth extraction, and conventional loading (type 2C) (Figure 3).

SURGICAL PHASE

Under local anesthesia, the maxillary right first and second premolars and the second molar were extracted (Figure 4). Healing progressed uneventfully. Eight weeks later, full-thickness buccal and palatal flaps were raised in the maxillary right premolar segment, revealing healing extraction sockets with intact residual bone walls. Two implants were placed in the first premolar (Narrow CrossFit [NC] Bone Level SLActive implant, 3.3 × 10 mm, Strauman) and the second premolar (RC Bone Level SLActive implant, 4.1 × 10 mm, Straumann) sites. Residual marginal defects were grafted with locally harvested autogenous bone chips. Healing abutments were attached to the implants and the flaps adapted around the healing abutments for transmucosal healing. Healing progressed uneventfully. Ten weeks after surgical placement, the implants were integrated and the patient returned to the prosthodontist for the next phase of treatment.

PROSTHODONTIC PHASE

Following the initial healing of the surgical site, the maxillary right first molar was prepared and evaluated and a direct provisional crown placed. Subsequently, direct screw-retained implant impression posts were placed and a conventional polyvinyl silicone impression was made of the implant sites and the prepared molar tooth using an open-tray technique.

The resulting casts were digitized using a laboratory scanner and customized all-ceramic zirconia abutments and coronal coping forms for the RC and NC implants designed and sent to Straumann for manufacture.

The implant single crowns had the external contour and color completed using a conventional application of veneering ce-

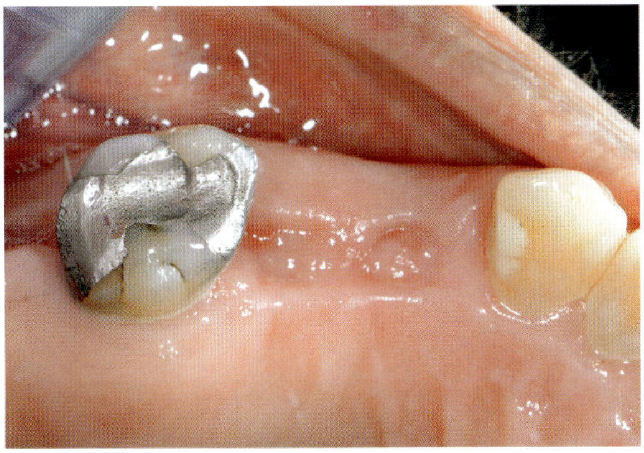

Fig 4a. Occlusal view of the maxillary premolar sites 8 weeks after extraction.

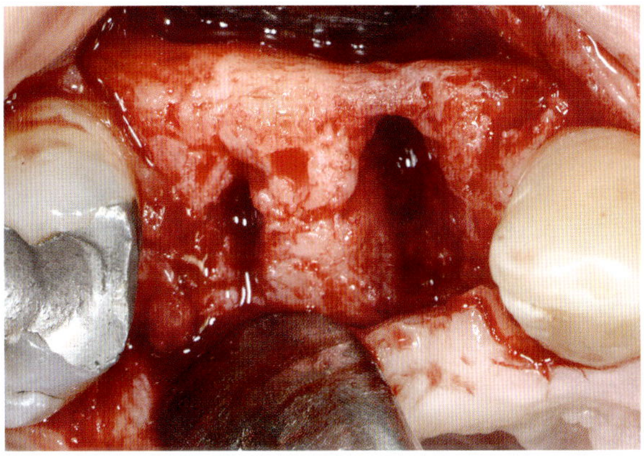

Fig 4b. Following reflection of full-thickness buccal and palatal flaps, the residual socket defects were visualized.

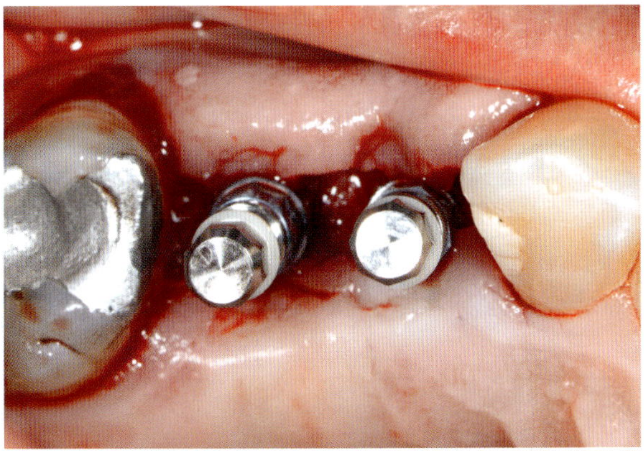

Fig 4c. Two implants were placed in the premolar sites. The occlusal view of the implants with the implant mounts attached shows the axial orientation of the implants.

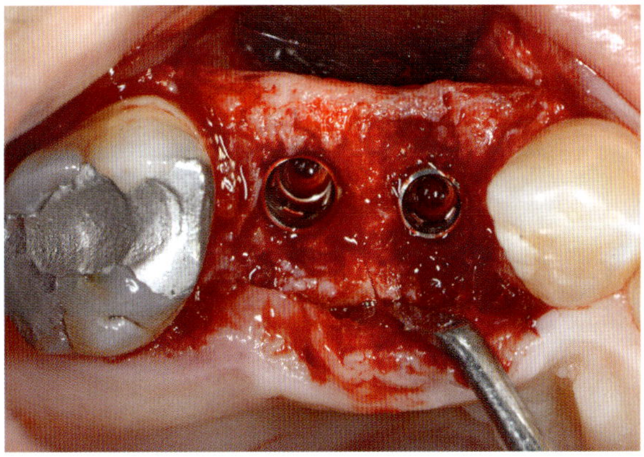

Fig 4d. Locally harvested autogenous bone chips were used to fill the peri-implant defects.

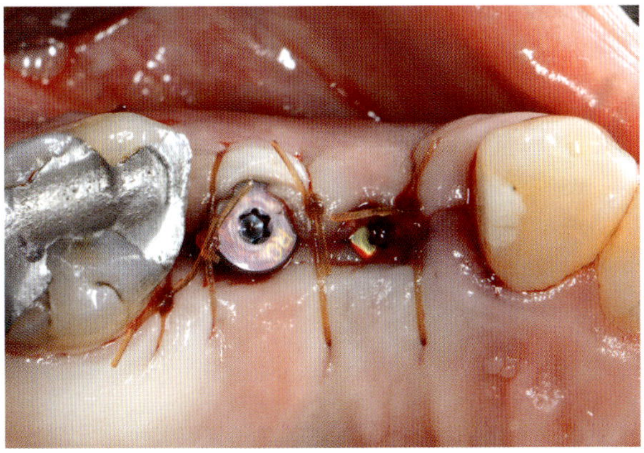

Fig 4e. Healing abutments were connected to the implants and the flaps adapted for transmucosal healing.

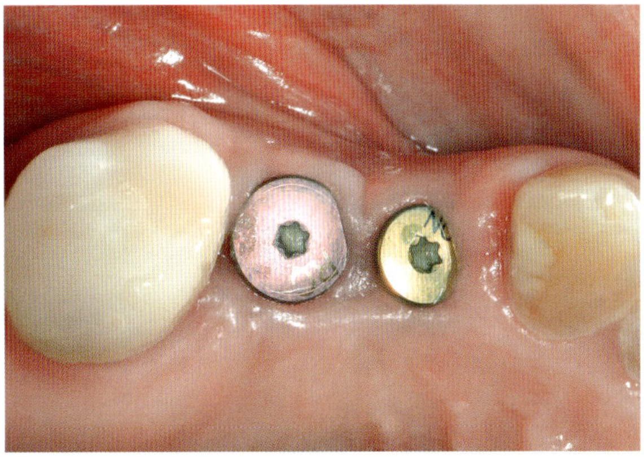

Fig 4f. Eight weeks later, the peri-implant soft tissues were healthy.

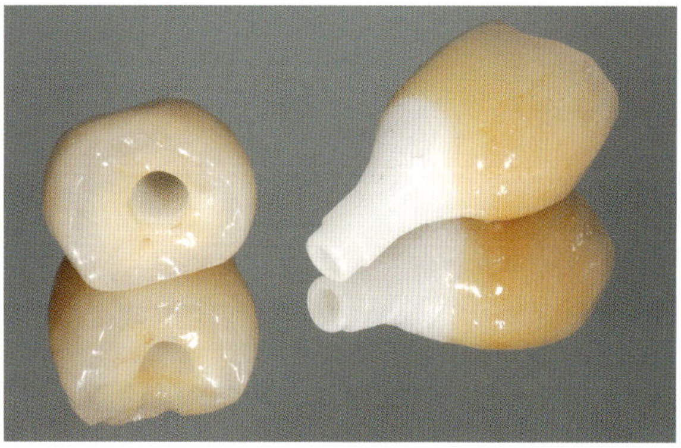

Fig 5a. The implant crowns had the external contour and color completed using a conventional application of veneering ceramic directly to the milled zirconia abutments.

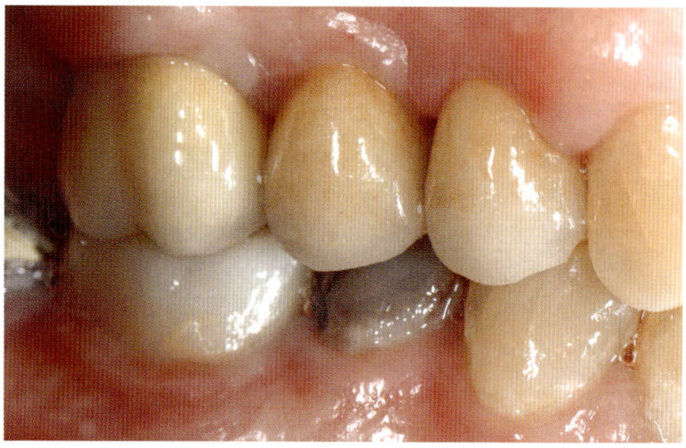

Fig 5b. Buccal view of the completed implant restorations.

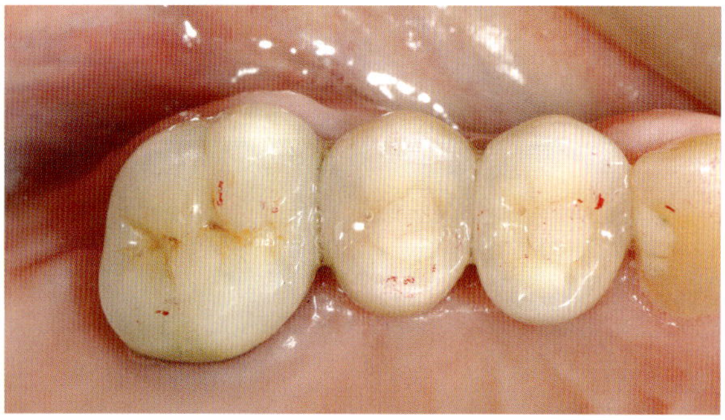

Fig 5c. Occlusal view of the completed implant restorations.

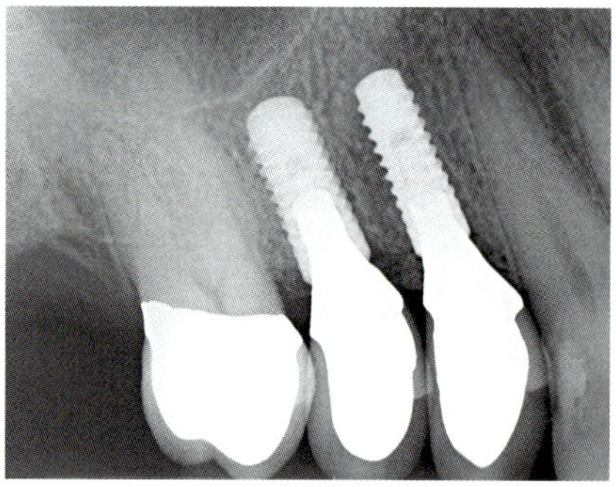

Fig 5d. Radiographic control of the implants following insertion of the definitive implant single crowns.

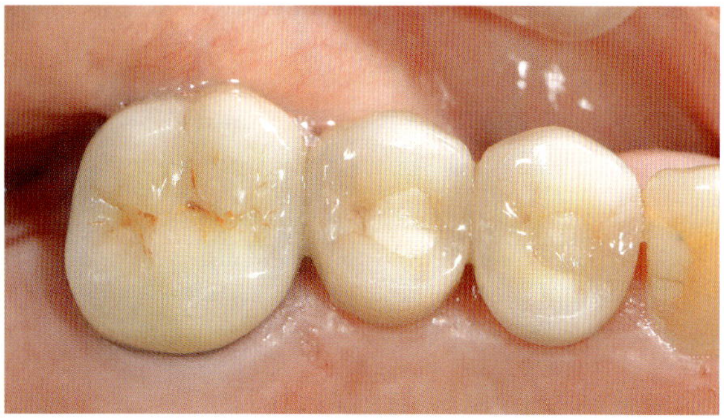

Fig 5e. Occlusal view 3 years after treatment.

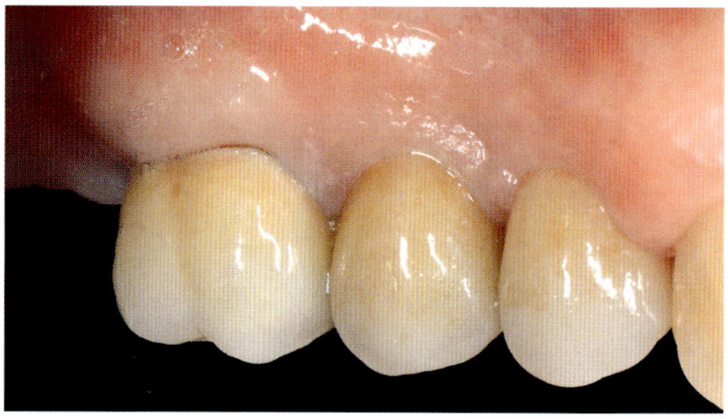

Fig 5f. Buccal view of the implant crowns 3 years after treatment.

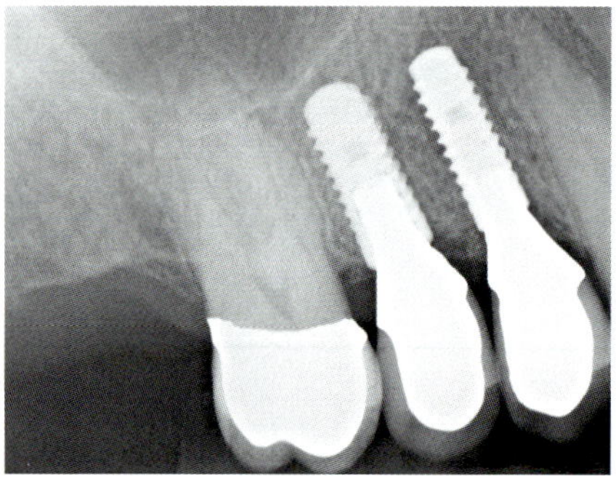

Fig 5g. Radiograph of the implant 3 years after treatment.

ramic directly to the milled zirconia abutments (Figure 5a). The design allowed for direct occlusal access to the basal screw.

The restorations were then fitted intraorally and finally placed with the manufacturer's basal screws on each implant crown torqued to 35 Ncm using the standard Straumann torque wrench (Figure 5b and c). The heads of the screws were covered with a white Teflon tape and the access sealed using a modified glass-ionomer restorative material.

A 2-week postoperative radiograph serves as the baseline record (Figure 5d). Further clinical reviews demonstrated continued good clinical function and soft tissue health at 3 years (Figures 5e and f). A periapical radiograph confirms a stable healthy bone response at the 32-month interval (Figure 5g).

REFLECTION AND DISCUSSION

The principle underpinning the treatment plan was to provide the patient with a long-term predictable outcome with minimal risk. With respect to the timing of implant placement, two options were considered. First, an immediate implant placement (type 1) approach could have been considered given the anatomy of the roots (uniradicular) and sufficient apical bone to achieve primary stability. This approach, however, would have resulted in wide marginal defects both on the buccal and palatal aspects of the implant due to the difference in dimension and geometry of the implants in relation to the root sockets. There would also have been a relative lack of soft tissue for primary closure, requiring adjunct procedures to facilitate soft tissue closure. The second option of early implant placement would ensure healing of any apical pathology present, and would also allow for spontaneous regeneration and increase thickness of the soft tissues over the ridge. Furthermore, after 8 weeks postextraction, a degree of bone regeneration within the sockets could be expected. Thus, an early implant placement approach was selected to simplify the surgical procedure and to minimize the surgical risks. In relation to the loading protocol, the option of immediate implant placement and immediate loading (type IA) was considered. However, the patient's esthetic demands were low, and she was unconcerned about the gap in the premolar region during the healing phase. Therefore, no pressing esthetic concerns were present to warrant adoption of the type IA approach. A conventional loading approach was recommended to the patient, as this is recognized as a low-risk loading protocol.

The treatment progressed uneventfully both surgically and prosthodontically. Both the patient and clinicians involved were satisfied with the outcome.

5.7 Implants for Restoration of Short Edentulous Spaces: Areas of High Esthetic Risk

5.7.1 Adjacent maxillary incisors

P. CASENTINI, M. CHIAPASCO

A 29-year-old woman was referred for a consultation and requested evaluation for a possible implant treatment in the esthetic zone. The dental history included the extraction of the maxillary central incisors and one lateral incisor for endodontic complications after a trauma 3 years before. Meanwhile, the edentulous area had been treated by means of a removable partial denture that did not satisfy the esthetic expectations of the patient. The patient was interested in a fixed prosthesis with better esthetics, but at the same time she was afraid about possible esthetic complications of an implant-supported reconstruction.

The patient was in good general health, she was not taking any medication, and was not a smoker.

CLINICAL EXAMINATION

In an extraoral view, the patient showed a high smile line, with exposure of the transition between the frontal teeth and the soft tissues. Discolored resin retainers of the removable partial denture were clearly identifiable on the adjacent teeth (Figure 1).

The intraoral examination showed a healthy oral cavity, free from caries lesions or periodontal pathologic conditions, with an adequate standard of oral hygiene and normal interarch relationships. The three missing teeth had been replaced by a removable partial denture with a metal palatal extension, metal interdental retainers in the posterior area, and buccal resin retainers on teeth 13 and 22.

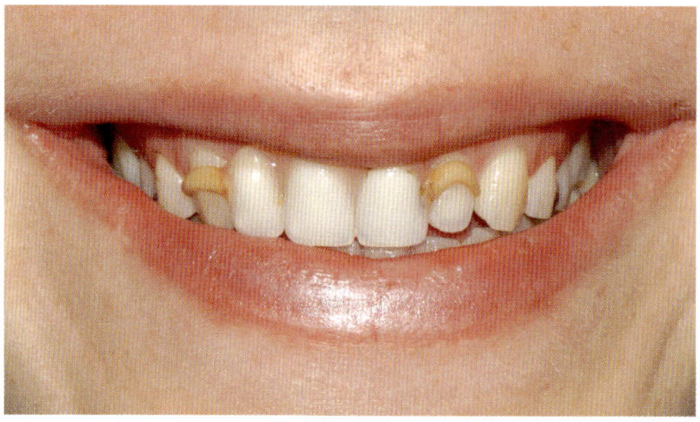

Fig 1. Extraoral view of the patient's smile.

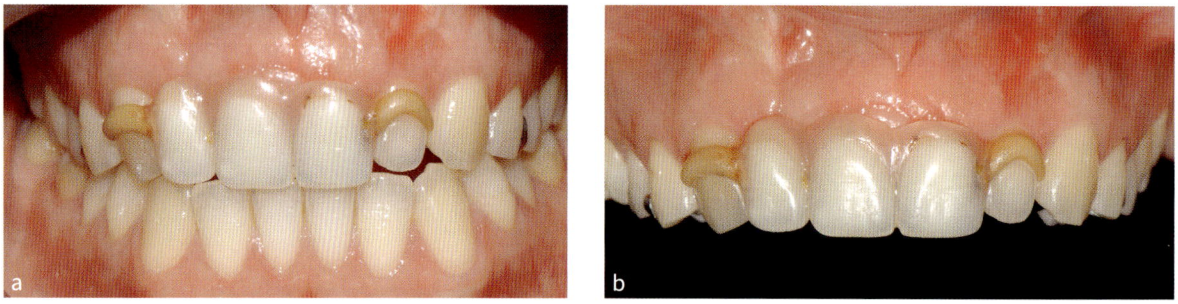

Fig 2 a-b. Intraoral view of the removable partial denture.

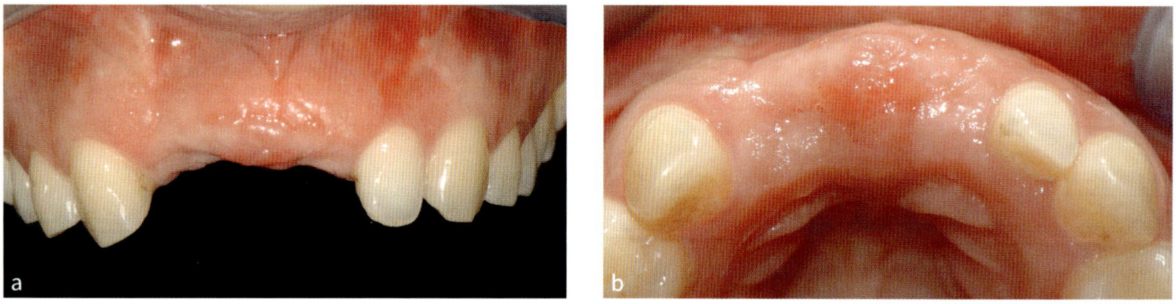

Fig 3 a-b. Frontal and occlusal view of the edentulous ridge.

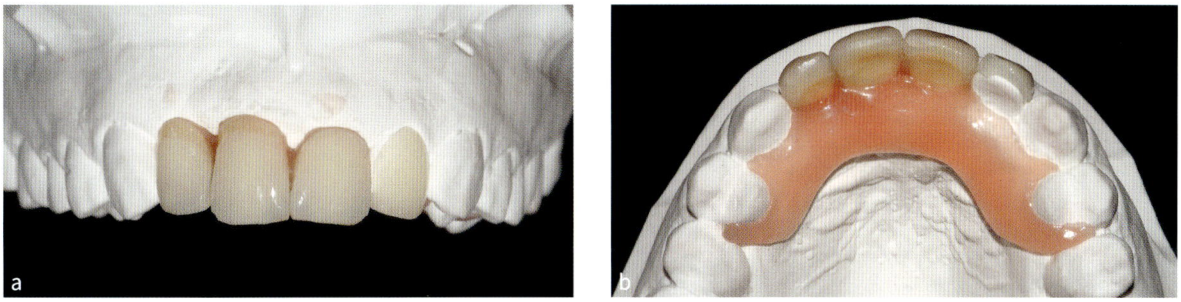

Fig 4 a-b. Frontal and occlusal view of the removable mock-up on the cast.

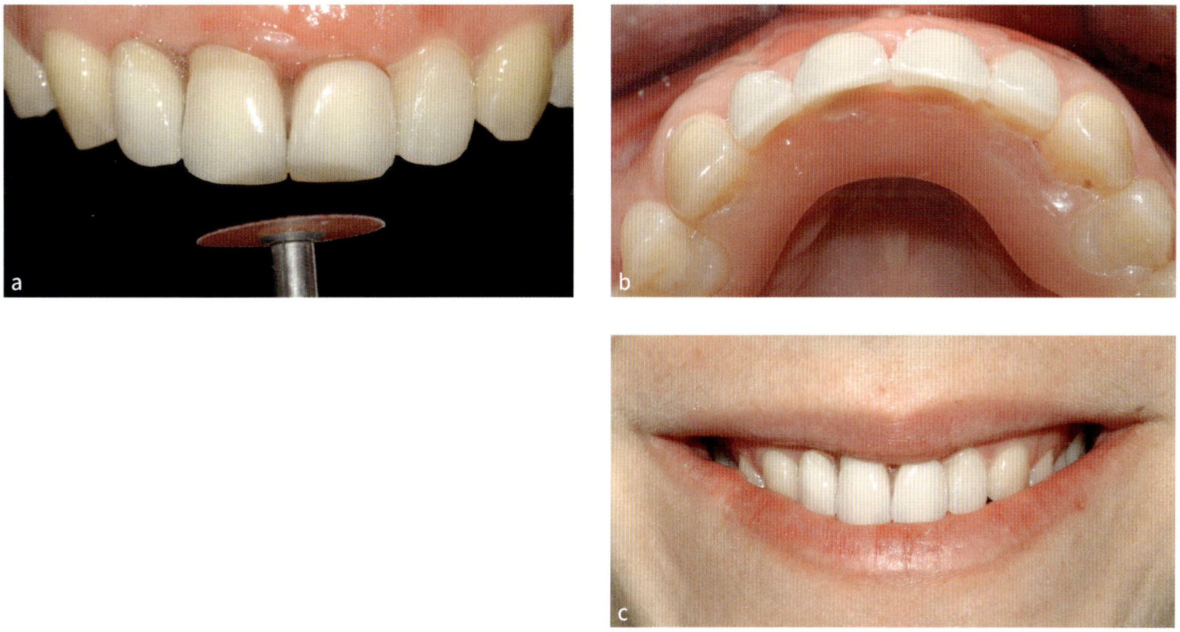

Fig 5 a-c. Intraoral and extraoral view of the diagnostic mock-up.

The resin retainers appeared discolored, with a different chromatic aspect compared to the adjacent teeth. A pink resin flange was replacing the apical and interdental areas of the prosthetic teeth.

The more critical aspects of the front teeth from an esthetic point of view were identifiable in the resin retainers and the asymmetry of the two lateral incisors that presented a different length of the clinical crown (Figure 2).

Once the partial denture was removed, the edentulous ridge presented a moderate atrophy and a visible horizontal defect in site 12 (Figure 3). The quantity of keratinized tissue was adequate, and tooth 22 appeared migrated in a palatal position compared with an ideal line of the incisal edges of the anterior teeth.

DIAGNOSTIC PROTOCOL

In order to define a precise prosthetic project, impressions were made, and the dental laboratory was asked to produce diagnostic casts and a wax-up of the missing teeth. A mock-up was also evaluated as an important step in order to previsualize the treatment outcome and motivate the patient to treatment (Figure 4). Therefore, the dental laboratory produced a removable resin mockup based on the wax-up. A resin veneer on tooth 22 was also included in the project to achieve a better display of the anterior teeth.

During the following visit, the mock-up was applied in the oral cavity and adjusted following the patient's requests in order to achieve the patient's approval of the previsualized treatment outcome (Figure 5).

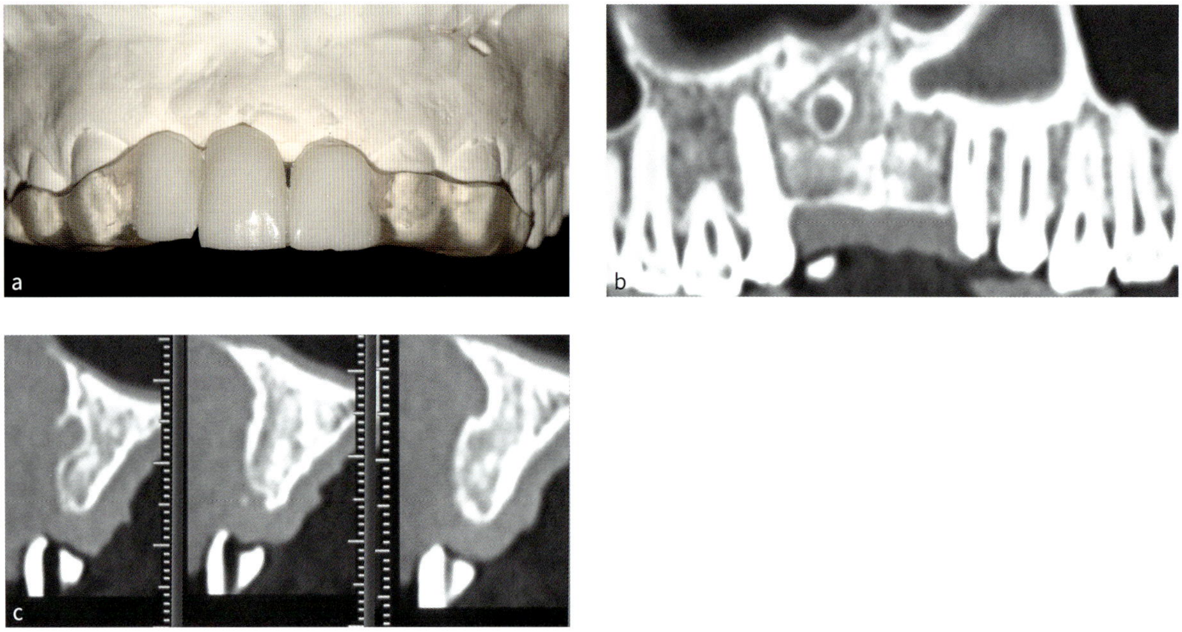

Fig 6 a-c. Diagnostic template with radio-opaque teeth and CBCT of the investigated area.

Once the prosthetic project was approved, the mockup was duplicated with a radiopaque material in order to investigate the bone anatomy and to verify the surgical feasibility of implants. Thereafter, the patient was sent to a radiology center for a CBCT scan. The CBCT scan revealed an adequate height of the bone crest combined with horizontal atrophy and a residual defect in the apical region in position 12 (Figure 6). Implant placement in combination with a simultaneous horizontal bone augmentation was defined possible.

TREATMENT RISK PROFILE

The treatment risk profile was assessed with the SAC Assessment Tool to define specific esthetic, surgical, and prosthetic risk factors (Figure 7).

From the esthetic point of view, the case was evaluated complex, with a high esthetic risk profile. Indeed, the patient has a high smile line and has realistic but high expectations for treatment. Edentulism is involving three adjacent teeth, and the natural teeth facing the edentulous area are surrounded by a thin buccal bone. Moreover, the distance between the flat bone crest and future restorative contact points is probably more than 6 mm. Main favorable factors are represented by the presence of adjacent unrestored teeth, rectangular shape of teeth, and thick and intact soft tissues with an adequate quantity of keratinized tissue.

Main surgical risk factors are represented by the need for horizontal bone augmentation and the need to achieve a perfect prosthetically driven implant position of multiple implants for a future screw-retained reconstruction. Surgical manipulation of delicate soft tissue at adjacent teeth also needs to be considered.

Prosthetic risk factors are related to the need to achieve a soft tissue architecture, including papillae starting from a flat shape of the edentulous ridge, the need for an interim prosthesis that does not interfere with bone augmentation, and the need to satisfy a patient with realistic but high expectations. Finally, an anterior incisal guide should be obtained by the prosthetic reconstruction.

TREATMENT PLANNING

Based on the clinical and radiologic situation, the following treatment plan was proposed:

- Prosthetically driven placement of two implants in positions 12 and 21, and simultaneous bone augmentation by means of GBR performed with autogenous bone combined with a xenograft and a collagen membrane. Submerged healing of implants was planned.
- Temporary, noncompressive removable prosthesis during the osseointegration phase.
- Reopening of implants after 4 months of healing.
- Provisional fixed screw-retained reconstruction to create an adequate soft tissue architecture. A temporary veneer on tooth 22 was also planned in this phase of treatment.
- Definitive screw-retained three-unit fixed reconstruction, realized in zirconia, veneered with porcelain and a feldspathic ceramic veneer on tooth 22.

The patient agreed to the proposed treatment, providing her written informed consent.

Fig 7. Overall treatment classification: Esthetic Risk = high; Surgical classification = advanced to complex; Prosthodontic classification = complex.

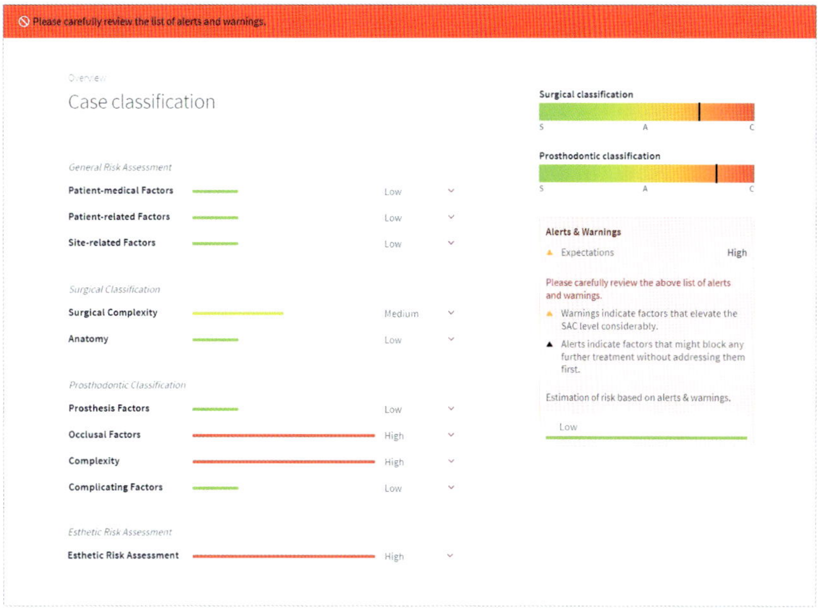

SURGICAL TREATMENT: IMPLANT PLACEMENT AND SIMULTANEOUS GBR

Implant placement in combination with bone augmentation was performed with local anesthesia in combination with intravenous sedation, and with the assistance of an anesthesiologist.

Autogenous bone was preliminarily harvested from the region of the mandibular ramus.

After elevating a full-thickness mucoperiosteal flap, with vertical releasing incisions, implant site preparation was guided by the same diagnostic template utilized for the CBCT and modified to act as a surgical template. An implant axis compatible with a screw-retained reconstruction was achieved.

Two Straumann Bone Level Implants were inserted after implant site preparation in position 12 (3.3 × 12 mm) and in position 21 (4.1 × 12 mm).

An hydrophilic implant surface (SLActive) was preferred in order to optimize osseointegration in a complex anatomical situation. The implant in position 12 presented an apical fenestration, as anticipated from the CBCT (Figure 8).

After implant placement, a first layer of autogenous bone chips was placed to cover the fenestration and to increase the thickness of the buccal bone. The autogenous bone was covered with a xenograft represented by DBBM (Bio-Oss) (Figures 9a and b). Finally, a collagen membrane (Bio-Gide) in a double layer was used to protect and stabilize the graft (Figure 9c).

A tension-free flap adaptation was achieved, sectioning the periosteal internal layer of the flap, and a primary intention closure was obtained with a combination of single and horizontal mattress 5-0 sutures (Figure 9d).

During the surgery, an intravenous steroidal medication was administered to reduce postoperative swelling.

Antibiotics were prescribed to the patient for 6 days (amoxicillin + clavulanic acid 1 g every 12 hours), chlorhexidine 0.2% mouthrinses were prescribed for 2 weeks together with ibuprofen 600 mg for pain relief. The patient was advised to avoid brushing the operation sites for 3 weeks.

After the operation, the patient reported swelling and the presence of a cutaneous hematoma, but pain was almost absent and easy to control with analgesics.

The sutures were removed at 15 days, and no complications were recorded.

PROVISIONAL REMOVABLE PROSTHESIS

One week after surgery, the patient was allowed to use a removable temporary prosthesis based on resin teeth contained in a vacuum-formed retainer (Figure 10). The design of the retainer and the temporary teeth allowed the patient to avoid any pressure over the grafted area.

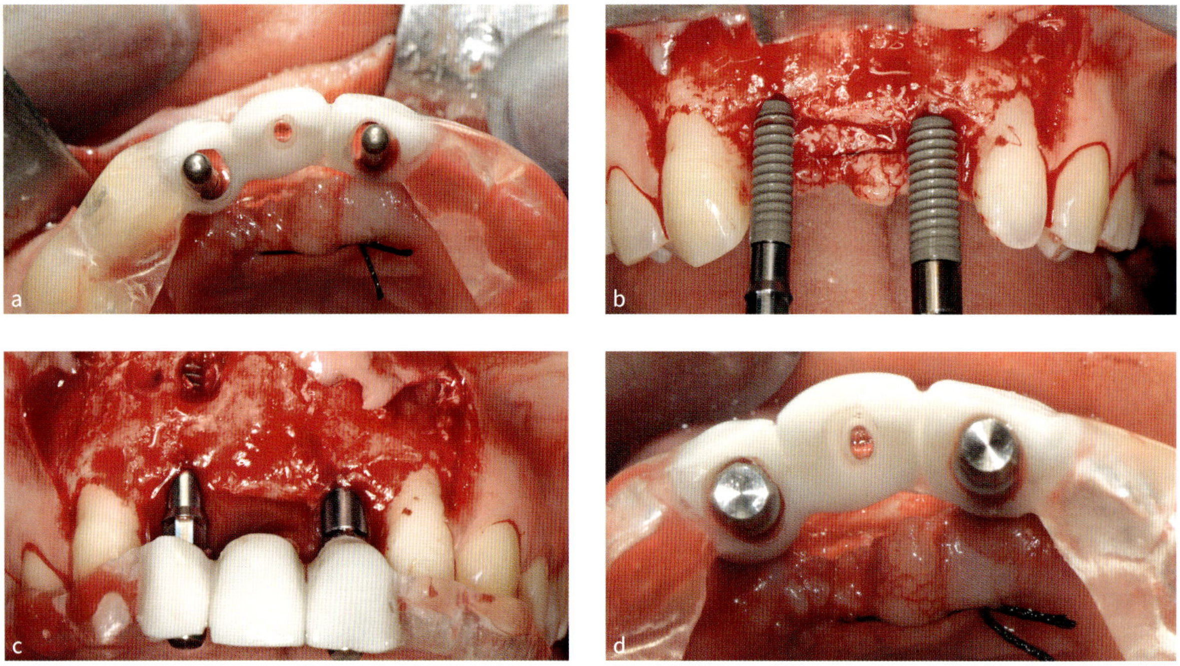

Fig 8 a-d. Prosthetically driven implant placement.

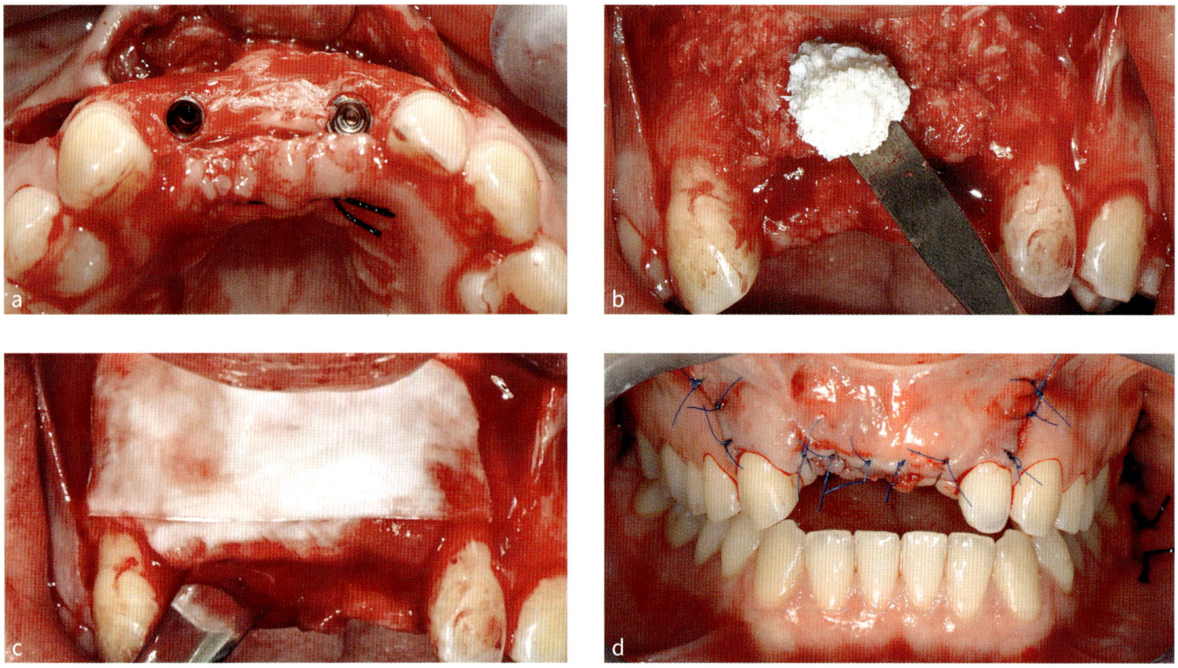

Fig 9 a-d. GBR procedure after implant placement.

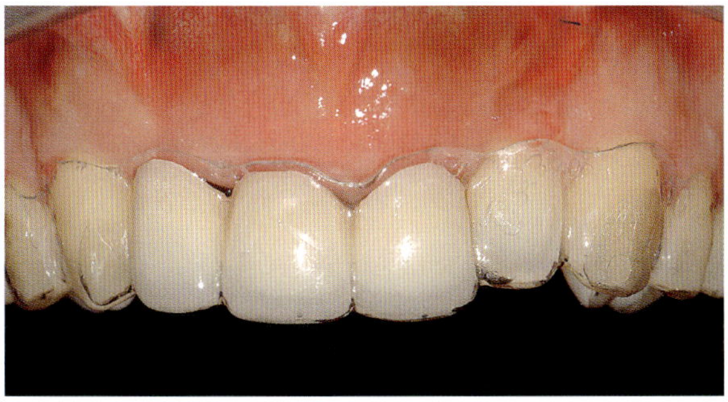

Fig 10. Temporary removable prosthesis.

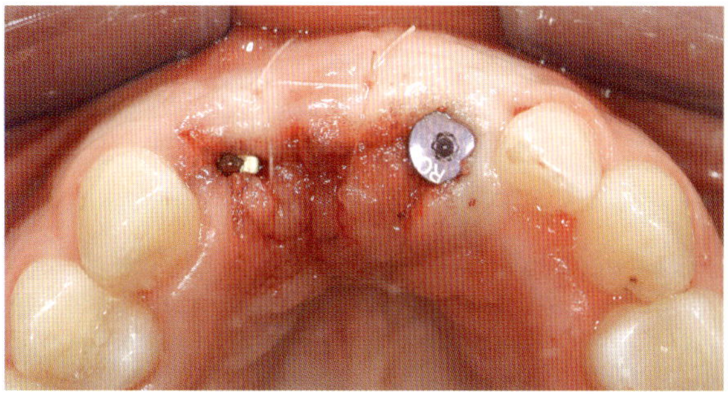

Fig 11. Occlusal view after healing abutment connection.

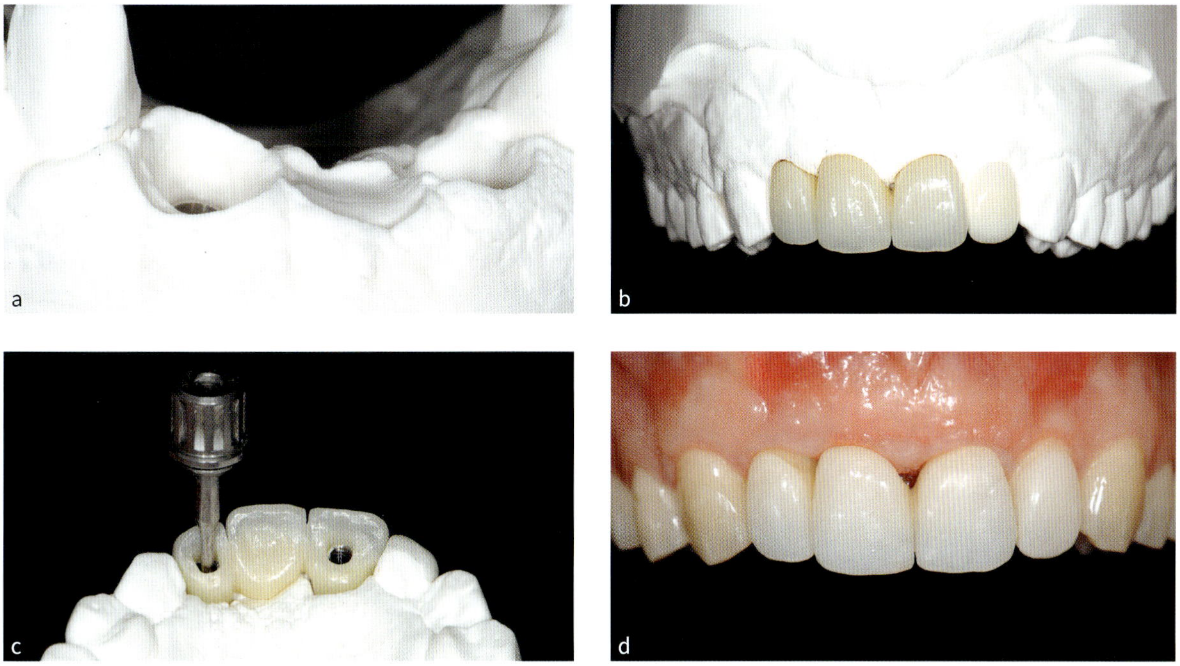

Fig 12 a-d. The provisional fixed reconstruction on the cast and after delivery in the oral cavity.

IMPLANTS UNCOVERING

Reopening of implants was performed after 4 months of healing, with small linear incisions without involving the adjacent papillae. After removal of the closure screws, transmucosal healing screws were connected to the implants (Figure 11).

PROVISIONAL SCREW-RETAINED RECONSTRUCTION

Two weeks after suture removal, the restorative phase was started. A polyether (Impregum) open-tray impression was taken after connecting metal transfer to the implants. Tooth shade information was also transferred to the dental laboratory. A three-unit screw-retained partial denture in resin, based on temporary titanium abutments, and a temporary resin veneer on tooth 22 were produced by the dental laboratory. Light reduction and shaping of the plaster model was completed by the dental technician to provide gentle pressure to the peri-implant soft tissues and start soft tissue conditioning (Figure 12).

In the weeks after the delivery of the provisional partial fixed prostheses and veneer, relining procedures based on the addition of flowable composite resin in the transmucosal and the pontic area allowed the patient to achieve gradual conditioning of the peri-implant soft tissues. During temporization, home-bleaching of the canines was also performed.

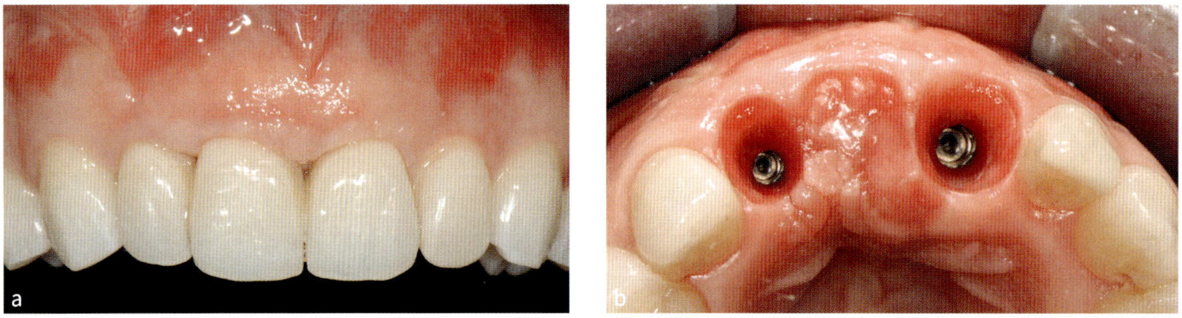

Fig 13 a-b. Frontal view of the provisional reconstruction after 4 months of soft tissue conditioning.

DEFINITIVE PROSTHETIC RECONSTRUCTION

After 4 months of temporization, soft tissue conditioning was evaluated adequate, and impressions for the definitive reconstruction were performed (Figure 13).

Definitive preparation for the veneer of tooth 22 was also done, and subsequently, a polyether (Impregum) open-tray impression was taken after connecting metal transfer to the implants (Figure 14). An extraoral silicon impression of the provisional screw-retained bridge was also taken to capture the exact soft tissue shape after conditioning.

The dental laboratory produced a three-unit hybrid partial denture: A precise connection to the implants was ensured by original titanium abutments, and the selected restorative material for the bridge was zirconia veneered with porcelain. The fixed partial denture and the titanium abutments were bonded extraorally by the dental technician with a dual cement to create a screw-retained reconstruction. A feldspatic ceramic veneer on tooth 22 was also produced (Figure 15).

After the try-in and approval by the patient, the internal cavity of the implants was disinfected with a 1% chlorhexidine gel, and the definitive reconstruction was screwed on the implants with a controlled torque of 35 Ncm. A periapical radiograph confirmed the precise fit of the crown. The access holes to the screws were sealed with Teflon tape and flowable composite.

The veneer was subsequently cemented with heated composite resin after isolation of the field with rubber dam (Figure 16). The view of the restoration after the delivery demonstrates how the implant-supported partial denture and the veneer achieved a positive biomimetic integration in the surrounding tissues and in the smile of the patient.

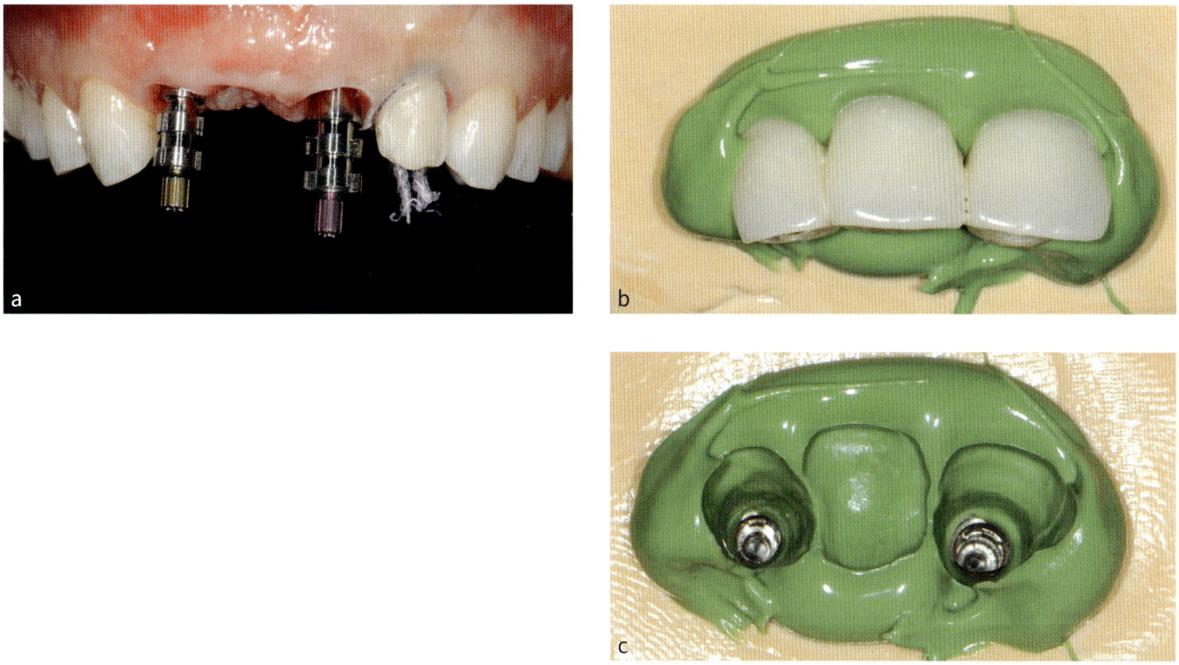

Fig 14 a-c. Precision impressions for the definitive reconstruction.

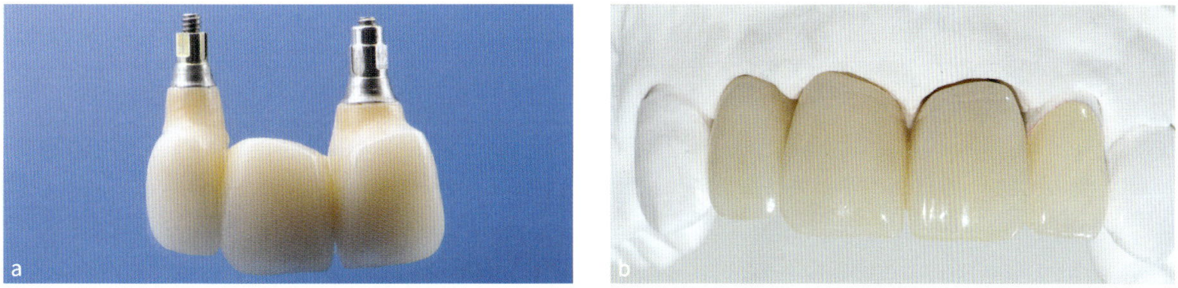

Fig 15 a-b. Definitive prosthetic reconstruction before delivery.

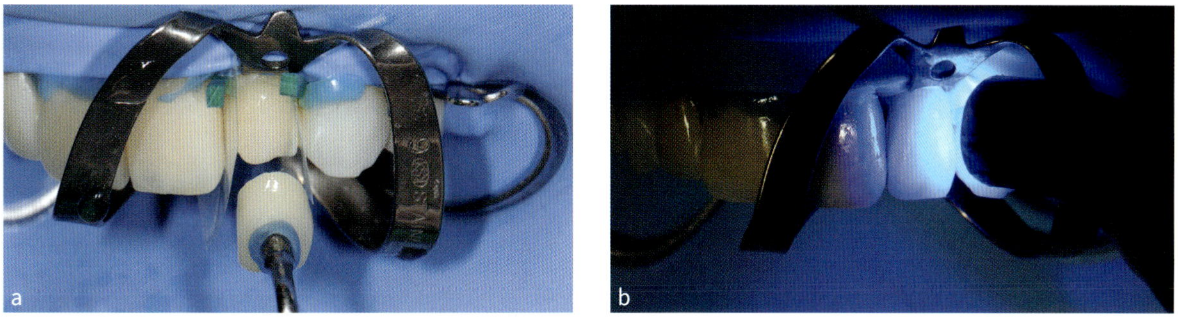

Fig 16 a-b. Adhesive cementation of the veneer on tooth 22.

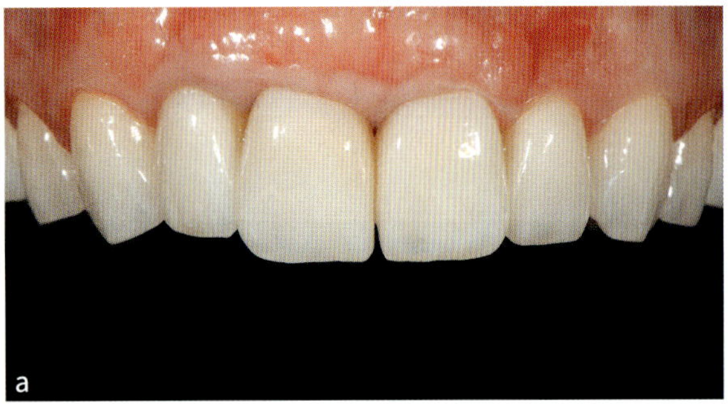

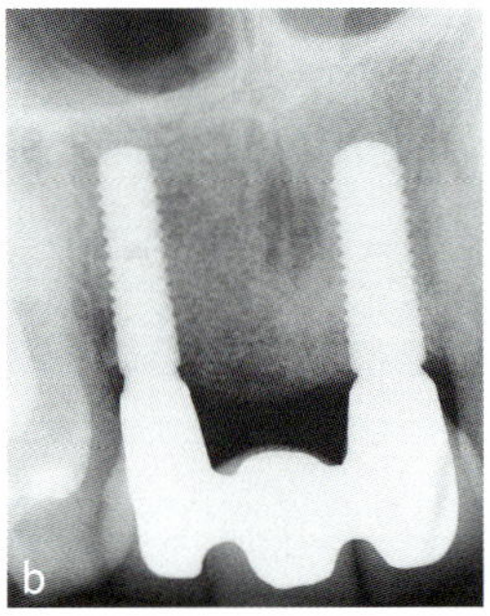

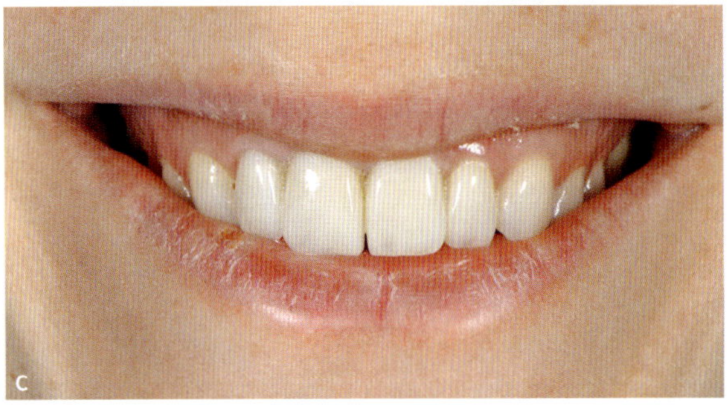

Fig 17 a-c. Intra- and extraoral view of the definitive prosthetic reconstruction and periapical radiograph.

The patient declared her esthetic expectations had been completely satisfied by the treatment outcome (Figure 17).

FOLLOW-UP

The patient was seen approximately once per year for professional oral hygiene and clinical check, and she always demonstrated a high standard of maintenance. After 10 years, the prosthetic reconstruction maintained an optimal integration in the surrounding tissues. The implant partial denture was disconnected in order to document the status of the underlying soft tissues, which demonstrated a total absence of inflammation (Figure 18).

DISCUSSION

When the edentulous ridge includes multiple missing teeth, implant treatment in the esthetic area always represents a challenge for the clinician. In this case, the high smile line and esthetic expectations of the patient and the presence of bone defects represented further complicating factors.

In this clinical scenario, a step-by-step prosthetically driven approach that starts with a precise and approved prosthetic project is mandatory to reduce risks and achieve a positive final result. After previsualization and approval from the patient, the prosthetic project will allow the creation of a diagnostic template that should verify bone volumes and implant feasibility. The same diagnostic template can be later transformed into a surgical guide that will assist precise implant placement. Nowadays, computer-guided surgery and digital impression can help the clinician to standardize a precise implant placement in similar cases, but when this case was treated, 10 years ago, a digital approach was not yet standardized. The case however demonstrates that a traditional nondigital approach is also able to guarantee an optimal result.

Treatment of this esthetic cases requires multiple steps. However, every step requires specific knowledge and skill. In the analyzed case, the prosthetic project included a porcelain bonded restoration in an adjacent tooth, and this represents another complicating factor, since preparation, laboratory procedures, and cementation of this delicate kind of restoration represent critical steps.

The "hybrid" design of the definitive restoration, with a combination of titanium prefabricated abutments bonded extraorally to a zirconia partial denture veneered with porcelain, could be considered experimental 10 years ago. The positive long-term follow-up of this, and many other cases, and recent literature demonstrates the predictability of this kind of prosthetic design.

Finally, the technical knowledge of restorative materials and artistic sense of the dental technician represent fundamental issues in order to achieve a biomimetic restoration.

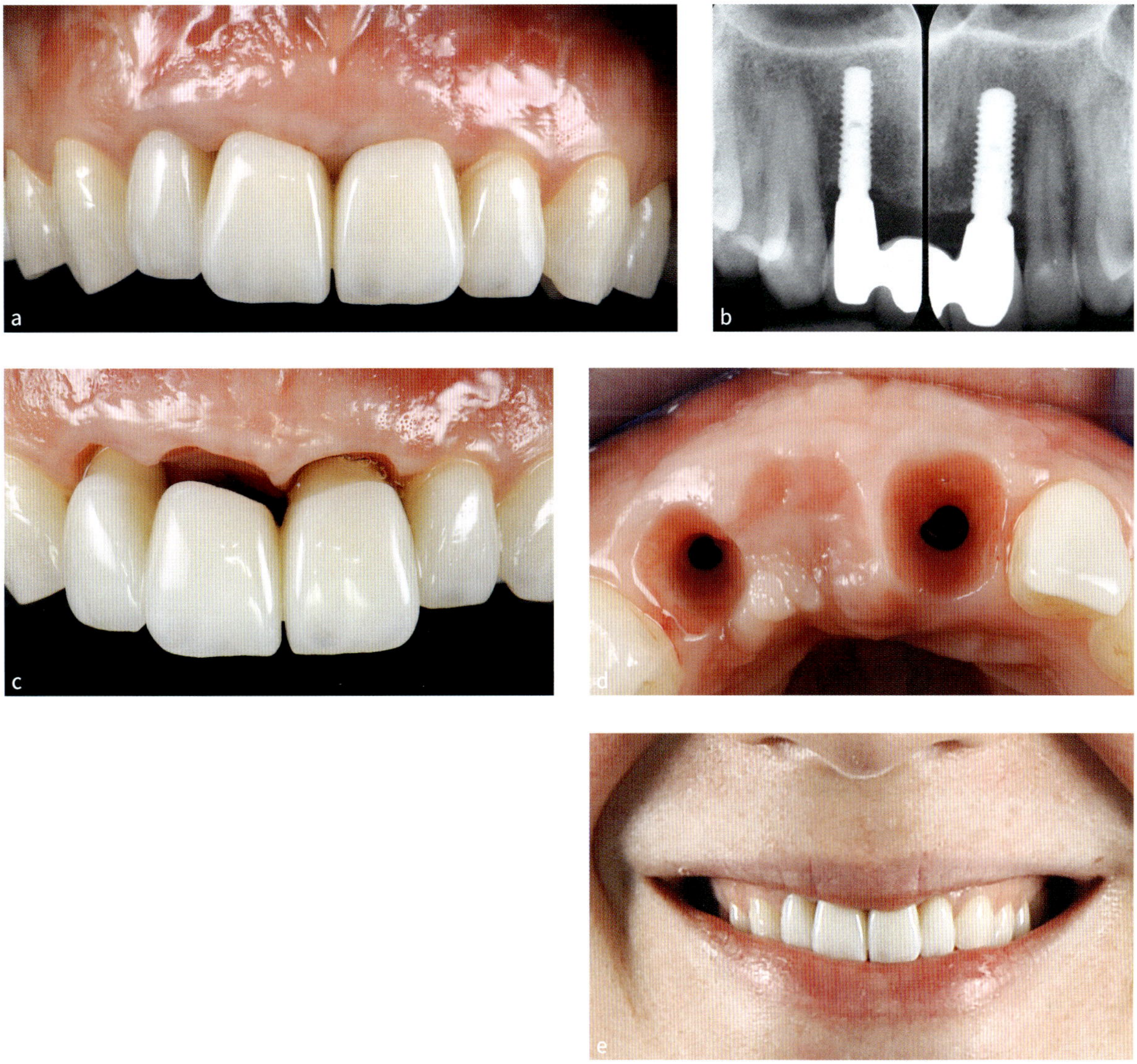

Fig 18 a-e. Clinical and radiographic 10-year follow-up.

The main clinical and technical steps in the workflow were represented by:

- Definition of the prosthetic project by a wax-up
- Mockup and previsualization
- Diagnostic template and CBCT
- Evaluation of surgical feasibility
- Transformation of the diagnostic template into a surgical template
- Prosthetically driven implant placement combined with GBR
- Provisional, noncompressive prosthesis
- Second surgery
- Provisional implant-supported prosthesis
- Soft tissue conditioning
- Impressions for the definitive reconstruction
- Delivery of the definitive reconstruction

Treatment team:
Surgery: Dr. Paolo Casentini and Dr. Matteo Chiapasco
Prosthetics: Dr. Paolo Casentini
Laboratory: Alwin Schoenenberger & Giuseppe Voce

5.8 Implants for Restoration of Long Edentulous Spaces: Areas of High Esthetic Risk

5.8.1 Maxillary lateral and central incisors

A. TREVIÑO SANTOS

A healthy 34-year-old woman had dental mobility caused by small roots in the maxillary central and lateral incisors due to poor orthodontic treatment. The patient wished to replace the teeth with implants, improving the esthetics and comfort. It is important to take into consideration that the patient has gingival display at full smile (Figure 1), all involved four teeth have a triangular shape (Figure 2). All these factors classify this clinical case as high level of risk.

A review of her past medical history showed no contributing factors that would prevent routine surgical and restorative treatment. Clinical and radiographic examination (Figures 3 and 4) of the region presents soft tissue anatomy intact with medium-scalloped gingival phenotype, but the characteristics of the bone present a vertical bone deficiency with 5.5 to 6.5 mm contact points at adjacent teeth.

TREATMENT PLANNING

Utilizing the information from the clinical and radiographic examination aligned with the evidence in the literature, an immediate implant placement approach was selected with the delivery of an interim restoration at the time of surgery (type 1A) (Figure 5).

SURGICAL PROCEDURE

A flapless surgery with minimal trauma extractions was performed to keep the facial bone intact and to be able to place the implants with the least tissue inflammation (Figure 6). The osteotomy for the implant bed preparation was made slightly palatal following the workflow for immediate implant placement (Figure 7), allowing for placement of a slow resorption xenograft in the gap between the implant and the facial bone. Meanwhile, in the fresh extraction sockets of teeth 11 and 21, a nonresorbable hydroxyapatite graft (Tissum, BOS-HA, Argentina) was placed to maintain bone volume (Figure 8).

Whenever possible to facilitate the prosthodontic work, it is important that the implants are as parallel as possible and leveled (Figure 9). The implants were left to heal for 3.5 months, not just for osseointegration but rather to allow the maturation of the soft tissue.

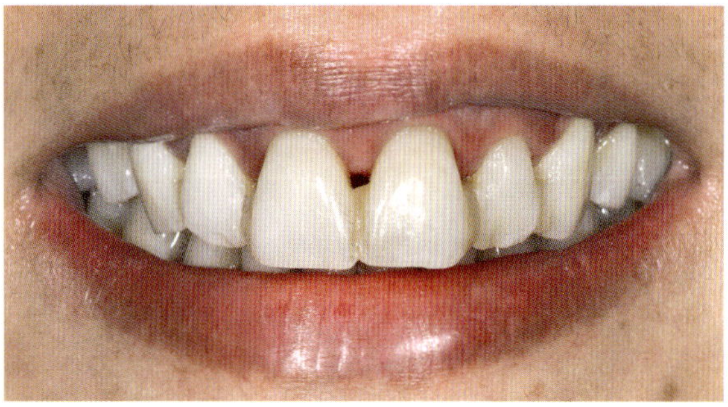

Fig 1. Gingival display at full high smile.

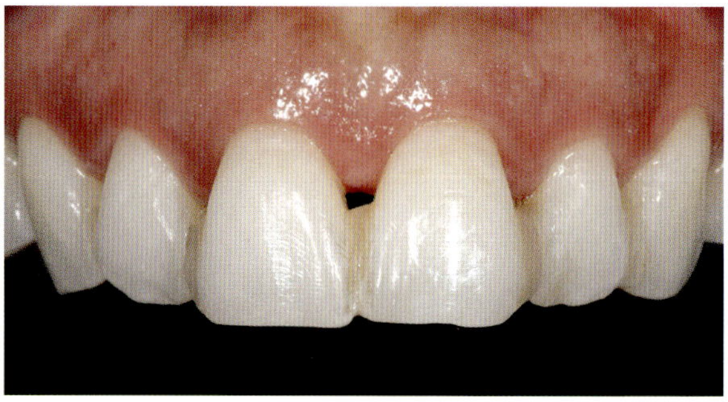

Fig 2. Frontal view, maxillary central and lateral incisors with triangular-shaped teeth.

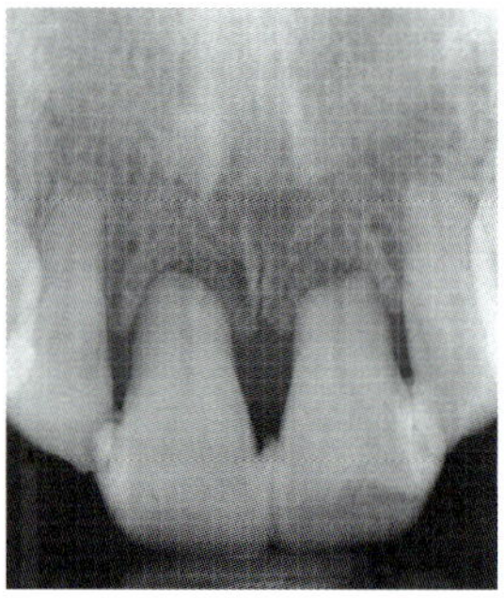

Fig 3. Initial radiograph.

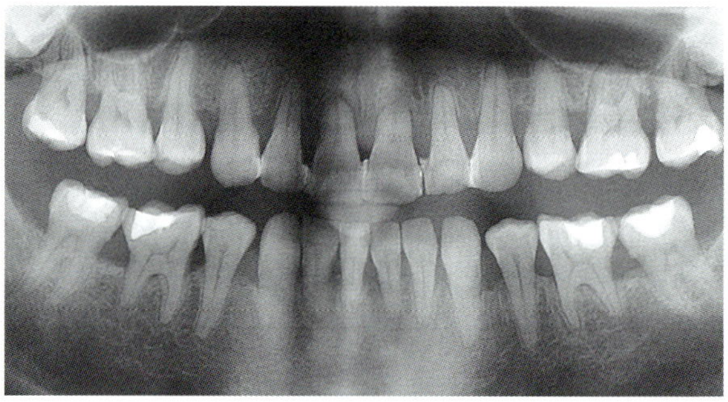

Fig 4. Panoramic radiograph.

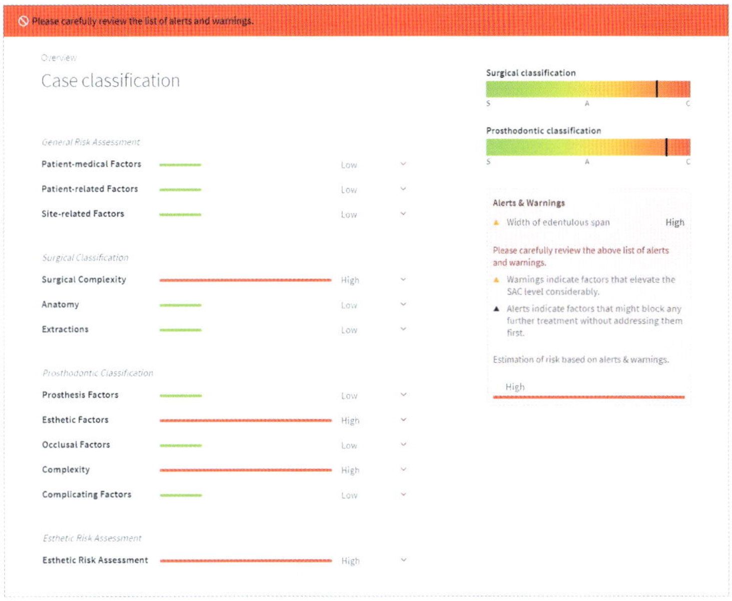

Fig 5. Overall treatment classification: Esthetic risk = High; Surgical classification = complex; Prosthodontic classification = complex.

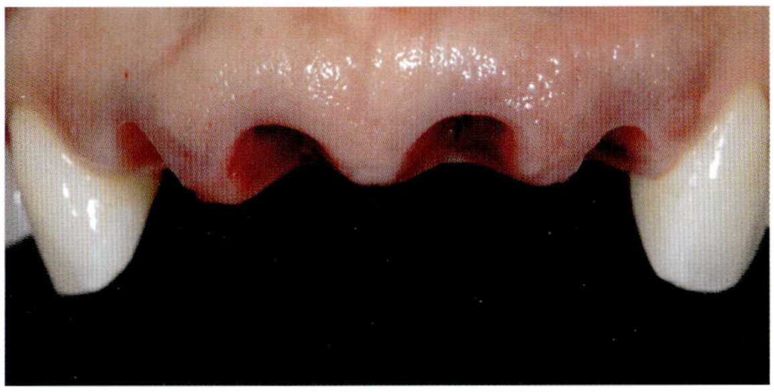

Fig 6. Post-extraction frontal view.

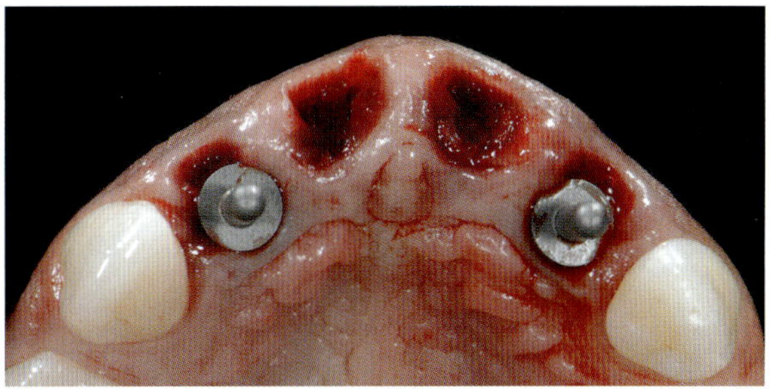

Fig 7. Osteotomy slightly palatal.

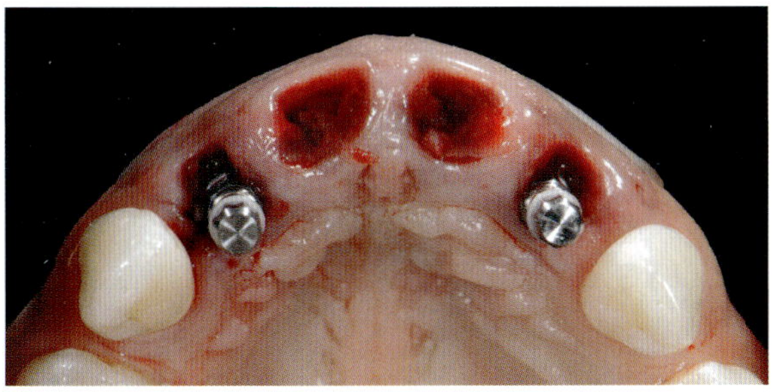

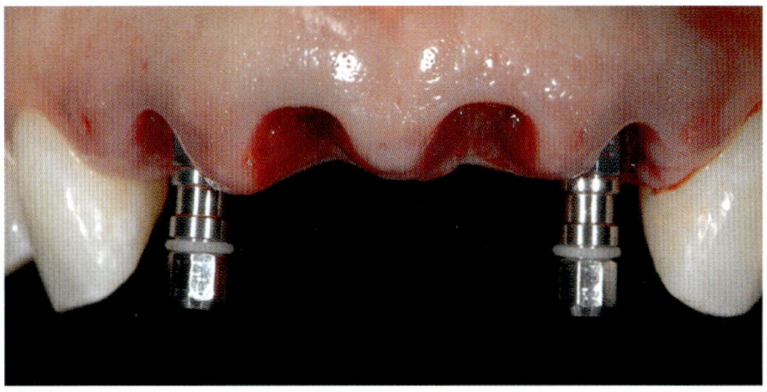

Figs 8 and 9. Occlusal and frontal view of immediate implant placement.

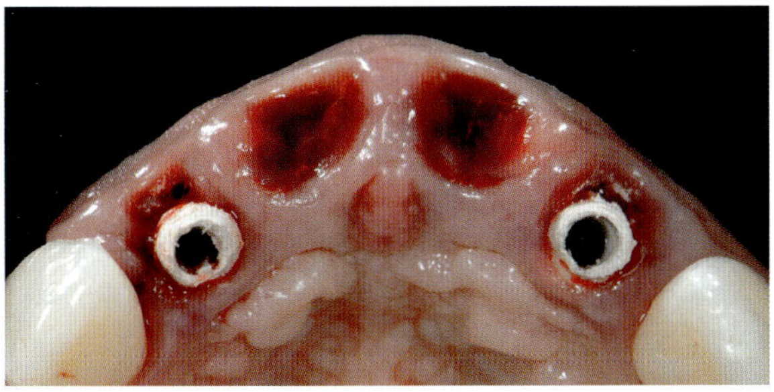

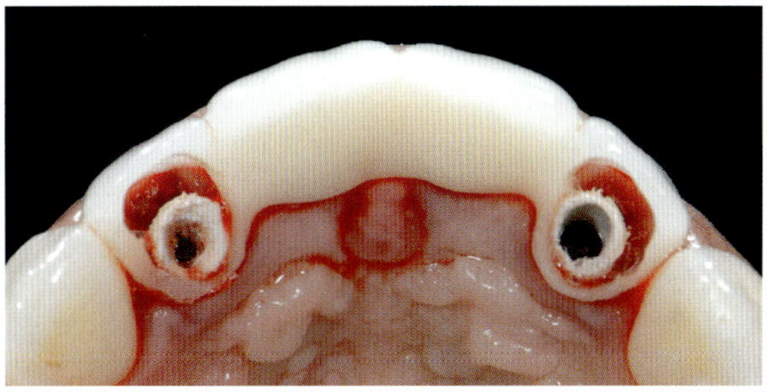

Figs 10 and 11. Provisional abutments and provisional restoration.

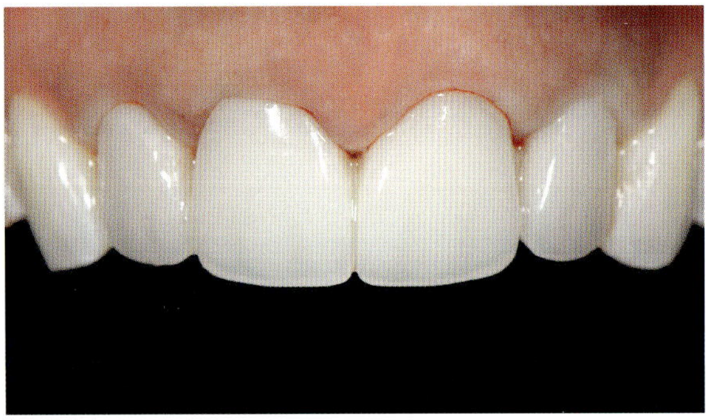

Fig 12. Frontal view of immediate provisional restoration.

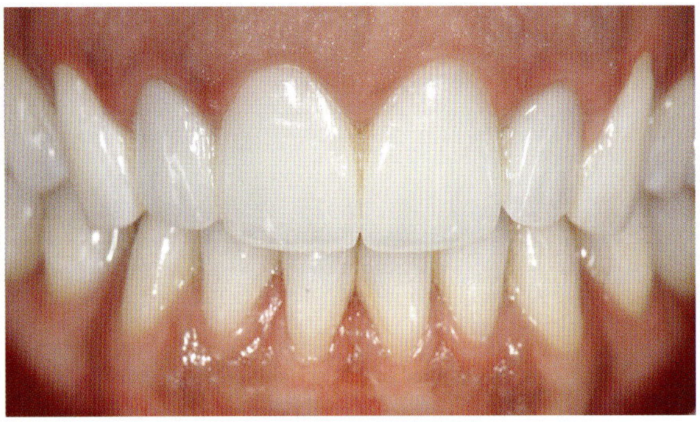

Fig 13. Frontal view 3.5 months postoperative.

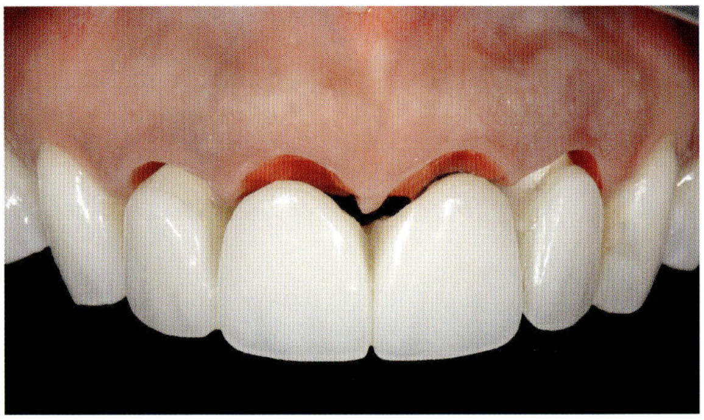

Fig 14. Provisional restoration removed.

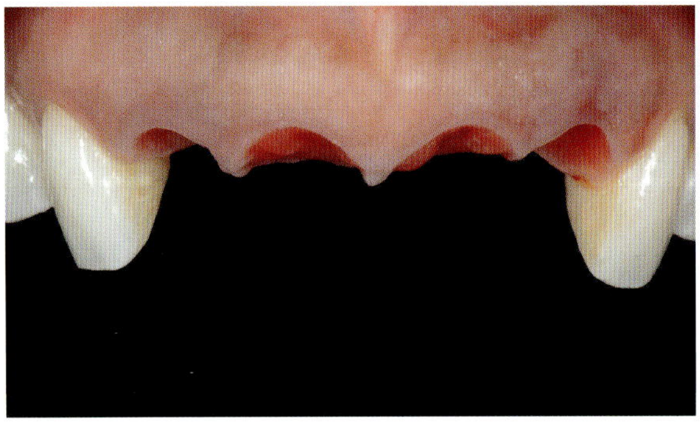

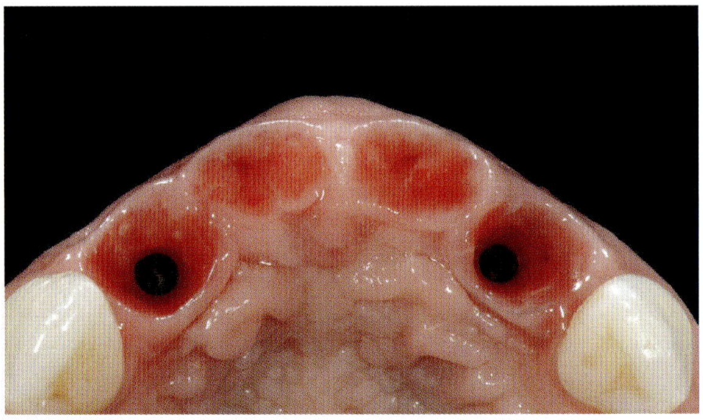

Figs 15 and 16. Conformation of the transition zone and emergence profile.

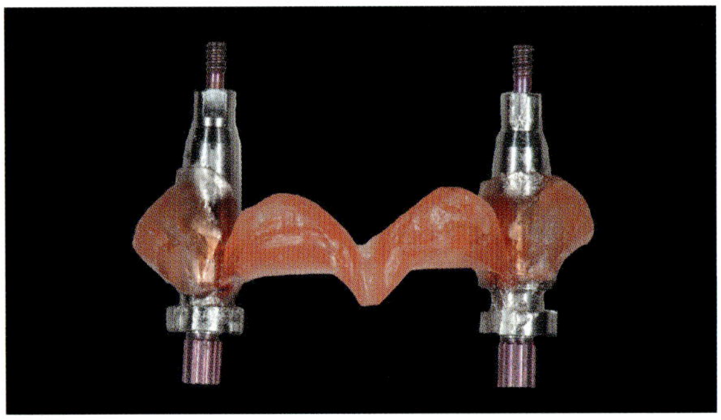

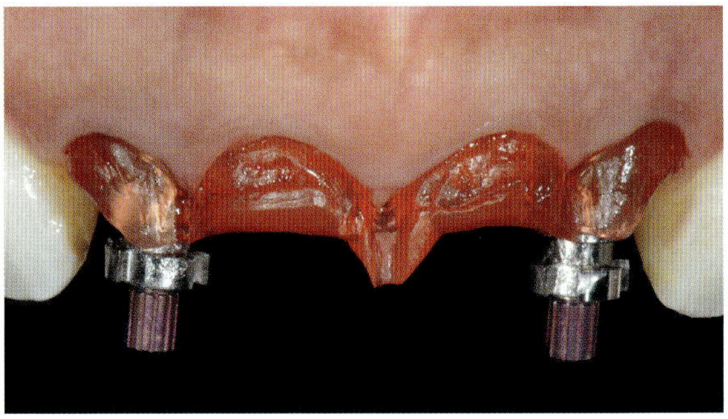

Figs 17 and 18. Customized impression posts: splinted technique.

SURGERY AND PROSTHETIC PROCEDURE

After confirmation of implant stability, the prefabricated provisional abutments were placed (Figure 10). It is important to already have the provisional prosthesis to be easily attached to the abutments (Figure 11) in order to focus on the conformation of the ovoid pontics in sites 11 and 21 as well as the emergence profile of the implants placed in sites 12 and 22 (Figure 12), avoiding contacts in all excursive movements.

PROSTHETIC PROCEDURE

Three and a half months after implant placement, the soft tissue healed perfectly with keratinized gingiva (Figure 13). The provisional restoration was removed (Figure 14), and 1 month later there were optimal conditions regarding the transition zone and emergence profile (Figures 15 and 16).

A customized impression technique was utilized (Figures 17 and 18) with polyvinyl siloxane to copy the emergence profile of the provisional restoration.

In the process of fabricating the definitive restoration, we try to find an implant-supported fixed prosthesis design with a passive fit and that is stress free (Figures 19, 20, and 21) to avoid the induction of unfavorable stress to the implant-prosthesis connection that may lead to loss of osseointegration and failure of prosthetic components. A passive fit is essential to maintain mechanical and biologic equilibrium and decrease loading on the abutment screws and supporting bone.

A screw-cemented implant-supported fixed prosthesis restoration was placed (Figures 22 and 23). It is important to verify that there is no cement residue (Figure 24).

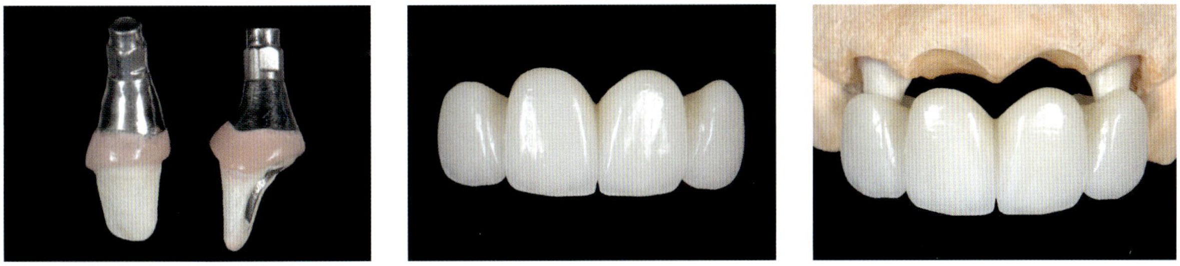

Figs 19, 20, and 21. Titanium abutments customized and ceramized to support a screw-cemented zirconia restoration.

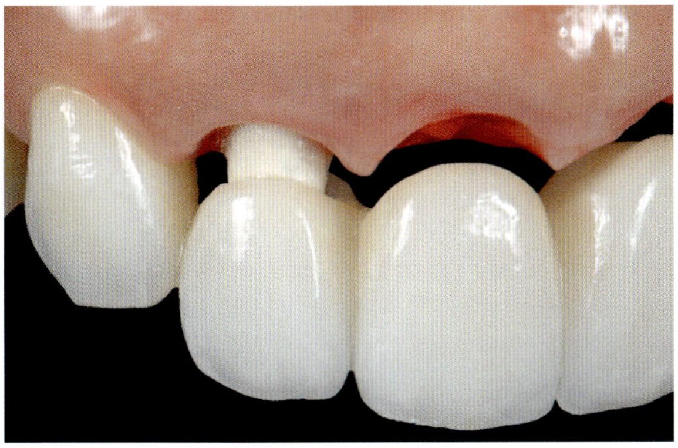

Fig 22. Frontal view before cementation.

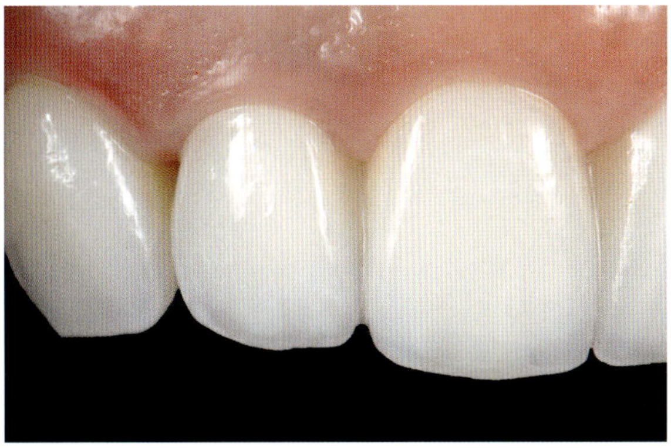

Fig 23. Frontal view with cemented definitive restoration.

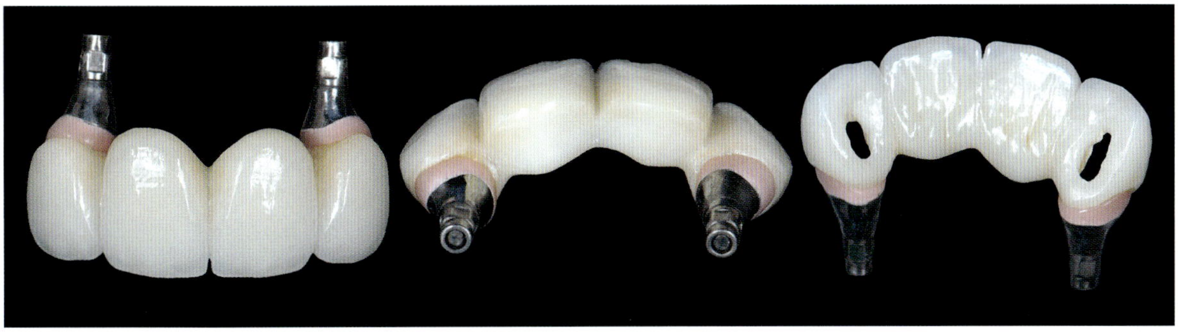

Fig 24. Multiple views of the definitive restoration.

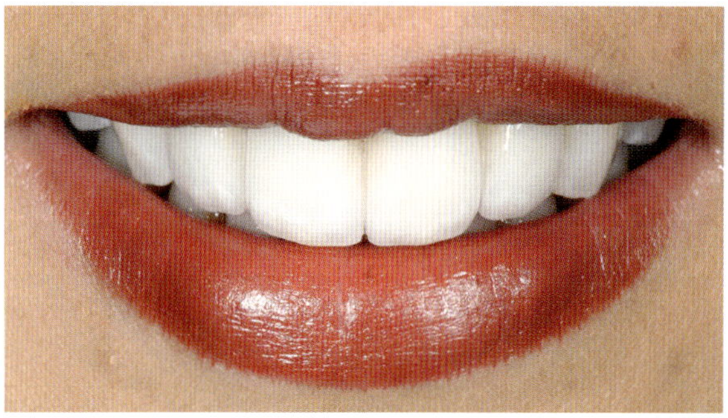

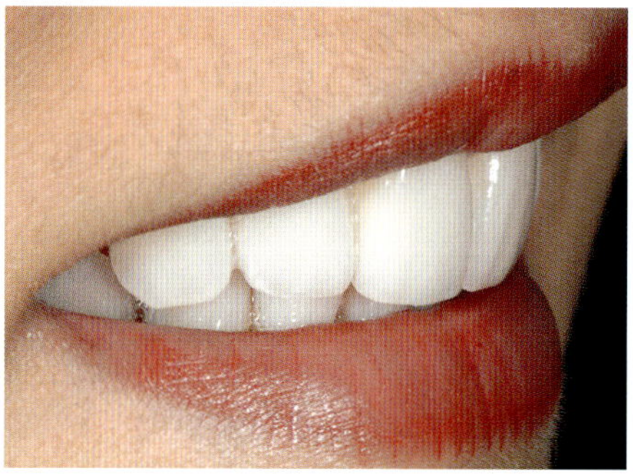

Figs 25 and 26. Final frontal and lateral view of the smile.

Esthetics and comfort were achieved (Figures 25 and 26), with pink esthetic score and white esthetic score values of 10.

CONCLUSIONS

Based upon the clinical evaluation, this patient was a good candidate for type 1A implants, recognizing that implants should be connected in a passive manner to avoid technical complications. Nonpassive interfaces between implants and restorations are considered as a possible cause of complications, ranging from porcelain and abutment fracture and connecting screw breakage to bone loss.

Treatment team:
Surgery and prosthetics: Alejandro Treviño
Laboratory: Thomas Graber, Estudio de Porcelana Suizo

5.9 Implants for Restoration of Long Edentulous Spaces: Removable Prostheses

5.9.1 Maxilla

C. STILWELL

A 63-year-old woman was seen in private practice with an interest in replacing her maxillary partial denture. The existing partial denture was 20 years old, and it was replacing a premolar on each side as well as the four incisors and the right canine. In the mandible, she had a shortened dental arch with five teeth either side of the midline (Figure 1).

The patient had been very happy with the partial denture from both an esthetic and functional perspective. She did, however, recognize that it was getting older and looking worn, and that she was gradually showing less of the front denture teeth in her smile. The denture had also developed an increasing tendency to move anteriorly, and this could lead to moments of loss of denture privacy and embarrassment.

The patient had a history of successfully treated breast cancer, and after 15 years of no recurrence, she was no longer on any medication. She described herself as fit, able, and active and enjoying a happy family life with three generations as well as helping out in her local community.

The missing teeth had been lost many years before, and she had not lost any during the life of the maxillary partial denture. It was also many years since she last had a new filling. She had, however, had the maxillary right first premolar root treated and fitted with a crown. She occasionally experienced discomfort from the gingiva between her maxillary molars on both sides, which would be a prompt to see the dental hygienist.

The clinical examination demonstrated good oral hygiene and gingival health except for some minor inflammation in the interproximal spaces between the maxillary molars. The latter was likely related to the open contact points seen on the panoramic radiograph and occasional trauma from food impaction. The radiographic examination confirmed the clinical findings of good, stable marginal bone levels for the patient's age as well as absence of dental caries and periapical pathology (Figure 2). The panoramic radiograph also showed bilateral pneumatization of the maxillary sinuses in the edentate second premolar sites.

The vertical dimension of static occlusion was determined by the opposing natural first premolar teeth, and the only natural tooth anterior guidance was between the opposing

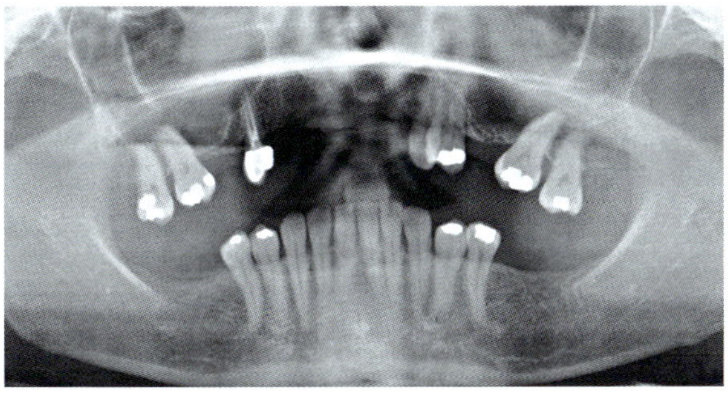

Fig 1. Baseline panoramic radiograph.

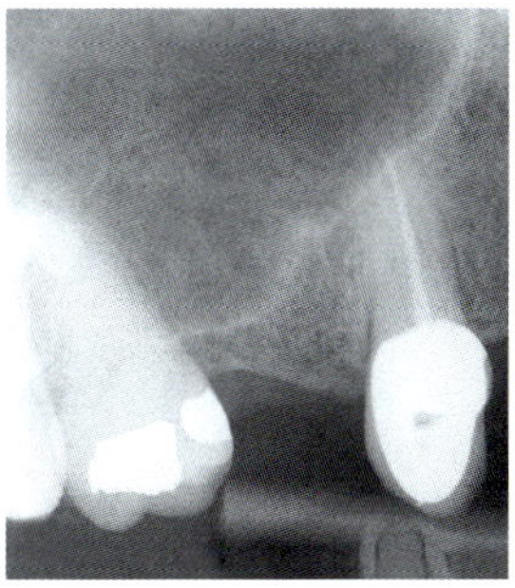

Fig 2. Periapical radiograph of the root-filled maxillary right first premolar showing satisfactory obturation and absence of periapical pathology.

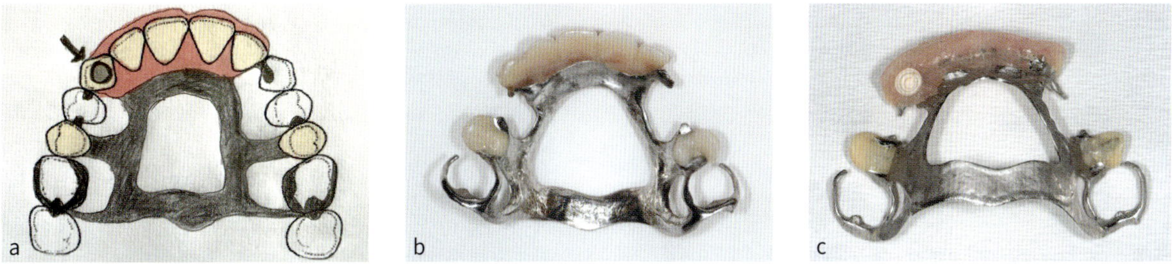

Fig 3 a-c. Schematic drawing of the proposed partial denture design and the actual prosthesis, improved by addition of rests for tooth support as well as planned use of single implant as an overdenture abutment with a stud attachment in the maxillary right canine site.

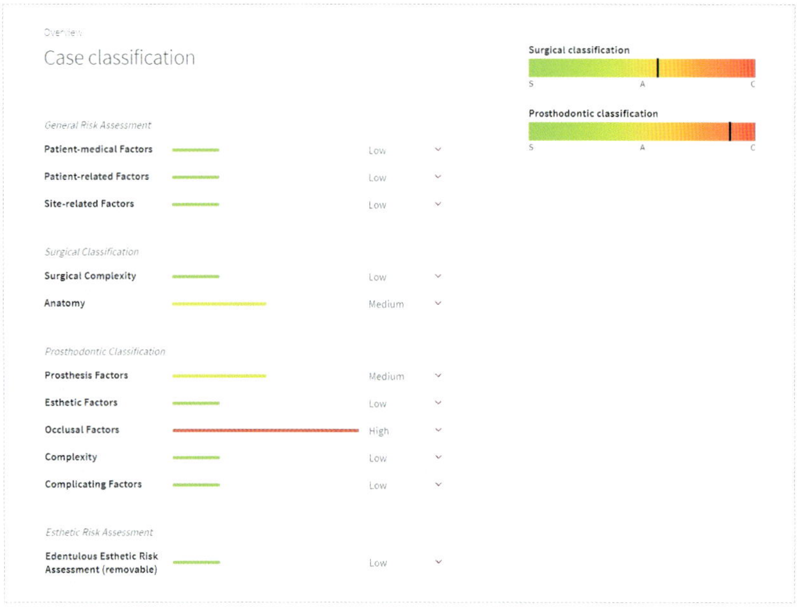

Fig 4. Overall treatment classification: Edentulous esthetic risk = low; Surgical classification = advanced; Prosthodontic classification = complex.

left canines. The partial denture had a cast metal framework with limited support from a few remaining occlusal rests on the posterior teeth but no support anteriorly to provide effective anterior guidance (Figure 3).

The other restorative options of fixed dental prostheses supported by teeth and/or implants were discussed, but the patient was very firm that she wanted a partial denture again and preferably with a very similar design to her old denture. It would be a bonus if the new denture was more retentive and thereby less likely to dislodge at the front. The patient would also like to achieve a definite if discreet show of front teeth.

Replacement of the missing mandibular molars via implant-supported crowns was discussed, but the patient felt she had managed well without. She did, however, express immediate interest at the suggestion of a strategically placed single implant in the maxillary right canine site. The implant would serve as an overdenture abutment for the long anterior denture saddle. Fitted with a stud attachment, this implant would provide both valuable support and retention and address the patient's wish to avoid movement and dislodging of the front denture teeth. A schematic drawing of the proposed new design can be seen in Figure 3. Note the addition of support for the anterior saddle from the proposed overdenture implant as well as the adjacent maxillary right first premolar and the left canine.

SAC RISK ASSESSMENT

General risk assessment

Under the general risk assessment, all patient- and site-related factors were low risk. It is important to note that, in spite of the significant tooth loss at a relative early age, the periodontal status of the remaining teeth as well as the patient's oral hygiene and compliance were very good. The patient was a nonsmoker, and the proposed maxillary right canine site had no preexisting concerns as a result of pathology or previous surgery. Importantly, the patient also had realistic expectations to the extent of benefit for the maxillary partial denture that could be derived from a single implant.

Surgical classification

From the risk factors considered in arriving at the surgical classification, only one was identified as a medium difficulty. The residual band of keratinized tissue was borderline at around 4 mm. So, to err on the side of caution, the moderate risk option was selected for this factor. The remaining risk factors (the planned single implant, placement without the need for adjunctive contour augmentation, adoption of a conventional loading protocol, good soft tissue quality, and little anatomical risk), all scored low difficulty in the surgical assessment (Figure 4).

Prosthodontic classification

Among the prosthodontic modifying factors, four factors were identified as potential concerns: Three medium-rated risk factors were identified (the anticipated minimal prosthetic volume, the interocclusal space at the planned implant site, and the ongoing mechanical and technical complications that might arise from these). Figure 6 shows the close relationship between the mandibular right canine and the opposing overdenture abutment. The implant was placed further apically to provide vertical flexibility, but a decision was made not to attempt to also move the level of the hard and soft tissues of the adjacent residual ridge further apically. The prosthetic volume and interocclusal clearance for the stud attachment was, therefore, still limited. Fortunately, an internal reinforcement of the denture through the cast metal framework and a horizontal offset between the attachment and opposing canine allowed all components to be accommodated without any fractures or pronounced esthetic compromise.

A fourth factor scored as a high risk was the role of the planned single implant in the maxillary right canine site to provide part of the anterior guidance (Figure 5). This ultimately elevated the prosthodontic classification to a high level. With the strategic placement of the implant seen in Figures 6 and 7, the aim was for the partial denture to be part of a mutually protected scheme with anterior canine lifts and even incisal rise; the latter is seen in Figure 8.

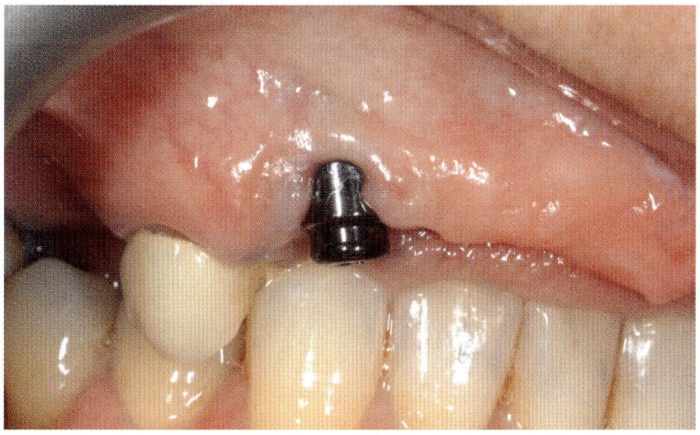

Fig 5. In this case, the keratinized tissue outcome was a 2-mm band that has remained stable for 7 years.

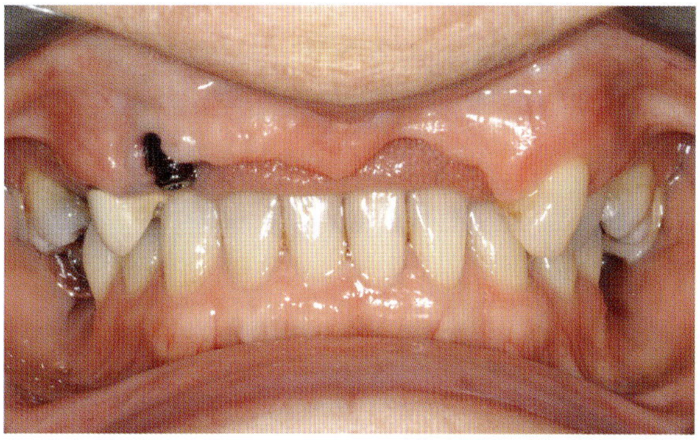

Fig 6. The close relationship between the mandibular right canine and the opposing ridge was evident from the outset. The implant was placed further apically to provide vertical flexibility. A decision was made not to move the level of the hard and soft tissues of the adjacent residual ridge further apically, and the prosthetic volume and interocclusal clearance for the stud attachment was therefore still limited.

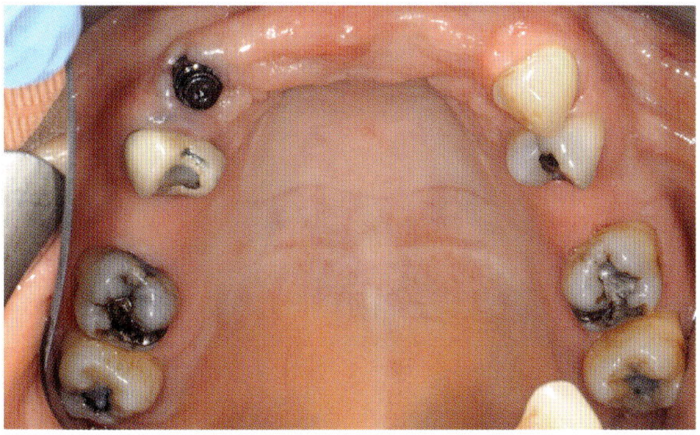

Fig 7. The strategic position from an occlusal perspective of the implant placed in the maxillary right canine site is evident in the clinical image here. The plan was therefore for the implant to be directly involved in enabling the anterior denture saddle to provide dynamic anterior guidance.

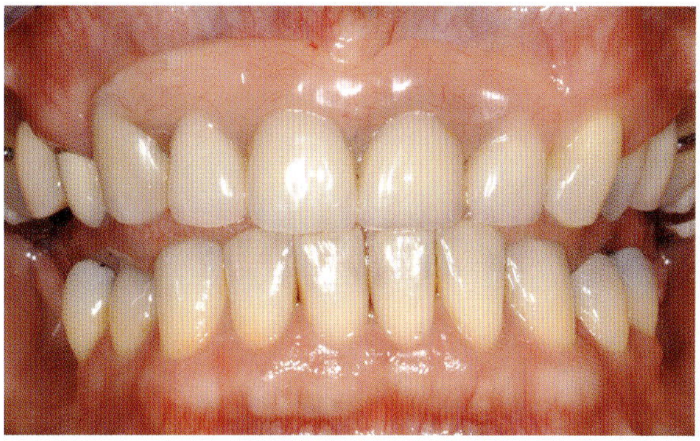

Fig 8. The maxillary partial denture is able to provide anterior guidance here demonstrated in protrusion by even incisal rise.

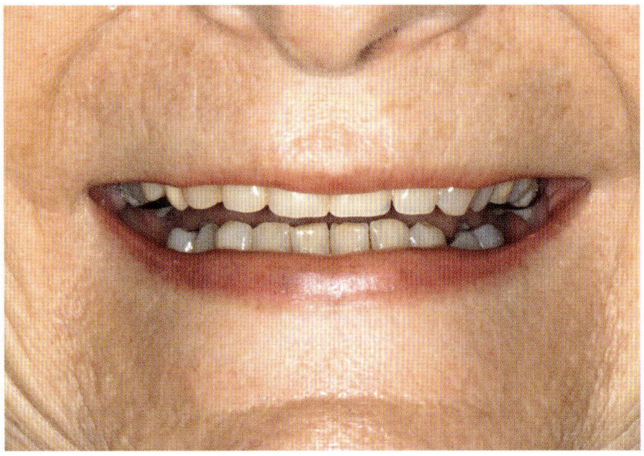

Fig 9. The esthetic outcome in a broad smile. The denture privacy is greatly assisted by a low smile line and long upper lip.

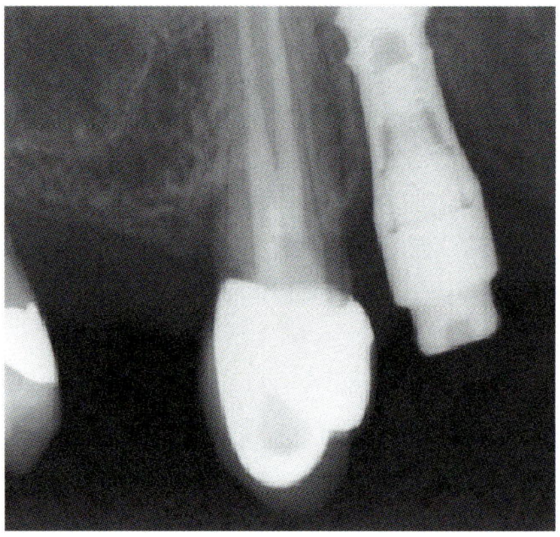

Fig 10. Intraoral radiograph confirming stable marginal bone levels 7 years after placement.

Edentulous esthetic risk assessment for removable dentures

With replacement of five anterior teeth by the planned maxillary partial denture, esthetic risk assessment is an important consideration even in the presence of modest and realistic patient expectations. In this case, the six modifying factors all scored as low, and the final smile can be seen in Figure 9.

REFLECTION AND FOLLOW-UP

The use of a single implant to enhance performance of removable partial dentures has gained increasing recognition over the past two decades (Mitrani et al 2003, Kaufmann et al 2009, Payne et al 2017). While the evidence is still limited, the advantages that a single implant can offer in terms of support, stability, and retention are described in the literature as an effective yet simple, economic, and less invasive use of the implant modality (Shahmiri et al 2010, de Freitas et al 2012, Zancopé et al 2015). The surgical aspects of this case were mostly low risk. However, while most of the prosthodontic factors scored as low risk, the combined anticipated issues related to prosthodontic space together with the critical involvement in occlusion increased risk and case difficulty.

The patient expressed immediate and continuing appreciation of the additional security offered by the implant and stud attachment against embarrassing dislodgement of the denture. She has also found daily oral hygiene of the overdenture abutment manageable, including the buccal mucosal margin contour seen in Figure 5. The identified potential mechanical/technical complications related to the limited prosthetic volume and interocclusal clearance has necessitated refitting of the stud attachment housing in the denture base on two occasions in the past 7 years with automatic renewal of the retentive insert at the same time. The Straumann Tissue Level standard 4.1 × 10–mm implant has maintained stable marginal bone levels for 7 years as confirmed by a recent intraoral radiograph (Figure 10). A 2-mm collar-height Straumann Locator implant stud attachment was used for the first 4 years. Thereafter, the attachment was changed to a Straumann Novaloc 2-mm collar-height stud attachment (seen in Figures 5, 6, and 7) as part of a case study series.

Acknowledgement:
Implant placed by Dr. Stephen Dover

5.10 Implants for Restoration of the Full Arch: Removable

5.10.1 Edentulous maxilla: Bar-supported overdenture

WS. LIN, D. MORTON

A 46-year-old woman presented to the clinic seeking implant-assisted treatment options. The patient described that she had lost all her teeth more than 20 years ago, and she disliked her current maxillary and mandibular complete dentures. The chief complaints were that she shows too much pink area of her dentures while smiling, and her teeth do not align properly (Figure 1). The extraoral examination showed high lip mobility and the need for denture extension for sufficient facial support. The intraoral examination revealed severely atrophic maxillary and mandibular alveolar ridges. The radiographic findings showed completely edentulous maxilla and mandible with minimal (maxillary anterior region), moderate (mandible), and severe (maxillary posterior) atrophy of residual alveolar ridge in the respective edentulous areas. The right maxillary sinus also showed signs of acute sinusitis (see Figure 1e).

TREATMENT RISK ASSESSMENT

The treatment risk for the maxillary milled bar overdenture was assessed using the SAC Assessment Tool highlighting key general health, full-arch esthetic, surgical, and prosthetic risk factors resulting in an overall treatment risk (Figure 2).

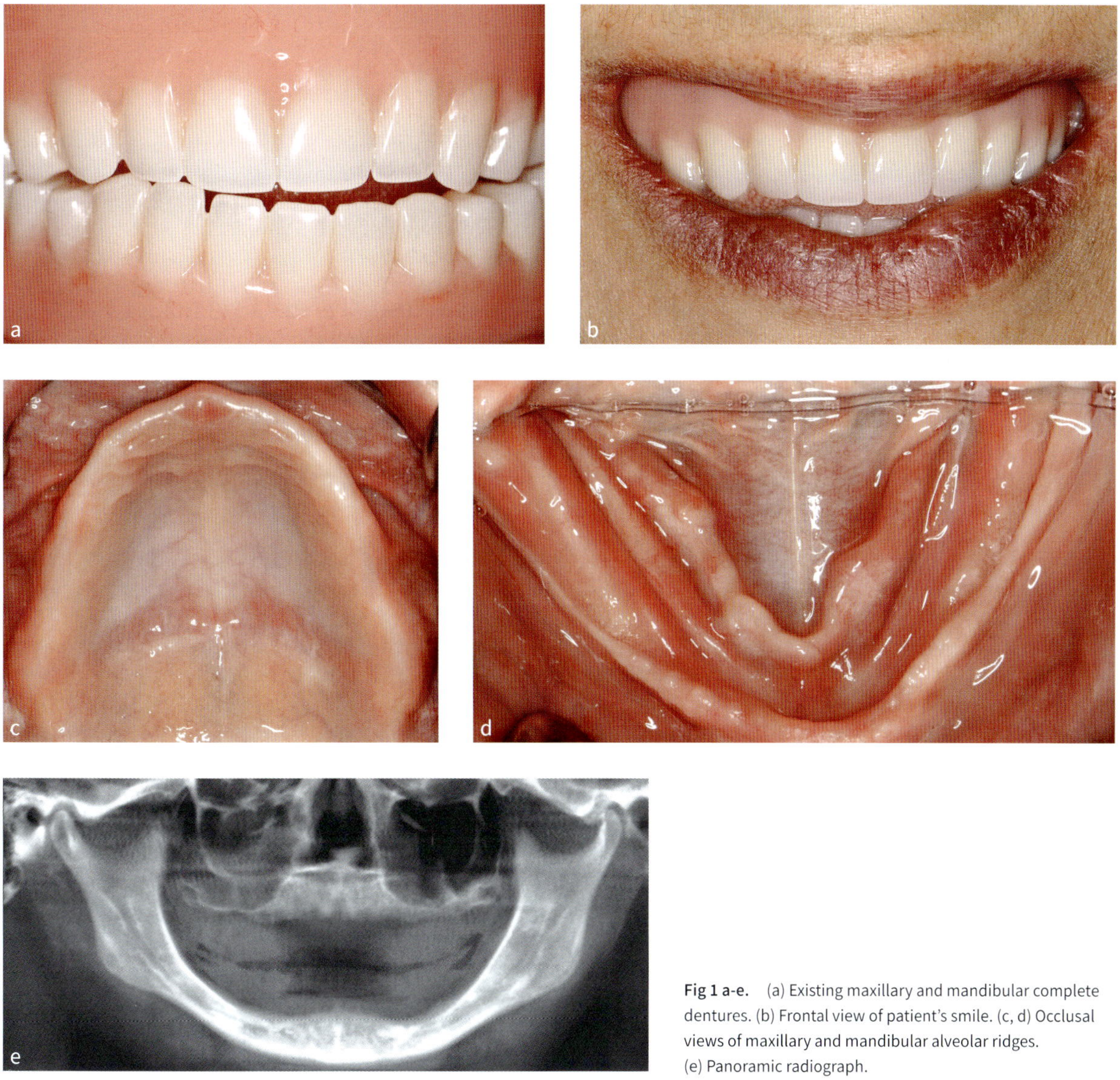

Fig 1 a-e. (a) Existing maxillary and mandibular complete dentures. (b) Frontal view of patient's smile. (c, d) Occlusal views of maxillary and mandibular alveolar ridges. (e) Panoramic radiograph.

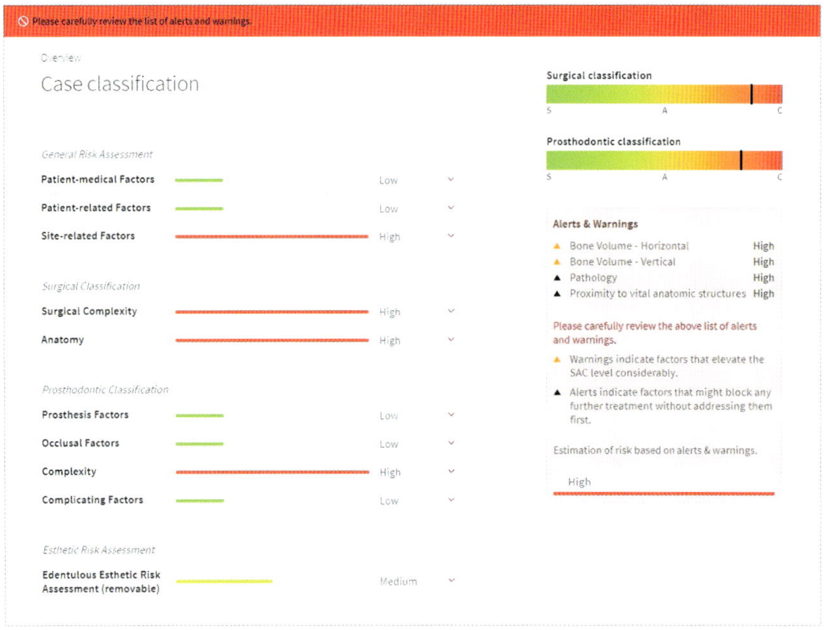

Fig 2. Overall treatment classification: Edentulous esthetic risk = medium; Surgical classification = complex; Prosthodontic classification = complex.

The patient's general health condition was not significant in the risk assessment. In the full-arch esthetic risk assessment, the patient's treatment has elevated risks due to the need for a maxillary implant-assisted prosthesis, short upper lip, excessive maxillary ridge display at full smile, and Class III maxillomandibular interocclusal relationship. The patient presented a realistic expectation of esthetic treatment outcomes but also significant surgical risks. The severely atrophic maxillary posterior alveolar ridge elevated the surgical risk with the need for bilateral sinus augmentations. The patient also required a larger number of implants to be placed. With the loss of soft tissue volume, prosthetic replacement of soft tissues was needed for both maxillary and mandibular prostheses. Full-arch maxillary and mandibular prostheses required special attention to the design of the occlusal scheme and anterior guidance. The need to splint multiple implants for the definitive prostheses also further increased the prosthetic treatment risk. Although the patient was highly motivated and compliant, a strict home care regimen and postoperative maintenance were critical factors to be with the patient during the treatment planning phase. Overall, this patient's treatment presented with high level of risk and degree of difficulty based on the full-arch esthetic risk, surgical risk, and prosthetic risk assessment.

PLANNING AND CLINICAL TREATMENT

Upon reviewing the patient's medical history, no contributing factors would contraindicate the patient for dental treatment, including routine surgical and restorative procedures. The patient reported no allergies and no prescription medication usage. Various implant-assisted treatment options were discussed with the patient, and she showed great interest in the fixed dental prostheses. The patient was informed that due to the high lip mobility and the need for denture extension for sufficient facial support, removable dental prostheses would be more suitable. An implant-supported milled bar overdenture assisted by six dental implants was proposed and accepted by the patient to achieve her desire for increased maxillary prosthesis stability. The patient also accepted a treatment plan of a mandibular implant-supported fixed complete denture supported by five dental implants.

Antibiotics were prescribed to the patient to manage the acute sinusitis, and bilateral sinus augmentations were performed. Six dental implants (Straumann Tissue Level Implants) were placed in the posterior maxilla, and five dental implants were placed in the anterior mandible (Straumann Tissue Level Implants). After the 3-month healing period, the patient returned to the prosthodontics clinic for definitive prostheses. Scan bodies were attached to the implants under 15 Ncm torque (Figures 3a-d). Intraoral scans were made for both maxillary and mandibular arches (Figure 3e). CAD/CAM dental casts were articulated with facebow transfer and the maxillomandibular relationship recorded on a semiadjustable articulator. Maxillary and mandibular trial teeth arrangements were made in a dental laboratory.

At trial insertion, the tooth arrangements were evaluated for esthetics, phonetics, occlusal vertical dimension, and centric relation. The denture extension was inadequate and distorted the facial appearance while smiling (Figures 4a, b). A wrinkle was noted below the patient's nose. Additional wax was added to the trial teeth arrangement to provide proper facial support (Figures 4c, d).

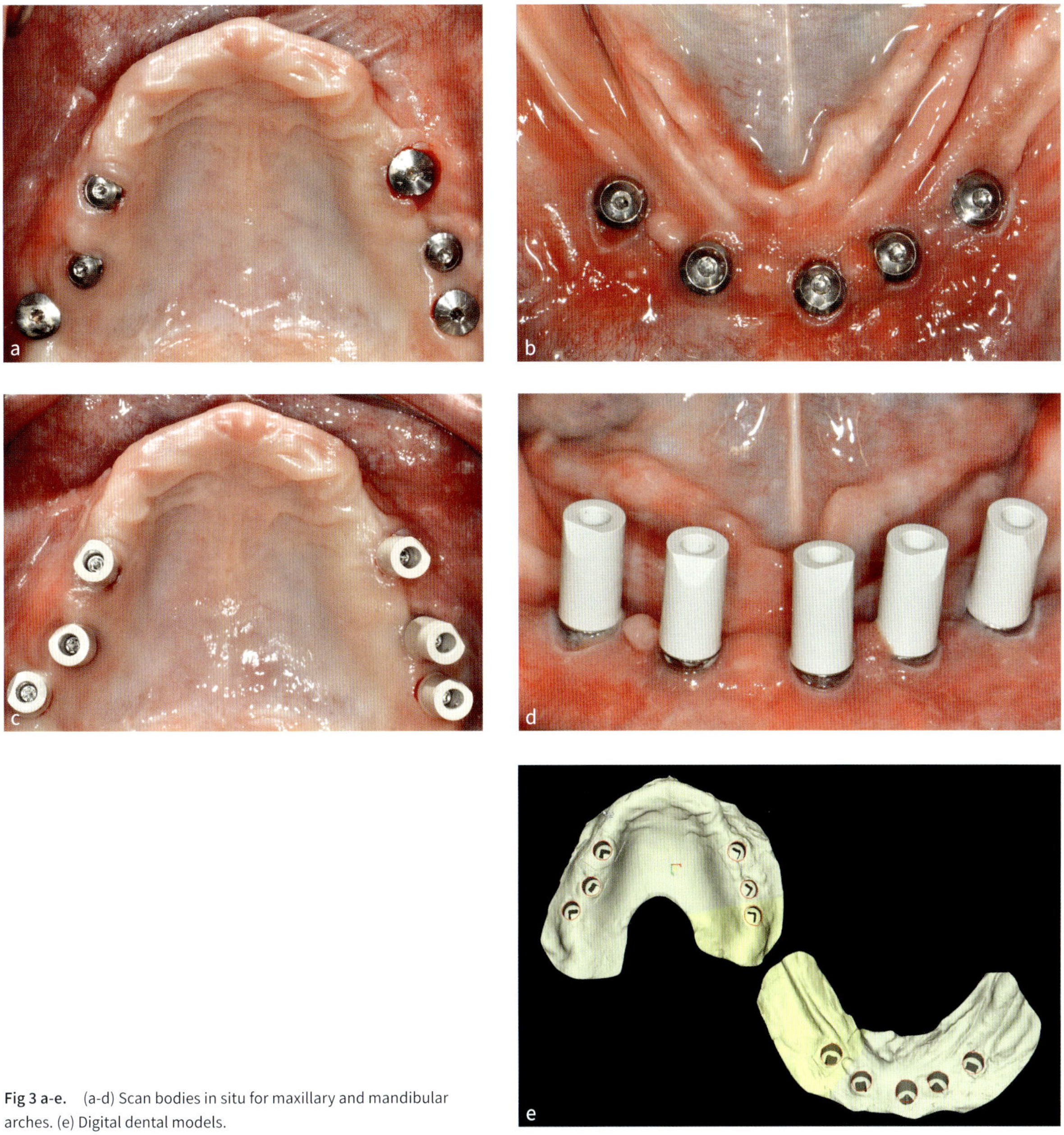

Fig 3 a-e. (a-d) Scan bodies in situ for maxillary and mandibular arches. (e) Digital dental models.

After the patient's approval for the trial tooth arrangement, the CAD/CAM dental casts and trial tooth arrangement were digitized with a dental laboratory scanner. The satisfactory tooth arrangements were used to assess the restorative space of the maxillary milled bar and mandibular implant-supported fixed complete denture. There must be 1 mm of space between the milled bar's intaglio surface and underlying soft tissue for adequate oral hygiene. Five-degree axial walls on both the lingual and facial sides of the milled bar were designed to provide proper resistance and stability of the overdenture. The tooth arrangement was also used to design the mandibular definitive CAD/CAM tissue-colored anodized titanium framework (AccuFrame IC, Cagenix) and all-ceramic restorations (Zenostar, Wieland Dental). A virtual design was achieved with a minimal 2-mm material thickness for the all-ceramic restorations, a minimum height of 4 mm for the simulated individual abutment structures on the titanium framework, and the minimum height of 3 to 4 mm for all the remaining areas on titanium framework (Figure 5a). The maxillary milled bar was positioned on the CAD/CAM dental cast and digitized with a dental laboratory scanner. The internal framework was designed and 3D-printed with direct metal printing (DMP) system (ProX DMP 200, 3D Systems) and Co-Cr metal alloy (LaserForm CoCr, 3D Systems) (Figure 5b). The contouring and characterization of the definitive all-ceramic restorations were completed in

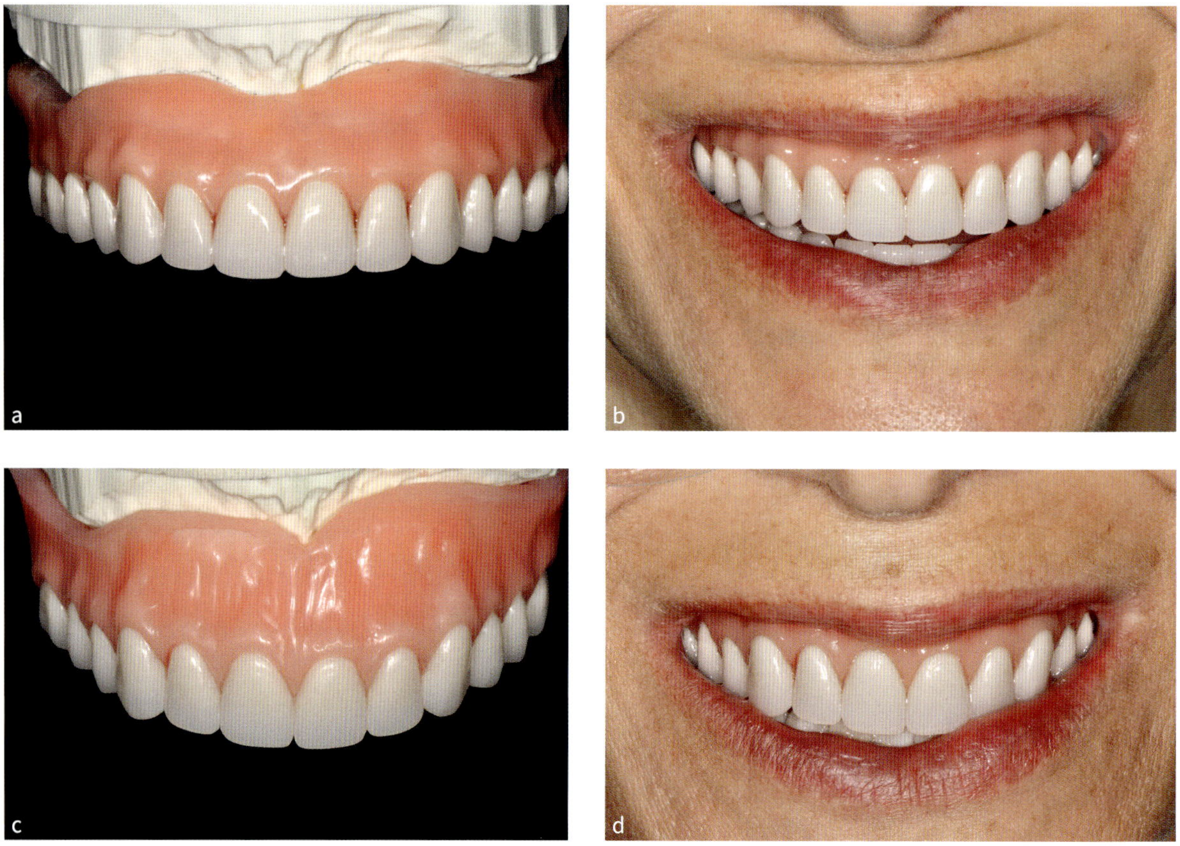

Fig 4 a-d. (a and b) Initial teeth arrangement with insufficient denture extension, causing a wrinkle while smiling. (c and d) Additional wax was added at the facial extension to provide proper facial support.

the dental laboratory with veneering porcelain (IPS e.max Ceram, Ivoclar Vivadent) and low-fusing nanofluorapatite glass-ceramic (IPS e.max Ceram Shades and Essences). The all-ceramic restorations were luted to the titanium framework with a resin luting agent (RelyX Unicem 2, 3M). The maxillary milled bar and mandibular titanium framework and all-ceramic restorations were evaluated clinically and radiographically (Figure 5c).

The waxing procedure for the definitive prosthesis was completed to mimic missing soft tissue. Autopolymerizing injection-molded acrylic resin (Ivobase High Impact, Ivoclar Vivadent) was used to complete the processing procedure. The definitive maxillary milled bar overdenture and mandibular implant-supported fixed complete denture were evaluated intraorally for the fit, functional and esthetic outcome, and adjustments were made with a diamond cutting instrument (Fine Diamonds, Brasseler) on the all-ceramic restorations and with laboratory carbide cutting instrument (Carbide Cutter, Brasseler) on the acrylic resin and denture teeth. The milled bar and implant-supported fixed complete denture were secured to the implants with 35 Ncm torque. Screw access openings in the definitive prosthesis were closed with cotton pellets and single-component resin sealing material (Fermit, Ivoclar Vivadent) (Figures 6a to c). The patient was provided with a mandibular occlusal splint and instructed on a home care regimen. Periodic maintenance appointments were scheduled in a 6-month interval. The patient was seen for a 1-year clinical and radiographic follow-up visit to confirm the conditions of the implants and prostheses (Figures 6d-f).

REFLECTION ON THE TREATMENT APPROACH AND OUTCOME

The biggest challenge during this patient's treatment was severely atrophic alveolar ridges and excessive display of maxillary ridge (caused by high lip mobility). The alternative treatment choice could be zygomatic implants instead of bilateral sinus augmentation in conjunction with regular dental implants. However, clinicians should have the proper expertise to plan and treat patients with zygomatic implants. The main concerns from the patient were the prosthesis stability and esthetic outcome. The prosthesis stability was achieved by offering the patient a fixed prosthesis option in the mandible and milled bar overdenture in the

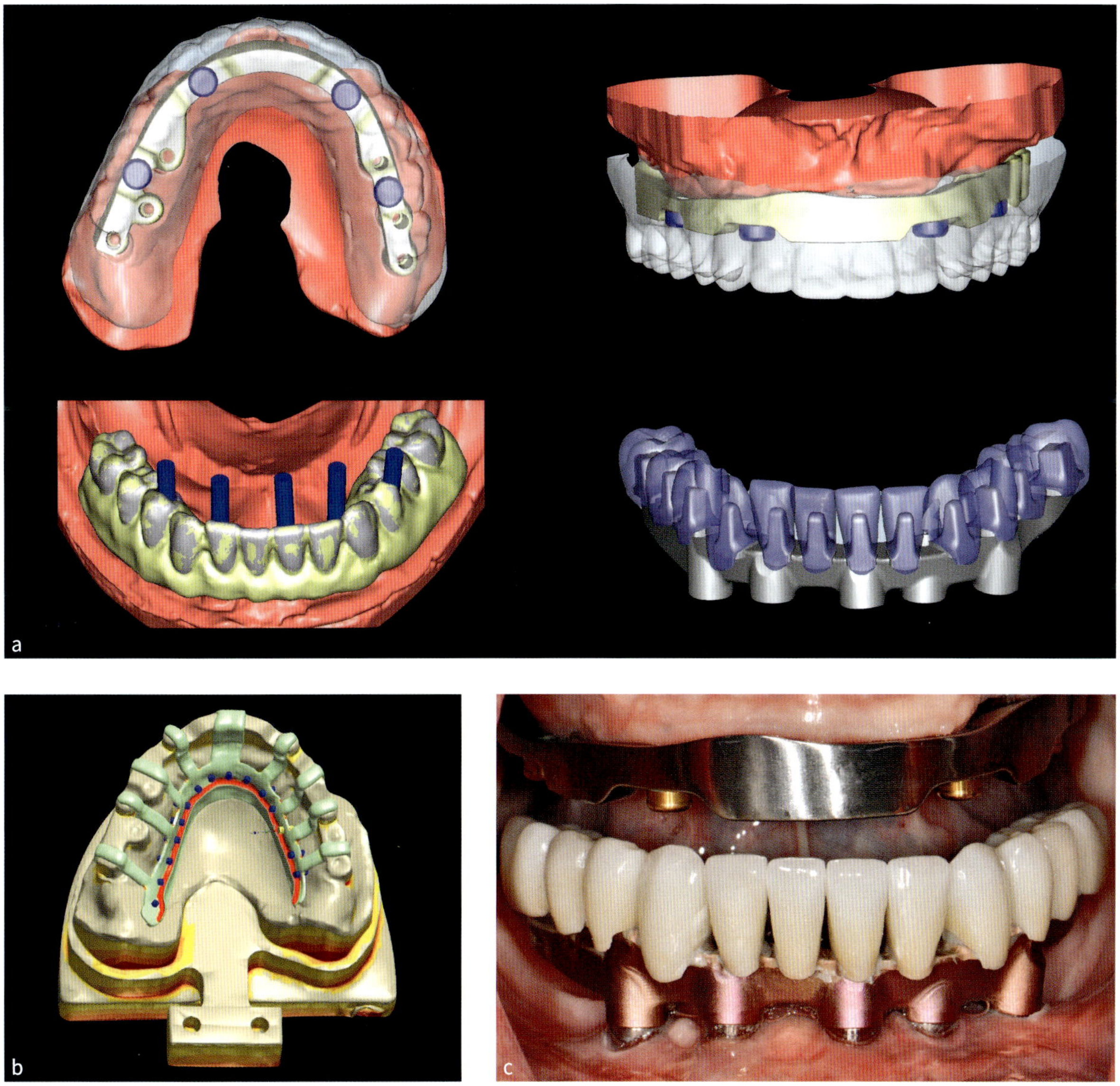

Fig 5 a-c. (a) Digitized tooth arrangement was used to assess available restorative space and design the CAD/CAM maxillary milled bar and mandibular implant-supported fixed complete denture. (b) Digital design of the internal framework for maxillary bar overdenture. (c) Trial insertion of the maxillary milled bar and mandibular titanium framework and crowns.

maxilla. Although a milled bar overdenture is still a removable dental prosthesis, the milled bar with carefully designed axial wall tapers and a flat occlusal surface can provide adequate stability to meet the patient's demand. The esthetic demand for a patient with excessive ridge display could be challenging. The overdenture with facial acrylic extension can facilitate the overall esthetic outcome by apically positioning visible prosthesis–soft tissue junction. One hurdle encountered during the patient's treatment was to determine the proper length of facial denture extension. When the facial denture extension was inadequate, although the prosthesis–soft tissue junction was still below the lip line, the patient's facial support was distorted while smiling. Facial denture extension should be carefully assessed during trial insertion to ensure that proper facial support is achieved. An occlusal splint should always be considered when treating edentulous patients with prostheses that may have persistent nocturnal occlusal contacts. In this instance, although the patient was instructed to remove overdenture at night, it is still possible for the mandibular implant-supported fixed complete denture to occlude to the milled bar in the maxilla. Excessive wear of prostheses could be expected if an occlusal splint was not provided and worn by the patient.

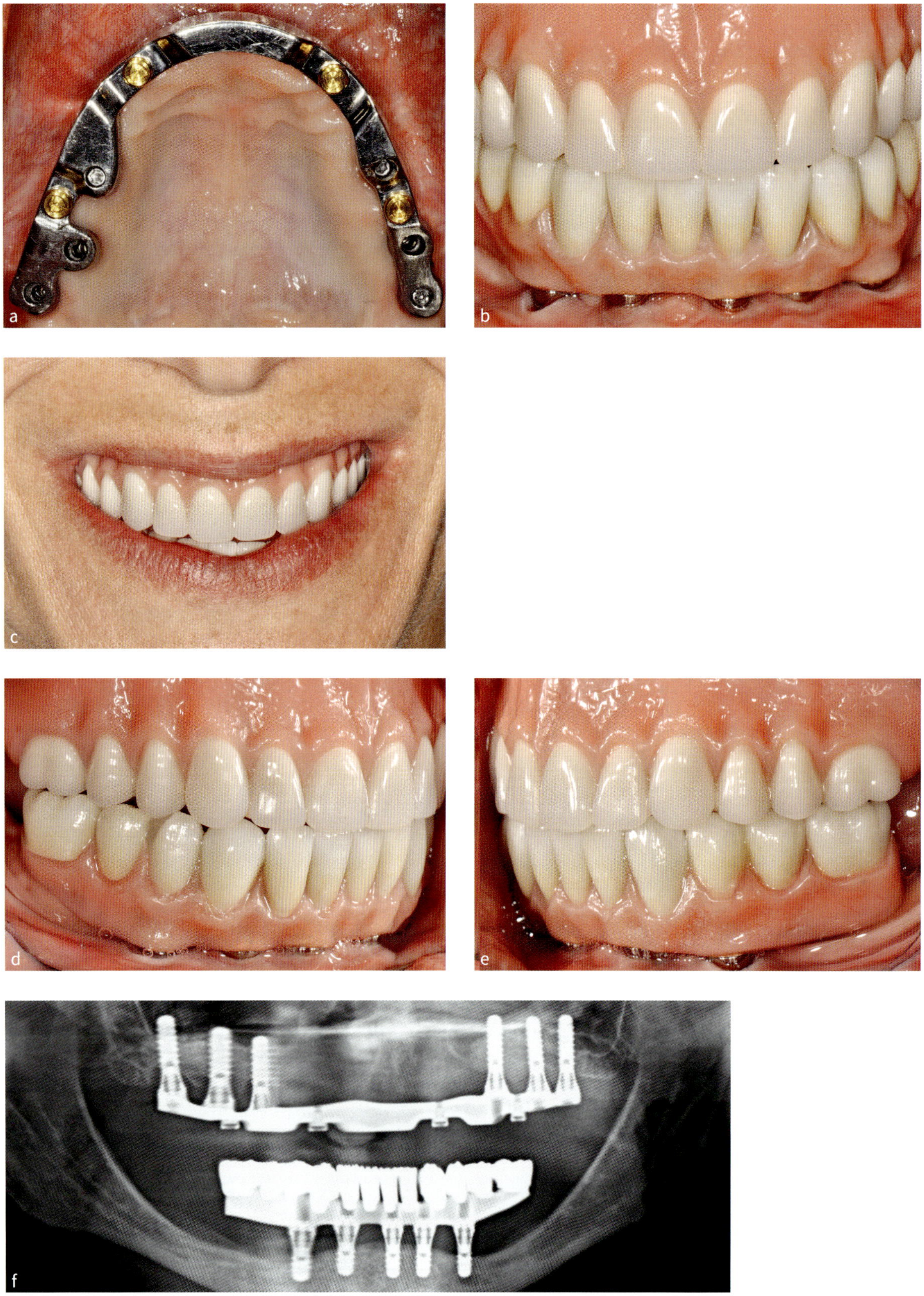

Fig 6 a-f. (a) Occlusal view of maxillary milled bar. Four locator attachments were used to provide retention of overdenture. (b) Frontal view of definitive prostheses. (c) Smile with definitive prostheses. (d-f) Postinsertion follow-up at 1 year.

5.10.2 Edentulous maxilla: Zygomatic implant bar-supported overdenture

W. D. POLIDO, WS. LIN

A 74-year-old woman presented to the oral and maxillofacial surgery clinic seeking implant-assisted treatment options. The patient described that she had lost all her teeth over 20 years ago, and she was not wearing any dentures, reporting having lost them. Her main complaint was that she wanted her teeth back, to be able to chew and smile. Extraoral examination shows a complete lack of support of the upper lip and midface when not wearing dentures (Figure 1). She had low lip mobility and a low smile line. She was also completely edentulous in the mandible.

Intraoral examination showed an extended intra-arch distance, but with a good arch form and adequate keratinized tissue, and absence of any scars from previous procedures. She denied having any implants or bone grafts placed in the past (Figure 2).

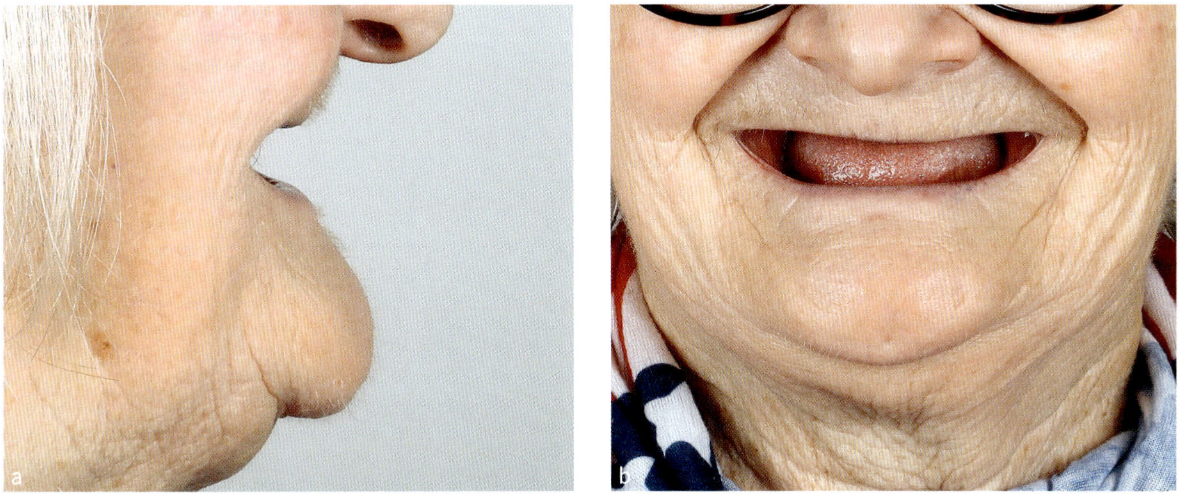

Fig 1 a-b. Observe lack of upper lip support and facial concavity when the patient is not wearing any dentures. No maxillary ridge is shown when smiling. The patient has a short upper lip and a low smile line.

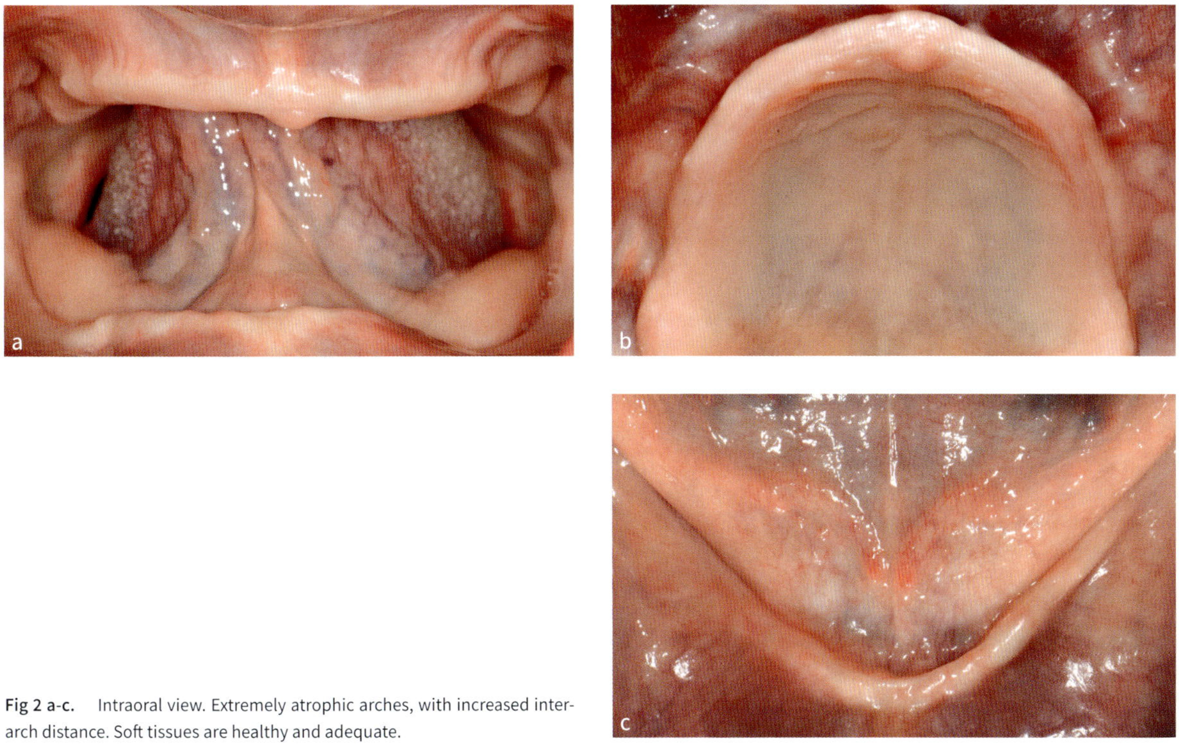

Fig 2 a-c. Intraoral view. Extremely atrophic arches, with increased inter-arch distance. Soft tissues are healthy and adequate.

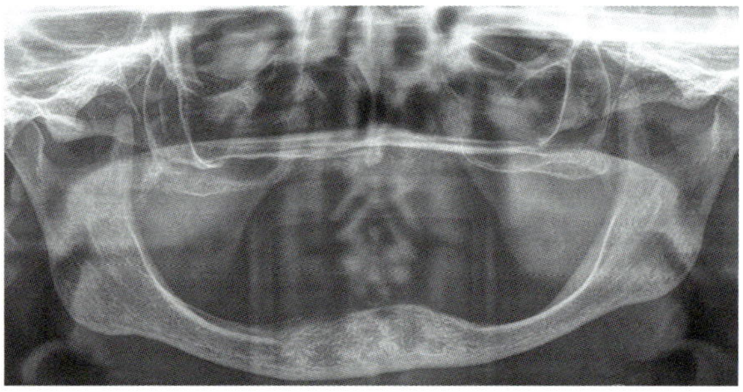

Fig 3. Preoperative panoramic radiograph. Note extreme resorption of the maxillary alveolar bone.

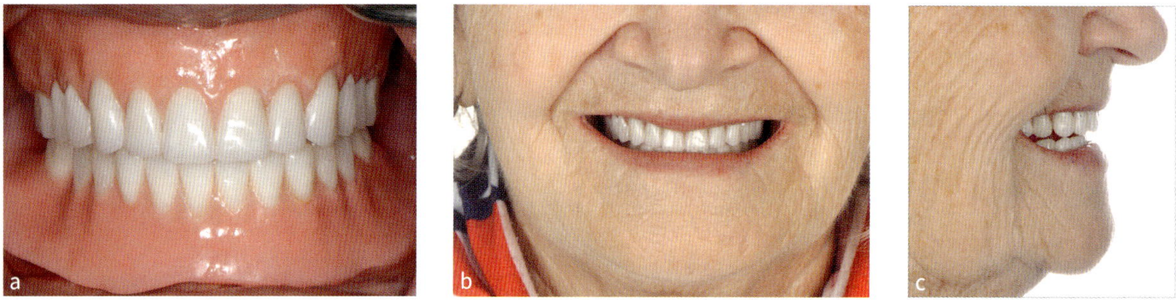

Fig 4 a-c. New dentures, in good occlusion, and providing adequate facial tissues and lip support.

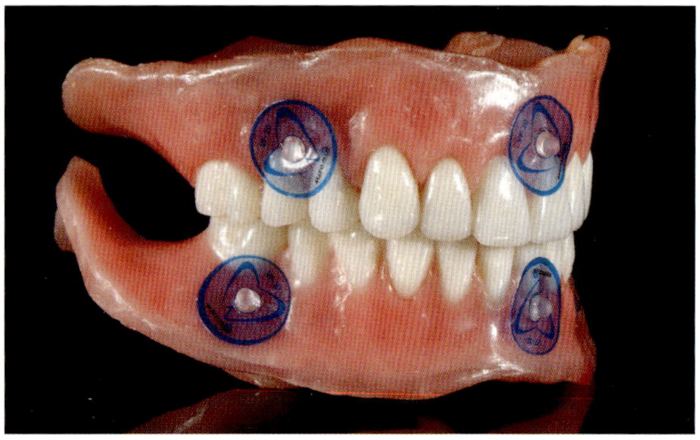

Fig 5. Dentures with radiopaque markers, prepared for dual scan on CBCT.

A review of her past medical history showed mild cardiovascular disease, controlled diabetes mellitus type 2, and previous history of a pituitary tumor, being monitored by the physician. A medical consult was sent to the primary care physicians, which cleared her health status for a surgical procedure under local anesthesia and intravenous moderate sedation. She was classified as an ASA 2 classification.

The initial panoramic radiograph showed an extremely atrophic maxilla, with no alveolar bone in the right and left posterior region, and advanced horizontal and vertical resorption in the anterior maxilla. Both maxillary sinuses were clear, without any sinus pathology (Figure 3).

A new set of interim dentures was fabricated, taking in consideration functional and esthetic prosthodontic parameters, like reestablishment of the occlusal vertical dimension (OVD), defining good occlusion, and restoring lip and facial tissue support (Figure 4).

After trial insertion and approval from the patient, radiopaque markers were placed in the dentures (Figure 5), and the patient underwent a dual CBCT scan.

Images of the denture were superimposed in the edentulous maxilla, using the radiopaque markers as references, on the coDiagnostiX software program (Figure 6).

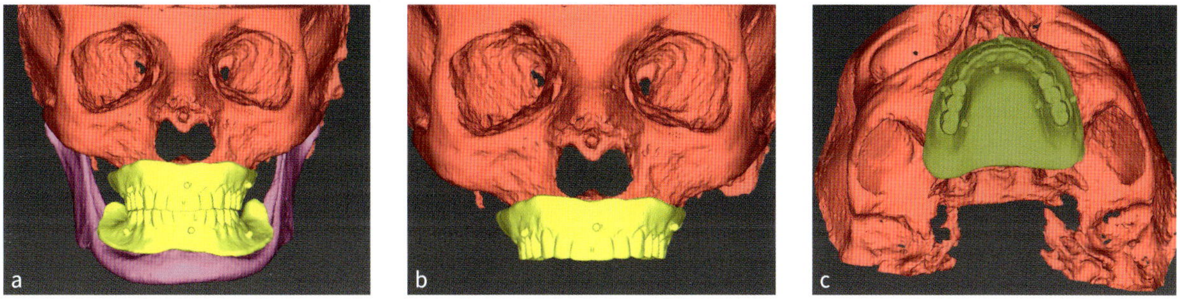

Fig 6 a-c. (a) Superimposition of maxillary denture, after dual scan, in occlusion. (b) Frontal view of maxilla. (c) Axial view of maxilla.

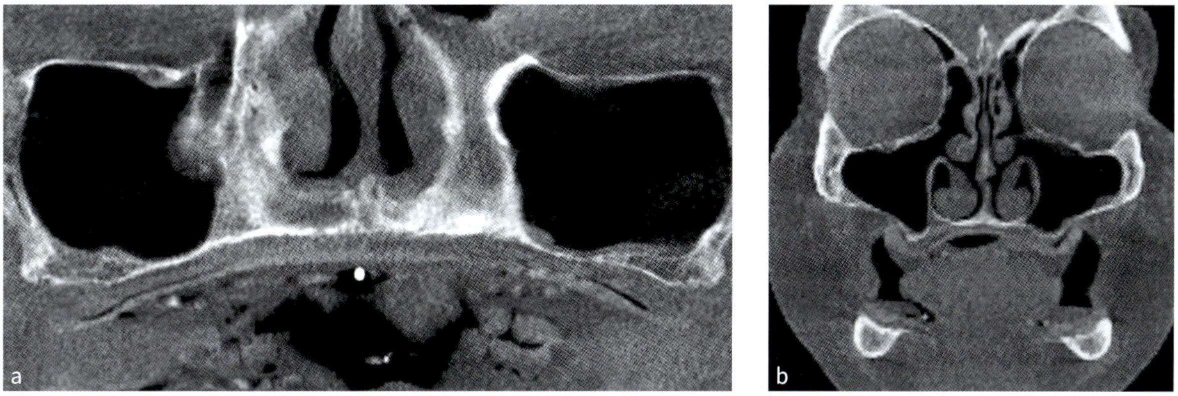

Fig 7 a-b. (a) Panoramic slice from CBCT showing maxillary atrophy. (b) Coronal CBCT slice, showing extreme posterior maxillary atrophy, clear and healthy maxillary sinus, zygomatic bone density, and relationship between the lateral maxillary wall and zygomatic bone.

CBCT scans confirmed extreme maxillary resorption. No alveolar bone was present in the posterior maxilla, distal to the canine region. The anterior maxilla (canine to canine) showed extreme resorption, with a buccal concavity in the region below the nasal fossa, but still minimum alveolar bone width. The sinuses were clear, without any signs of pathology or inflammatory diseases (Figure 7).

A complete risk assessment was performed utilizing the SAC Assessment Tool, addressing general risk, surgical risk, prosthodontic risk, and the edentulous esthetic risk assessment (Figure 8).

In the general risk assessment, she had a *medium risk* due to the medical condition of diabetes mellitus. However, that was very well controlled, and she could have surgery under sedation or even general anesthesia. Access was favorable, since she allowed good access to the instruments necessary to perform the proposed technique. The patient was compliant and had realistic expectations from the treatment, and was in acceptable overall health to undergo a surgical procedure.

Surgical classification was considered complex, due to the high risk associated with the placement of multiple implants and the proximity to anatomical structures, such as the orbits, infraorbital foramen, maxillary sinus, nasal cavity, incisal foramen, and posterior superior vascular complex. This treatment requires expertise in management of these structures and is usually performed by oral and maxillofacial surgeons.

Prosthodontic classification was considered to be complex, due to the technical and mechanical risk when dealing with multiple (and angled) implants to support a complete arch restoration. Prosthetic volume and interarch space were adequate, and conventional loading was chosen, without the need for an immediate interim prosthesis. The edentulous esthetic risk assessment (EERA) was considered medium once all esthetic factors could be managed with the planned restoration.

Overall SAC classification was considered to be complex.

After careful analysis of all risk factors and after discussing all risks and benefits of the alternatives with the patient, the decision was made to proceed with the detailed plan and execution of the quad zygomatic implant technique. The patient was informed that, due to the need for denture extension for sufficient lip and facial support, a removable dental prosthesis would be more suitable. An implant-supported bar overdenture assisted by four zygomatic implants was proposed and accepted by the patient to achieve the patient's desire for increased maxillary prosthesis stability.

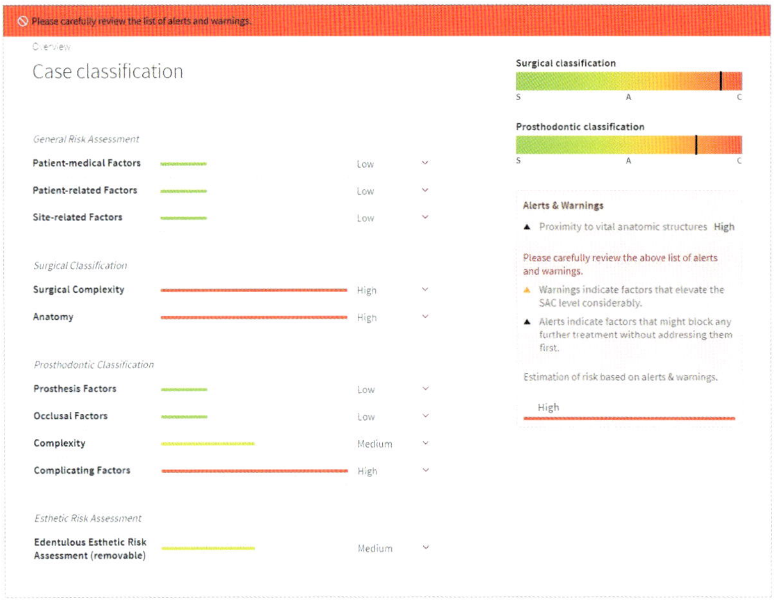

Fig 8. Overall treatment classification: Edentulous esthetic risk = medium; Surgical classification = complex; Prosthodontic classification = complex.

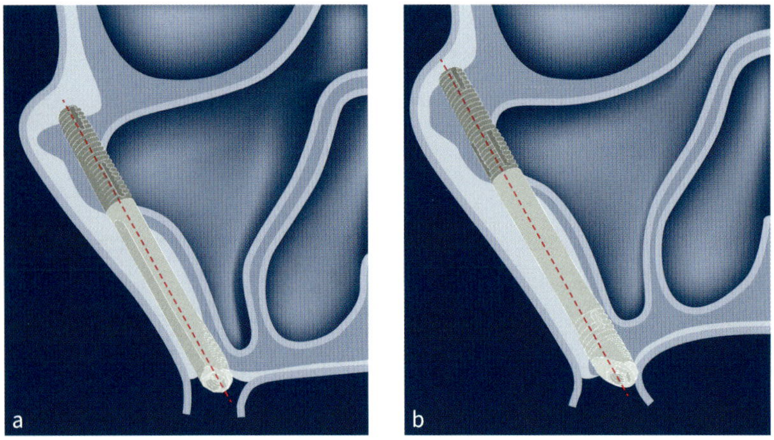

Fig 9 a-b. (a) ZAGA Type III, extrasinus path. (b) ZAGA Type IV, extramaxillary path. (Reprinted with permission from Aparicio [2017])

SURGICAL TREATMENT PLANNING AND PROCEDURE

Digital planning using coDiagnostiX software was undertaken, aiming at a combination of optimal bone anchorage on the zygomatic bone and an adequate position of the restorative head of the implant in order to achieve a good anteroposterior (AP) spread.

Anatomical configuration was considered to be a ZAGA Classification type III for the anterior region, and ZAGA type IV for the posterior region (Figure 9).

This classification allows for an anatomically guided decision about the implant position, type, and the surgical technique to be utilized (Aparicio et al, 2021).

In the posterior regions, a Straumann zygomatic implant with a Flat design was chosen, due to the extramaxillary path technique indicated for the ZAGA type IV regions. The correct angulation of the implant head is checked on the digital plan and transferred to the actual surgery using special direction indicators as a reference.

In the anterior regions, a Straumann zygomatic implant with a Round design was chosen, since the anterior alveolar bone had a buccal concavity, allowing the implant head to be fully covered by bone. The technique chosen was an extrasinus path, ZAGA type III. An estimate of the implant length was determined based on the digital planning (Figure 10).

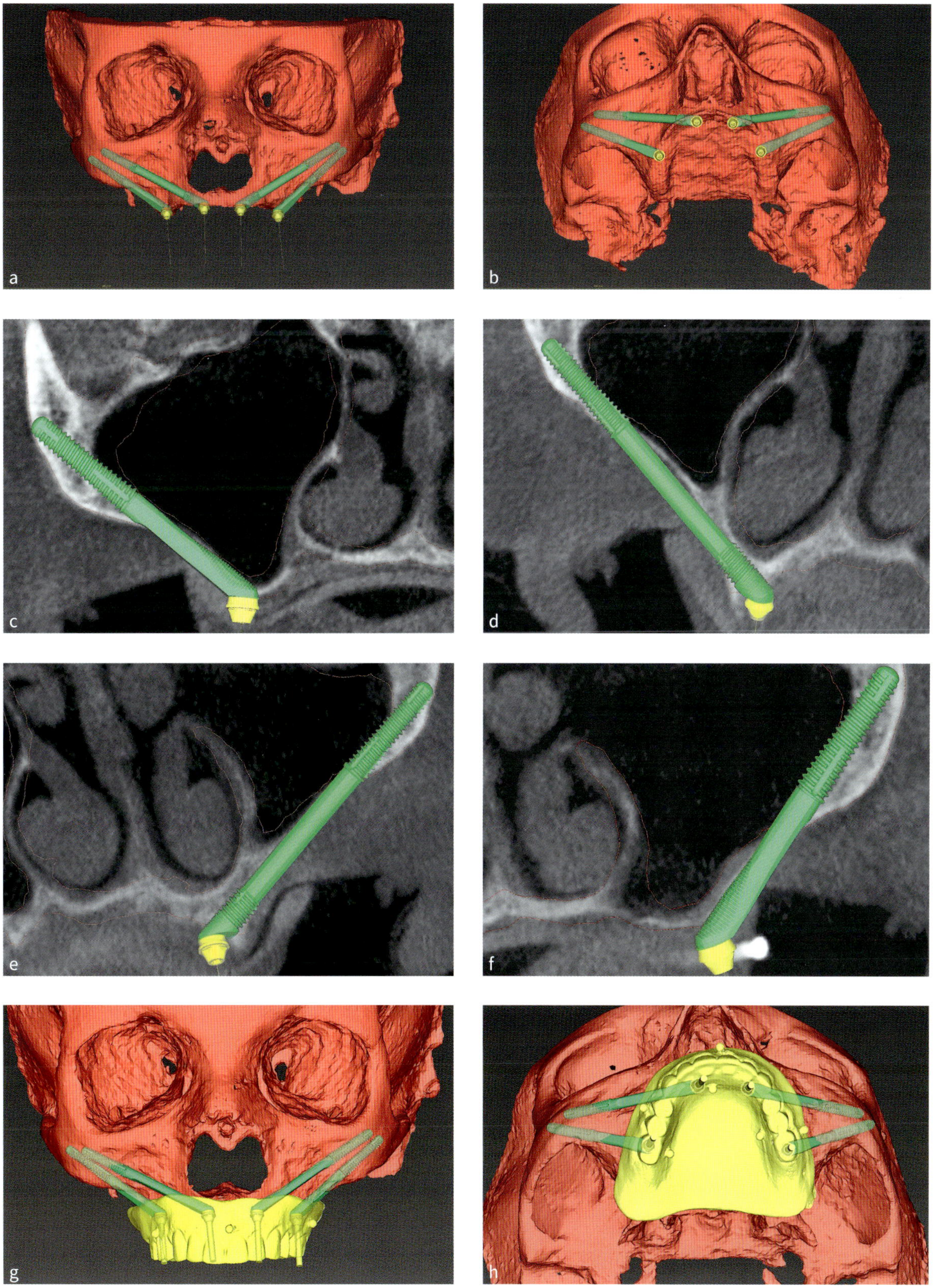

Fig 10 a-h. Virtual surgical plan. (a, b) Frontal and inferior view; note apical and coronal position of implants. (c-f) Virtual plan, four zygomatic sites: posterior right (ZAGA 4, Straumann Flat), anterior right (ZAGA 3, Straumann Round), anterior left (ZAGA 3, Straumann Round), posterior left (ZAGA 4, Straumann Flat). (g, h) Inferior and frontal views of planned implant positions in relation to the future prosthesis.

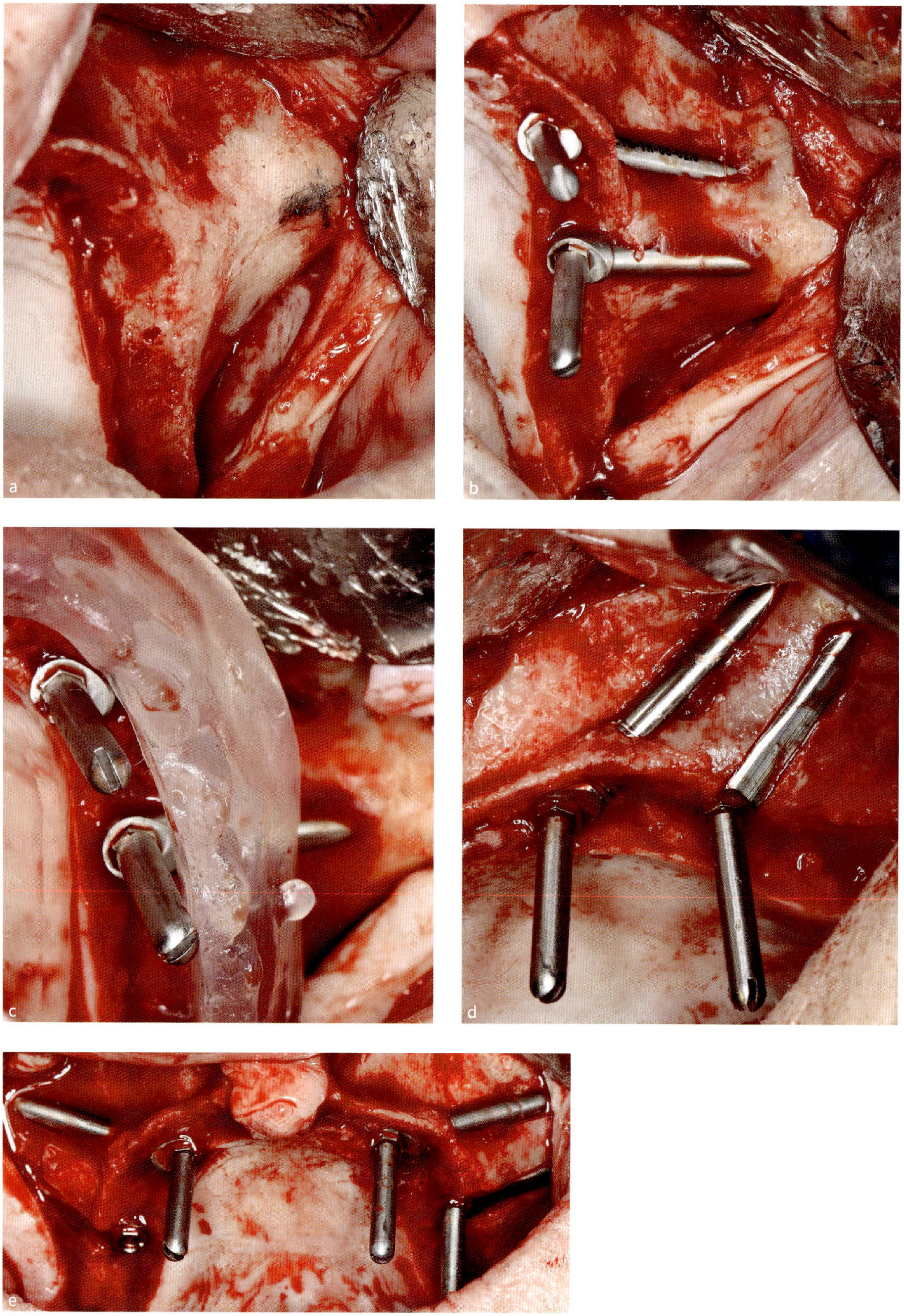
a
b
c
d
e

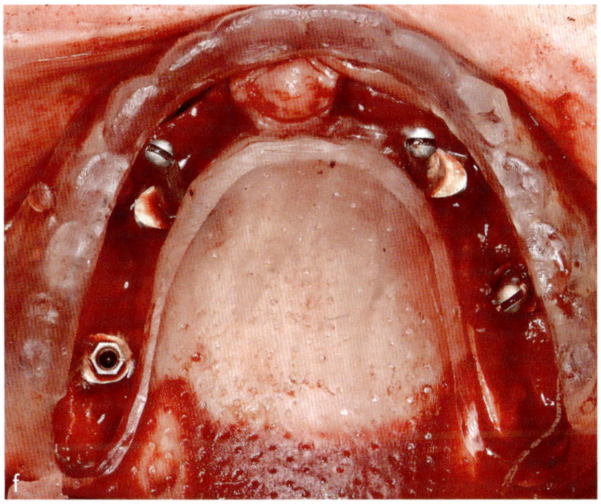

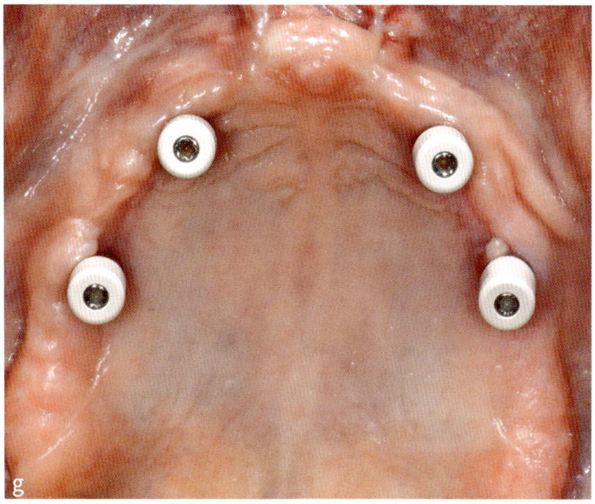

Fig 11 a-g. (a) Intraoperative image, left side. Note the mark where posterior zygomatic entrance should be directed. (b) Direction indicators with implant head: left anterior and posterior implants. (c) Direction indicators and restorative template: left anterior and posterior implants. (d) Implants positioned, with direction indicators screwed into implant head: left anterior, Round, coming through alveolar bone; left posterior, Flat, coming lateral to the sinus. (e) Intraoperative image of the four implants with direction indicators, buccal view. (f) Occlusal view: checking implant distribution in relation to restorative template. (g) Occlusal view at 2-month follow-up.

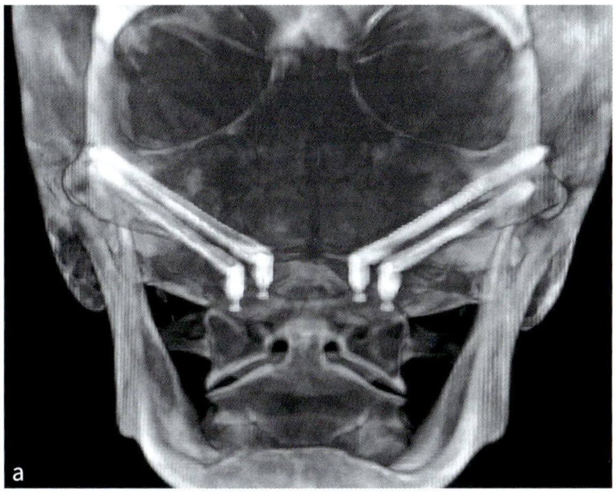

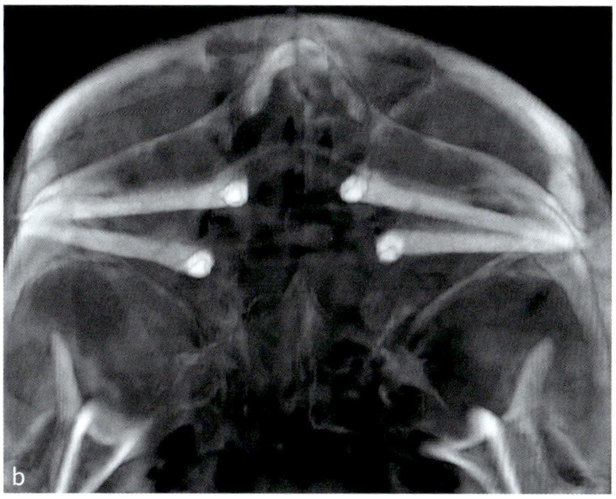

Fig 12 a-b. (a) Immediate postoperative CBCT, coronal view. (b) Immediate postoperative CBCT, axial view.

SURGICAL TREATMENT

Surgery was performed under local anesthesia and moderate intravenous sedation, in an office setting.

An incision was made on the top of the crest, slightly to the palatal, in order to obtain a thick keratinized tissue around the implant neck and abutment at the end of the procedure. The incision was carried first on the left side, preserving the midline. Using a duplicate of the denture as a template, implant insertion points were defined. Surgical drilling was then carried out, using the technique described by Aparicio (2017) and Aparicio et al (2021). An extrasinus pathway was used for the anterior implants and an extramaxillary path for the posterior implants.

A 40-mm-long Straumann Zygomatic Flat was placed on the posterior left, and a 47.5-mm long Straumann Zygomatic Round implant was placed on the anterior left. On the anterior right, a 52.5-mm long implant was utilized, and on the posterior right, a 42-mm long implant was used. Surgery was performed as planned, without any deviations from the proposed technique. Straumann screw-retained abutments (SRAs) were placed, and suturing was performed leaving abutments exposed, in a one-stage technique, without immediate loading. Healing was uneventful (Figure 11).

Postoperative CBCT scans show implant position comparable to the digital plan (Figure 12).

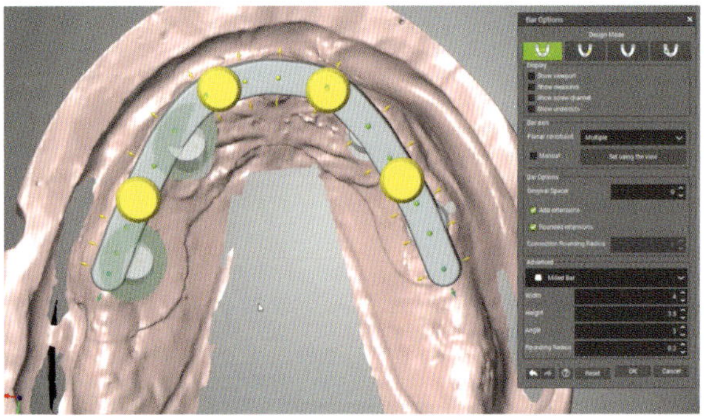

Fig 13a. CAD of milled bar splinting implants.

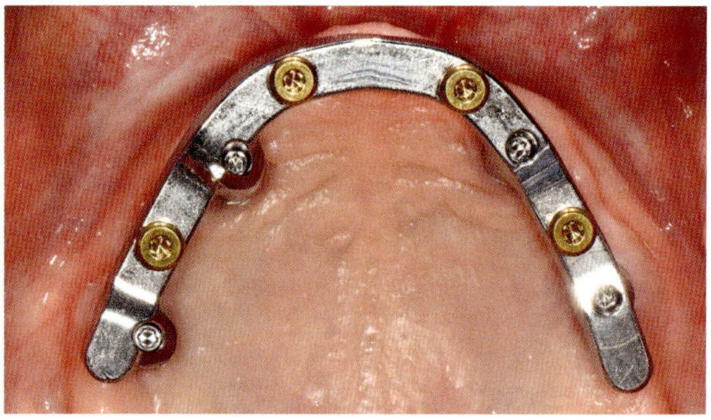

Fig 13b. Screw-retained milled bar splinting implants, with Novaloc abutments for retention of palate free maxillary removable denture.

After the osseointegration period of 3 months, impressions were made, and implants were splinted with a bar. A bar-supported overdenture was screw-retained, and a palate-free denture delivered (Figure 13).

REFLECTION ON THE TREATMENT APPROACH AND OUTCOME

The presented treatment illustrates a SAC complex situation on the surgical and prosthodontic aspects.

When addressing extremely resorbed maxillae, the surgeon usually has to decide between two possibilities: grafting versus nongrafting techniques.

Grafting has to be done in two stages, since there is no remaining bone to perform simultaneous implant placement. Any grafting procedure brings more risk factors associated with the grafts, in addition to extended treatment time and more costs. Considering the age and the medical condition of this patient, all grafting alternatives were ruled out.

Graftless solutions may include short implants, reduced-diameter implants, or a combination of both, placed in a parallel fashion. Implant placement requires a minimum bone height and width to stabilize the implants in key positions to allow for a good AP distribution.

Two implants placed in the anterior maxilla and two implants distally tilted along the anterior maxillary wall is another available graftless alternative. For both alternatives mentioned, implants always have to be splinted and may require simultaneous grafting ("graft less" approach). As described, in this patient there was no remaining alveolar bone to place any type of implants.

The remaining graftless alternative for this situation is the use of four zygomatic implants (quad zygoma technique), anchored in the zygomatic bone and tilted anteriorly, to allow for an optimal AP distribution. This procedure requires surgical expertise on dealing with the anatomical structures of the midface, and also brings risks related to the anatomy. However, there is sound scientific evidence about this technique, with over 90% survival rates after 10 years. They can be placed in only one stage and even be immediately loaded.

The use of recently developed designs of zygomatic implants, and an anatomically guided approach, gives surgeons an excellent tool to rehabilitate extremely atrophic maxillae. However, this case type is considered complex in both surgical and prosthodontic SAC classification and requires surgeons and prosthodontists with experience to perform all steps in an optimal manner, and also deal with potential complications.

Treatment team:
Surgery: Dr. Waldemar D. Polido
Prosthodontics: Dr. Wei-Shao Lin

5.11 Implants for Restoration of the Full Arch: Fixed

5.11.1 Edentulous mandible: Fixed dental prosthesis

P. CASENTINI

A 59-year-old woman came to our clinic for a recall visit. The patient had already been treated for periodontal disease and was used to visiting the clinic for professional oral hygiene every 4 months. The mandible had undergone treatment for advanced periodontal disease 12 years earlier. This included maintaining the first and second molars with root canal treatment and full metal crowns. The remaining teeth were hopeless, and were extracted and replaced with a removable partial denture stabilized by retainers on the molars. In the maxilla, periodontal treatment allowed the patient to maintain the anterior teeth, and three posterior teeth were replaced by implant-supported reconstructions that allowed a stable occlusion to be maintained.

During the recall visit, root caries were diagnosed underneath the crowns on the mandibular first molars.

Although the patient was satisfied by the previous removable reconstruction, she expressed the desire to evaluate the feasibility of a fixed prosthesis supported by implants, if this option was possible for her budget.

Anamnesis was negative for bruxism. The patient was not taking any medication, was not a smoker, and was in good general health.

CLINICAL AND RADIOGRAPHIC EXAMINATION

In the extraoral view, the patient had a limited exposure of the mandibular teeth during smiling, she had a normal profile, and the support to the extraoral tissues was evaluated as adequate.

During the oral examination, it was possible to confirm the presence of caries involving the roots and the furcation area of the mandibular first molars that were defined hopeless.

The partial removable prosthesis included eight teeth from first premolar to first premolar: occlusion was defined regular with normal contacts between the two arches. The resin teeth of the removable prosthesis and the maxillary teeth did not show significant signs of wear.

In the edentulous area, a certain degree of vertical atrophy with augmented interarch distance was clearly visible. The survival of the mandibular molars, however, contributed to maintain a stable vertical dimension and occlusion.

Palpation of the edentulous area highlighted the presence of a regular profile of the underlying bone crest, without the presence of undercuts. A narrow band of keratinized tissue was still present.

The periodontal conditions of the residual teeth that showed a certain degree of recession were stable, without pathologic

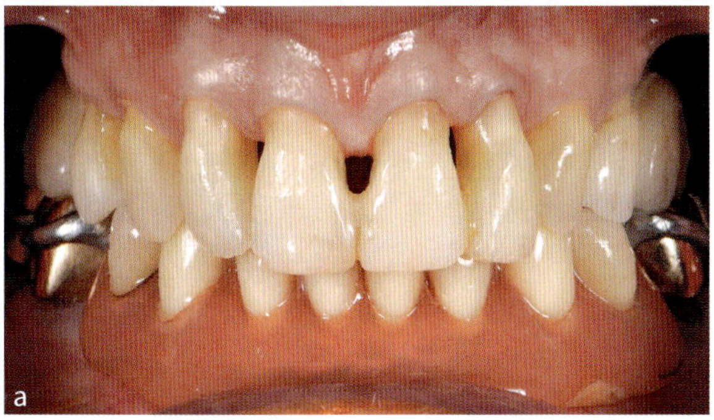

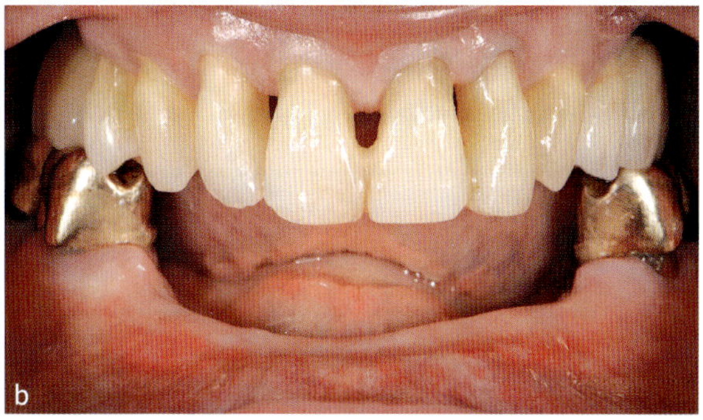

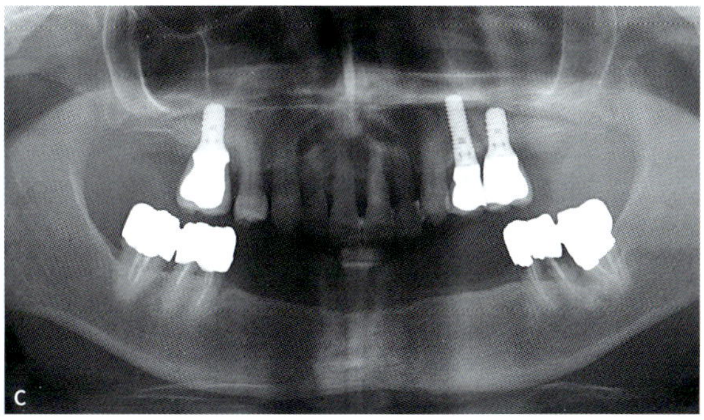

Fig 1 a-c. Intraoral view of the edentulous mandible with and without the removable prosthesis, and panoramic radiograph.

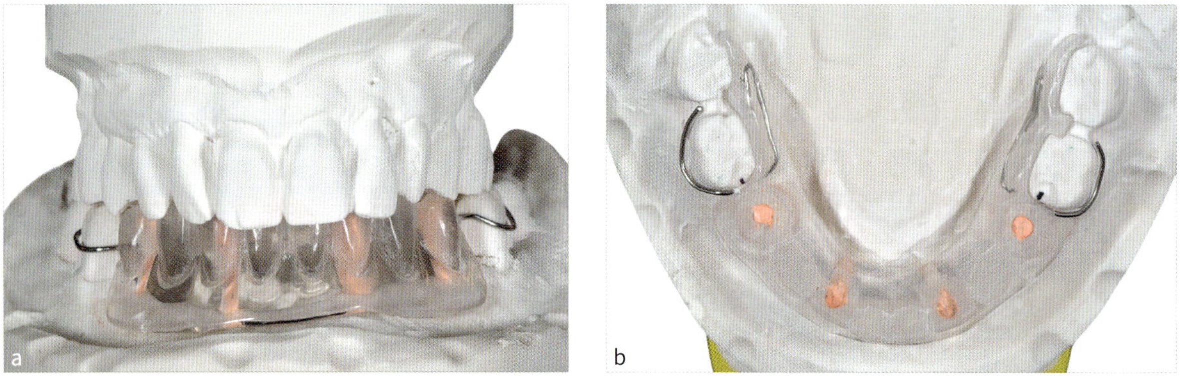

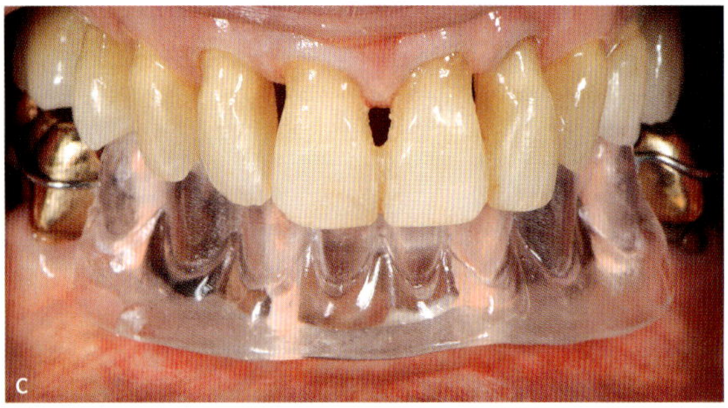

Fig 2 a-c. Diagnostic template on the model and inserted in the oral cavity.

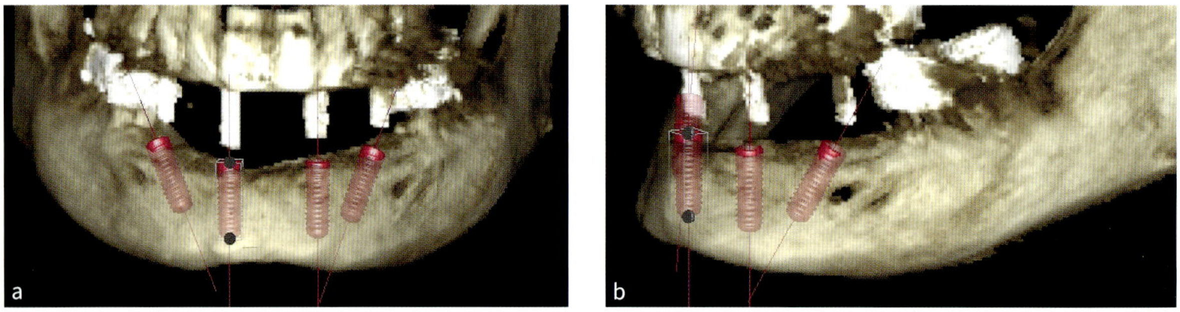

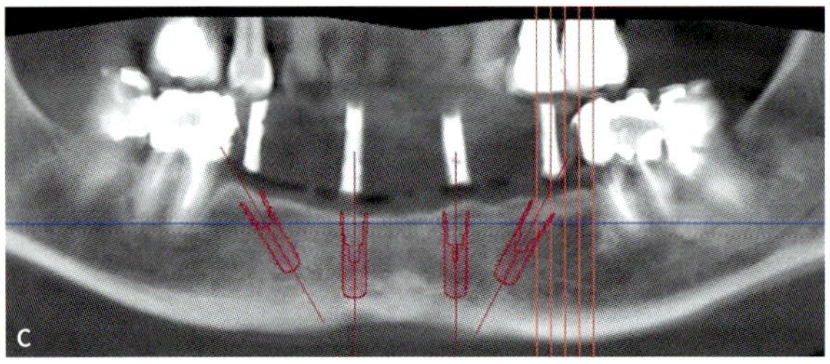

Fig 3 a-c. 3D visualization of the mandible and implant simulation.

probing or bleeding on probing. The maxillary implant-supported crowns also showed healthy peri-implant tissues (Figures 1a and 1b).

The panoramic radiograph confirmed the presence of caries underneath the previous crowns and demonstrated normal density and a certain height of the residual ridge (Figure 1c).

The mental foramina were not clearly identifiable.

DIAGNOSTIC PROTOCOL

A 3D radiographic examination was considered mandatory in order to evaluate bone volume and implant feasibility in the edentulous area. After impressions and bite registration were taken with a wax device, the dental technician created a resin diagnostic template with four radiopaque markers in the positions of the lateral incisors and first premolars, maintaining the same occlusal arrangement as the remov-

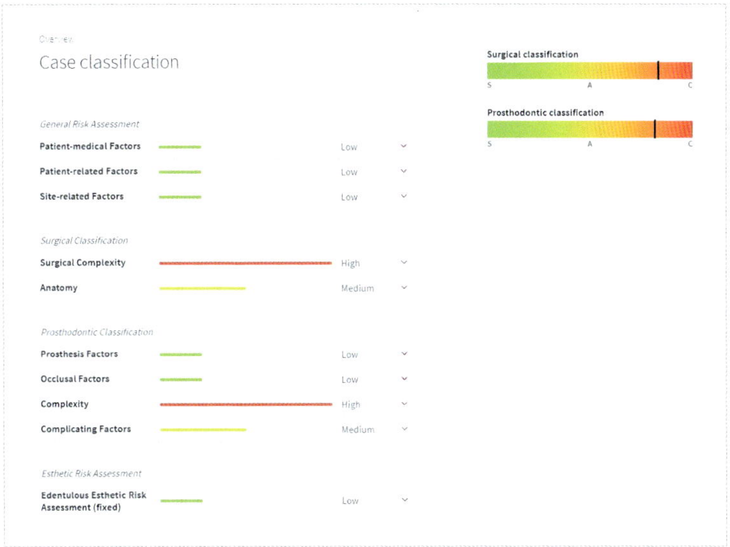

Fig 4. Overall treatment classification: Edentulous esthetic risk = low; Surgical classification = complex; Prosthodontic classification = complex.

able prosthesis. The diagnostic template was stabilized by metal retainers. After the try-in of the template, a CBCT scan was obtained (Figure 2).

The CBCT showed an adequate thickness of the residual alveolar ridge: mental foramina were instead localized in a mesial and superficial position.

Based on the current anatomical condition, traditional implant placement in the position of the premolars was not possible.

However, if the distal implants were tilted, it would be possible to achieve emergence in a more distal position, at the level of the distal radiopaque marker.

Implant positioning was simulated with a planning software (Figure 3).

TREATMENT RISK PROFILE

The treatment risk profile was assessed with the SAC Assessment Tool in order to define specific surgical and prosthetic risk factors (Figure 4).

Esthetic risk was judged low in this case, since the area of treatment is partially visible when the patient smiles. The only critical factor from an esthetic point of view was represented by the need for a prosthetic flange including pink restorative material in order to provide adequate support to the lower lip and allow placement of teeth with a correct length.

The expectations of the patient, from an esthetic point of view, were considered realistic.

The main surgical risk factors were represented by the superficial emergence of the mental nerves. Correct 3D implant placement of multiple implants requires exposure and delicate surgical manipulation in the proximity of the mental nerves. Preparation of distal tilted implant sites also requires visual control of the mental foramina and angulation control.

A second surgical risk factor was the reduced band of keratinized tissue that should be divided between the buccal and the lingual side of the surgical flap; once again, this will require a precise incision and a delicate elevation of the flap.

Finally, a third surgical factor that could be involved in the case of an immediate loading procedure is represented by the need to achieve primary stability and a prosthetically driven implant position in a complex anatomical situation. Multiple prosthetic risk factors should also be considered. One risk factor is the need to perform a certain amount of prosthetic replacement of the soft tissues in order to provide adequate support to the lower lip.

The future reconstruction will be fully involved in occlusion, since the contacts with the opposite arch will be completely provided by the prosthetic reconstruction that will need to reproduce an adequate occlusion.

Another risk factor is the need to manage tilted implants from a prosthetic point of view, since this treatment requires adequate knowledge and management of the specific prosthetic components.

A final, very important prosthetic risk factor is related to the loading protocol. Theoretically, an immediate loading protocol would be the first option in this case because the management of a removable provisional prosthesis would be difficult, uncomfortable for the patient, and increasing risk of failure during the osseointegration phase. On the other hand, immediate loading procedures increase the degree of the required prosthetic skill for the clinician and for the dental laboratory.

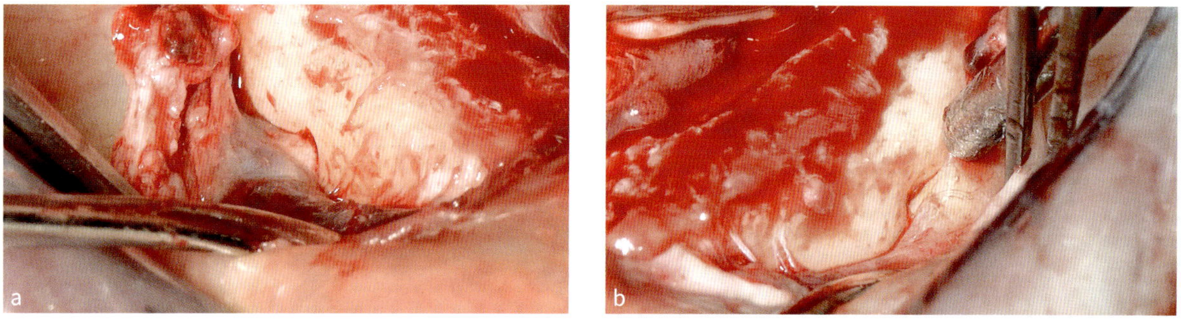

Fig 5 a-b. Exposure of the mental nerve bundle.

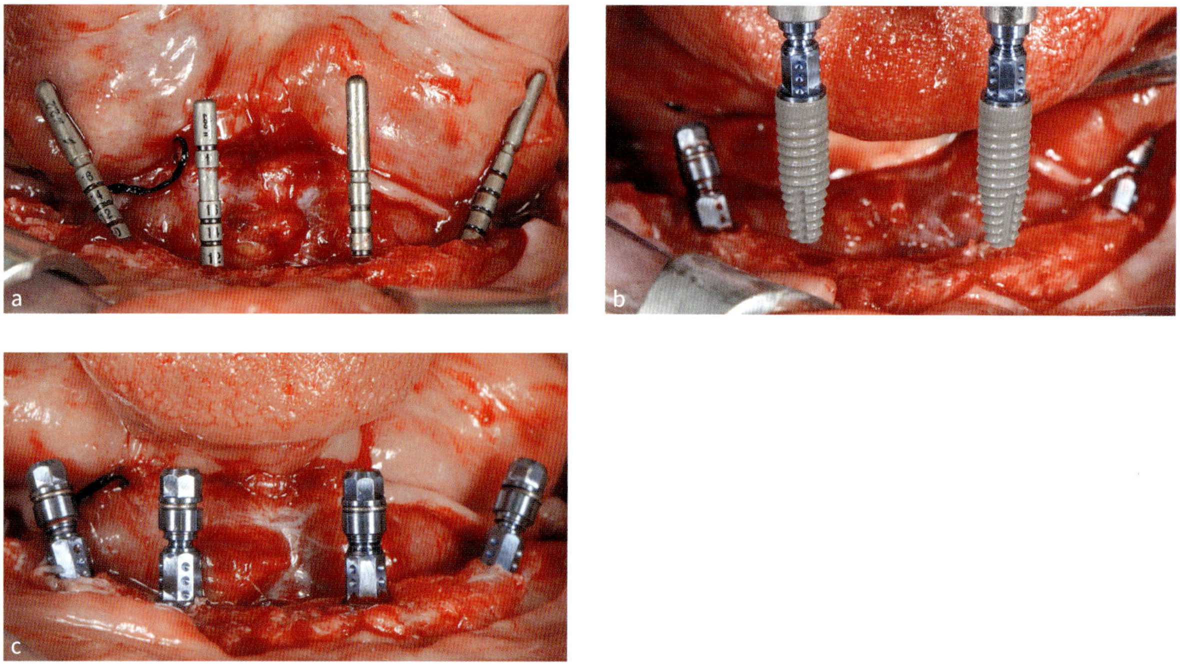

Fig 6 a-c. Different phases of implant site preparation and implant placement.

TREATMENT PLANNING

Based on the clinical and radiologic situation, the following treatment plan was proposed to the patient:

- Extraction of the first molars and placement of four implants between the mental foramina of the mandible.
- In case of adequate primary stability, immediate loading of the implants with the definitive fixed prosthesis, based on a titanium framework veneered with composite resin.
- In case of inadequate primary stability, the old removable partial prosthesis would be modified and relined with a soft material during the osseointegration phase. In this case, the definitive reconstruction would be placed after 12 weeks.

The patient agreed to the proposed treatment, providing her written informed consent.

SURGICAL TREATMENT

Extraction of first molars and implant procedures, including impressions for immediate loading, were performed under local anesthesia in combination with intravenous sedation, and with the assistance of an anesthesiologist.

After extraction of the molars, a flap was elevated, splitting the residual band of keratinized tissue between the buccal and the lingual flap.

The second molars, although they were not in occlusion with the opposite arch, were temporarily maintained to assist with the indexing procedures for immediate loading. Extraction of the second molars was delayed and planned for a second stage.

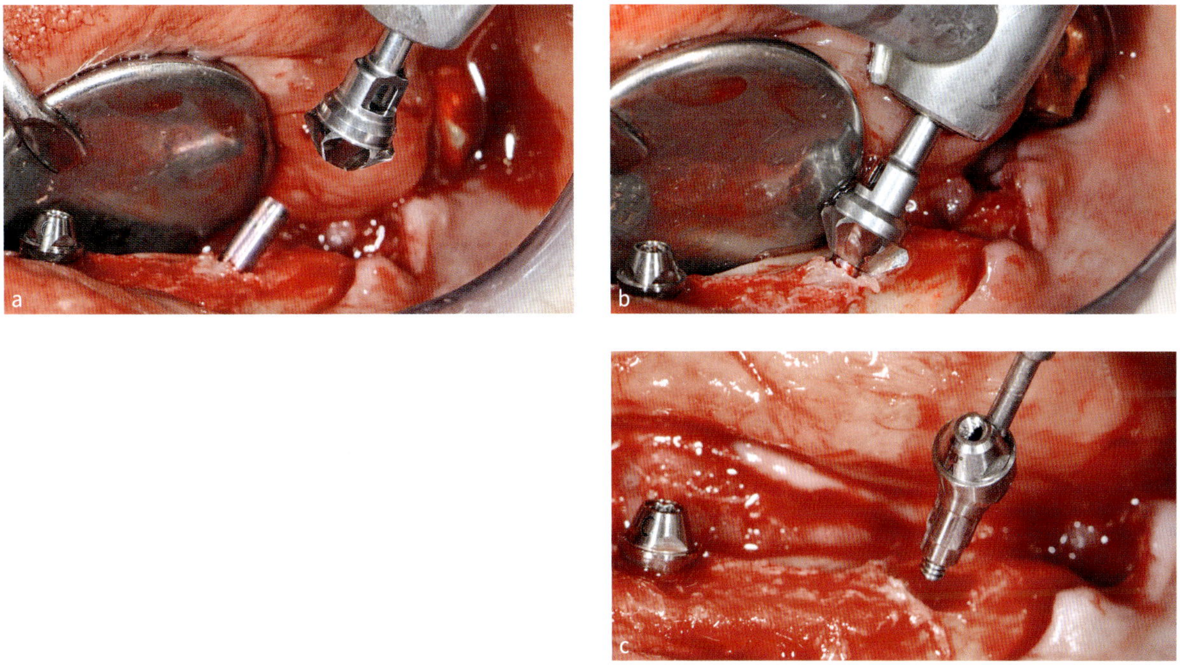

Fig 7 a-c. Use of the bone profiler drill at the distal implants to allow correct insertion of the SRA.

The mental foramina were exposed, and the implant sites were prepared (Figure 5).

Drilling of the distal sites was performed under direct visualization of the mental foramina in order to optimize control of position and angulation of the implants with respect to the nerve bundle. An angulation of approximately 30 degrees was selected for the distal implants (Figure 6a).

Four BLT implants (4.1 × 12 mm) were selected and achieved a high degree of primary stability with an insertion torque greater than 35 Ncm (Figures 6b and c).

Implants with a hydrophilic surface (SLActive) were preferred to shorten the osseointegration time in consideration of the loading protocol.

IMMEDIATE LOADING PROSTHETIC PHASES

Because primary stability of the implants was optimal, the immediate loading protocol was confirmed, and four titanium SRAs were immediately screwed on top of the implants and tightened with a torque of 35 Ncm. The height of the abutments was selected considering the soft tissues thickness. Two straight abutments were selected for the anterior implants, and two abutments with an angulation of 30 degrees for the distal ones. A specific bone profiler drill was used at the distal implants to create an adequate space for correct abutment placement (Figure 7).

Once the SRAs were in position, titanium copings were connected to them, and the flaps were sutured with a 6-0 resorbable sutures (Vicryl).

After isolating the soft tissues with the rubber dam, the implant position was later captured with a resin transfer-stent obtained from the diagnostic template and stabilized with retainers at the second molars. Autopolymerizing resin was used to connect the titanium coping to the transfer template. This indexing procedure allowed the implant position and the bite registration to be recorded in only one step (Figure 8).

After the indexing procedure, polyetheretherketone (PEEK) protection caps were placed on the SRAs to avoid coverage by the soft tissues (Figure 9). The index was immediately sent to the dental laboratory.

The postsurgical pharmacologic protocol included antibiotics for 6 days (amoxicillin + clavulanic acid 1 g every 12 hours), chlorhexidine 0.2% mouthrinses for 2 weeks, and ibuprofen 600 mg for pain relief. The patient was advised to avoid brushing the operated area for 2 weeks.

An appointment was scheduled after 2 days for the delivery of the fixed reconstruction.

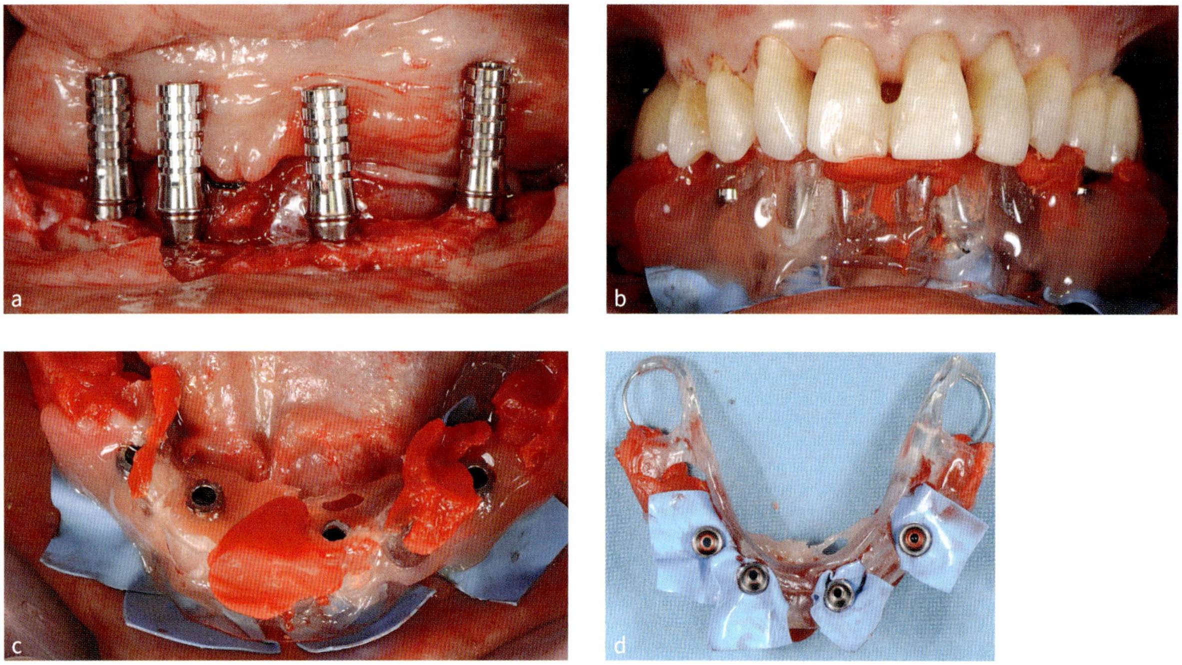

Fig 8 a-d. Titanium copings screwed on top of the SRAs. Indexing procedure was done to define implant position and interarch relationship.

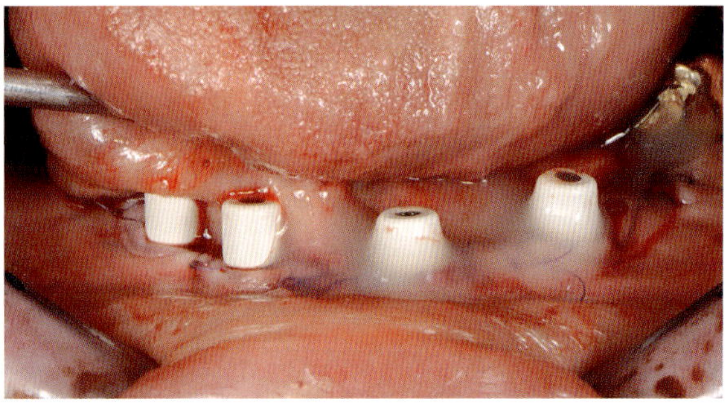

Fig 9. Plastic protective caps in place.

DENTAL LABORATORY PROCEDURES

The dental technician connected the analogs of the SRAs to the index and modified the mandibular model to host the prosthetic analogs.

At the end of the process, he obtained the mandibular model, including the exact position of the SRA, mounted in the correct interarch relationship with the opposite arch (Figure 10).

A screw-retained customized titanium framework was later obtained with a laser melting procedure that allowed the original titanium copings to be connected with bar segments. The titanium framework was subsequently veneered with dental and pink composite resin. The entire dental laboratory protocol required 48 hours, and after this time, the definitive reconstruction was ready for the delivery to the patient (Figure 11).

DELIVERY OF THE FIXED RECONSTRUCTION

After 2 days, the postoperative course was normal, and the patient presented with moderate swelling. The patient was able to achieve a complete control of pain with two ibuprofen tablets per day. The soft tissues had a normal aspect after 2 days of healing, and the sutures were still in place.

The wound was gently rinsed with a chlorhexidine 0.2% solution, and the protective PEEK caps were removed. The fixed prosthesis was positioned over the SRAs, and the fixation screws were gently tightened in order to verify the presence of a passive fit. Excessive compression on the soft tissues was excluded, and the patient did not report any discomfort (Figure 12).

Occlusion was carefully checked, and minimal adjustments were required.

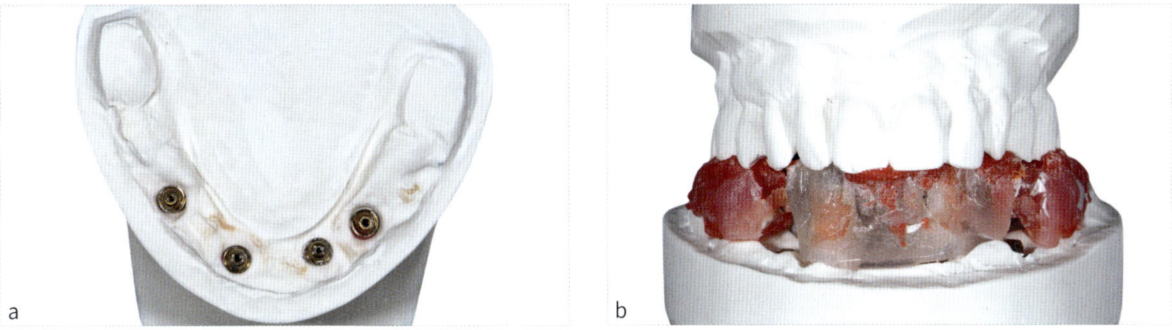

Fig 10 a-b. Mandibular model with implants in place mounted with the opposite arch.

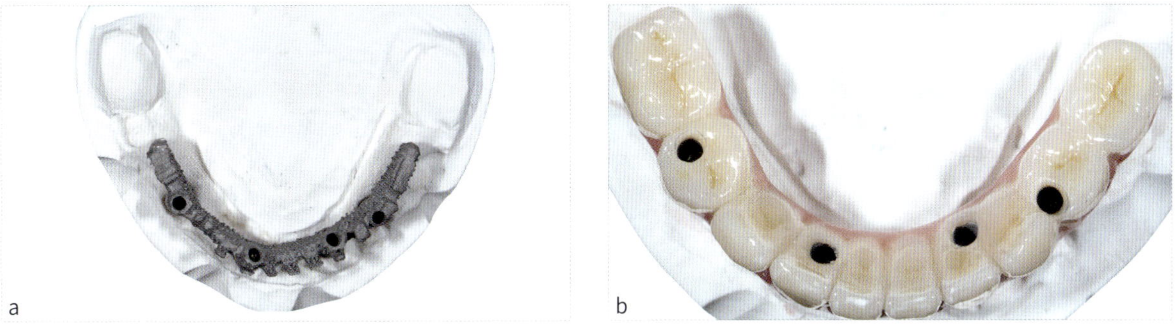

Fig 11 a-b. Titanium framework and definitive prosthesis on the model.

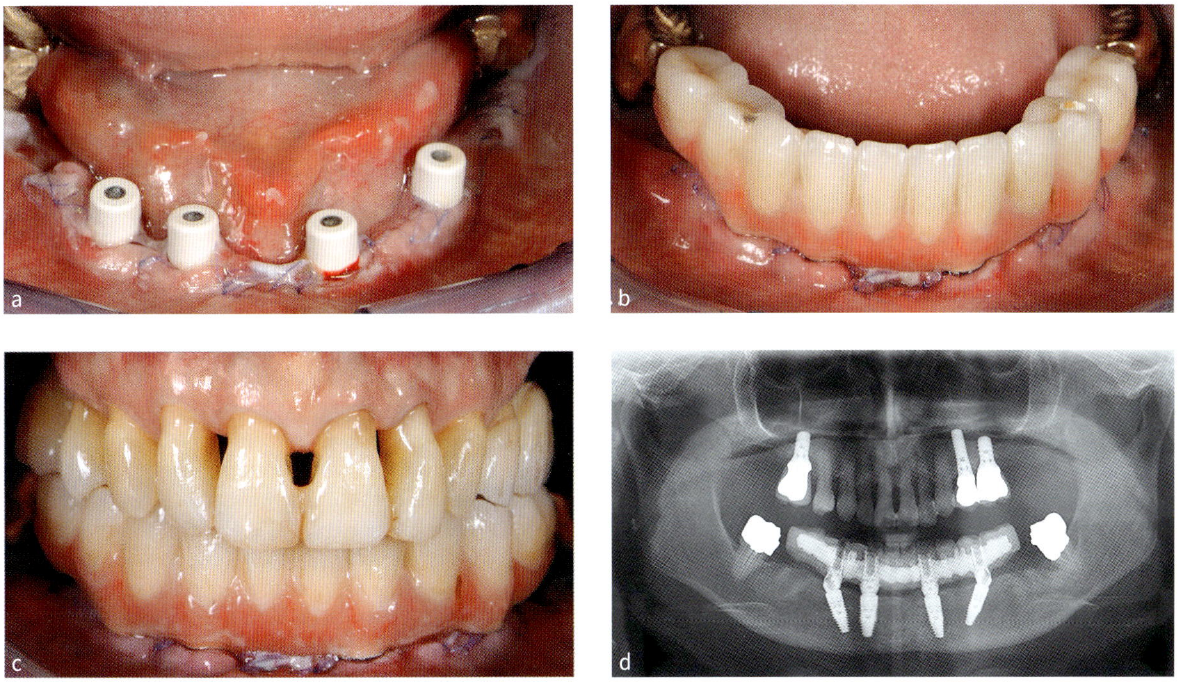

Fig 12 a-d. Delivery of the definitive fixed reconstructions 2 days after surgery, and radiographic control.

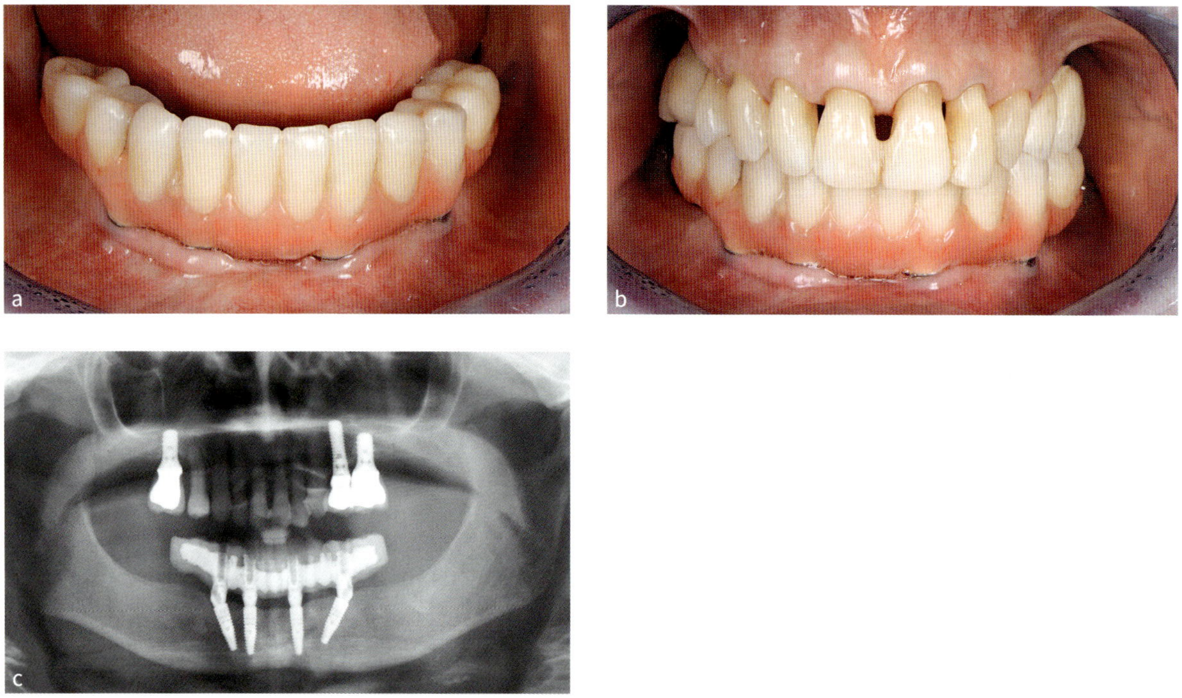

Fig 13 a-c. Five-year clinical and radiographic follow-up.

After the patient approved the esthetic appearance of the prosthetic reconstruction, the screws were activated with a controlled torque of 15 Ncm.

A panoramic radiograph confirmed precise fit of the full-arch reconstruction.

Subsequently, the access holes were sealed with packed Teflon tape and with a temporary filling material.

A soft diet was recommended to the patient for 6 weeks, and suture removal was planned after 2 weeks.

After suture removal, specific hygienic instructions were provided to the patient, and in particular the use of an interproximal brush and dental floss were recommended.

After 2 months, the implant-supported reconstruction was disconnected and reconnected after osseointegration of the implants was confirmed. No significant changes in the soft tissue profile could be recorded, and no relining procedure of the pink flange was necessary.

The access holes were again sealed with packed Teflon tape and with flowable composite resin.

The patient declared herself fully satisfied by the treatment outcome and reported a significant improvement in the ability to chew, and in her quality of life in general.

FOLLOW-UP

A 4-month recall for professional oral hygiene was maintained in consideration of the patient's susceptibility to periodontal disease. The patient always demonstrated a high standard of maintenance. No increased periodontal probing depth nor bleeding on probing were recorded on natural teeth and implant sites during the follow-up visits.

After 5 years, the occlusal surfaces of the fixed reconstruction did not show a significant wear.

The control radiograph after 5 years showed stable peri-implant bone levels.

The patient confirmed that her esthetic and functional expectations had been fully satisfied, and she was able to easily clean the treated area without any kind of discomfort (Figure 13).

DISCUSSION

Immediate loading of implants in an edentulous arch with the definitive reconstruction is not a routine procedure, and it can be applied only if specific conditions are present. In particular, a stable occlusion represents a mandatory condition.

An optimal primary stability of implants and a well-defined prosthetic and laboratory protocol are also fundamental requisites.

Specific limitations of this protocol can be identified:

- Because there will only be a definitive prosthesis and no provisional prosthesis will be used, during laboratory procedures that require 48 hours, the patient will remain edentulous.
- It is not possible to create a metal-ceramic framework in 48 hours. The protocol can be therefore applied if the planned definitive reconstruction will be a metal (titanium) and composite resin prosthesis.
- If significant remodeling of the soft tissues will take place during healing, a relining procedure of the pink flange could be necessary after some months.

On the other hand, this approach presents different benefits:

- Treatment time and chair time can be remarkably reduced because the entire process requires basically one diagnostic session, one surgical-prosthetic session, and one session for the delivery of the definitive reconstruction.
- The definitive reconstruction is delivered 48 hours after implant placement.
- No provisional prosthesis, removable or fixed, will be used.
- CAD/CAM procedures are not required, and the restorative materials are represented by titanium and composite resin. In the meantime, precise connection between the fixed reconstruction and the SRAs is guaranteed by the use of the original titanium copings.
- In consideration of all the previous aspects, the costs of this kind of reconstruction can be significantly reduced, and this allows this treatment to be offered even to patients with a limited budget.
- The SRAs are tightened to 35 Ncm immediately after implant placement and never disconnected; this procedure should prevent bone resorption around the head of the implants.
- Following the experience of the author, if a correct surgical and prosthetic protocol is applied, the predictability of the protocol is very high, and it allows a fixed reconstruction to be offered at a reasonable cost to more patients.

Based on these considerations and on the experience of many cases treated with success, the presented protocol can represent a further option in the treatment of the totally edentulous patients.

Treatment team:
Surgery and prosthetics: Dr. Paolo Casentini
Laboratory: Alessandro Giacometti

5.11.2 Edentulous maxilla and mandible: Implant-supported all-ceramic fixed complete dentures

D. MORTON, WS. LIN, W. D. POLIDO

A 56-year-old man presented requesting treatment for his deteriorating dentition. His chief complaints included an inability to chew and smile. He stated that he was embarrassed to socialize and understood that he was responsible for his oral condition and was highly motivated to make things better. The patient had seen a general dentist and had been referred for care due to the complexity of treatment options.

A review of his medical history identified no factors of significance to dental treatment, inclusive of implant surgery. He reported no allergies and no routine use of medications. He reported regular care by his medical care provider and denied use of tobacco, alcohol, or any recreational drugs. Extraoral examination revealed appropriate lip mobility, tissue tone, and health. The patient demonstrated moderate display of both the maxillary and mandibular teeth in repose and during function (Figure 1).

His missing teeth and occlusal plane disharmony were visible during speech and smiling. The patient demonstrated a short to medium maxillary lip length. During both speech and swallowing, he demonstrated lip competence without strain. His pretreatment panoramic radiograph revealed no evidence of pathology. Missing teeth, occlusal plane disharmony, periodontal compromise, and dental caries were noted. The alveolar ridges in the areas of missing teeth appeared to be of adequate height (Figure 2).

Intraoral examination revealed a deteriorating dentition. Dental caries was evident throughout, and many existing restorations were fractured or esthetically compromised. His oral hygiene was considered to be poor (Figure 3).

The patient expressed a strong desire to have his remaining teeth removed. He was presented with several treatment alternatives, including periodontal therapy and restoration of his teeth with missing teeth to be replaced by implant-assisted fixed prostheses or removable partial prostheses. Additional treatment options subsequent to tooth removal were implant-assisted overdentures and implant-assisted fixed metal acrylic or all-ceramic prostheses.

TREATMENT RISK ASSESSMENT

The SAC Assessment Tool was used to evaluate surgical, prosthetic, and esthetic risk factors and determine risk associated with the chosen treatment plan. For the maxilla, both the surgical and prosthodontic classifications were considered complex, and the estimation of risk based on

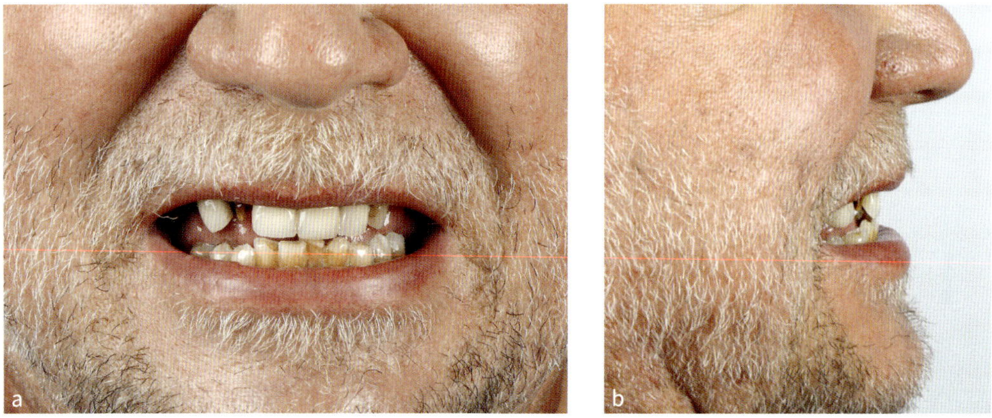

Fig 1 a-b. Frontal and lateral profile views, pretreatment.

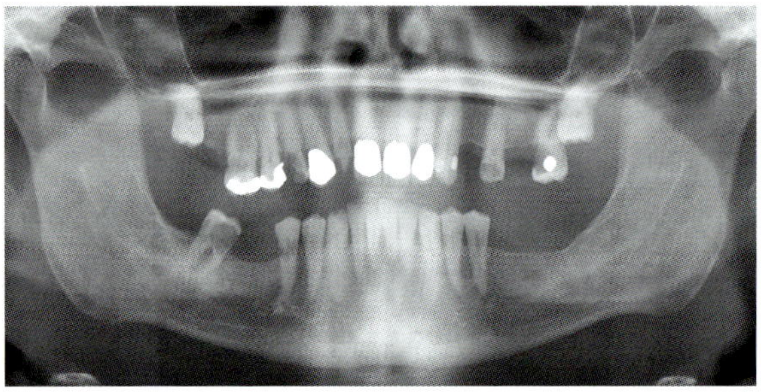

Fig 2. Panoramic radiograph, pretreatment.

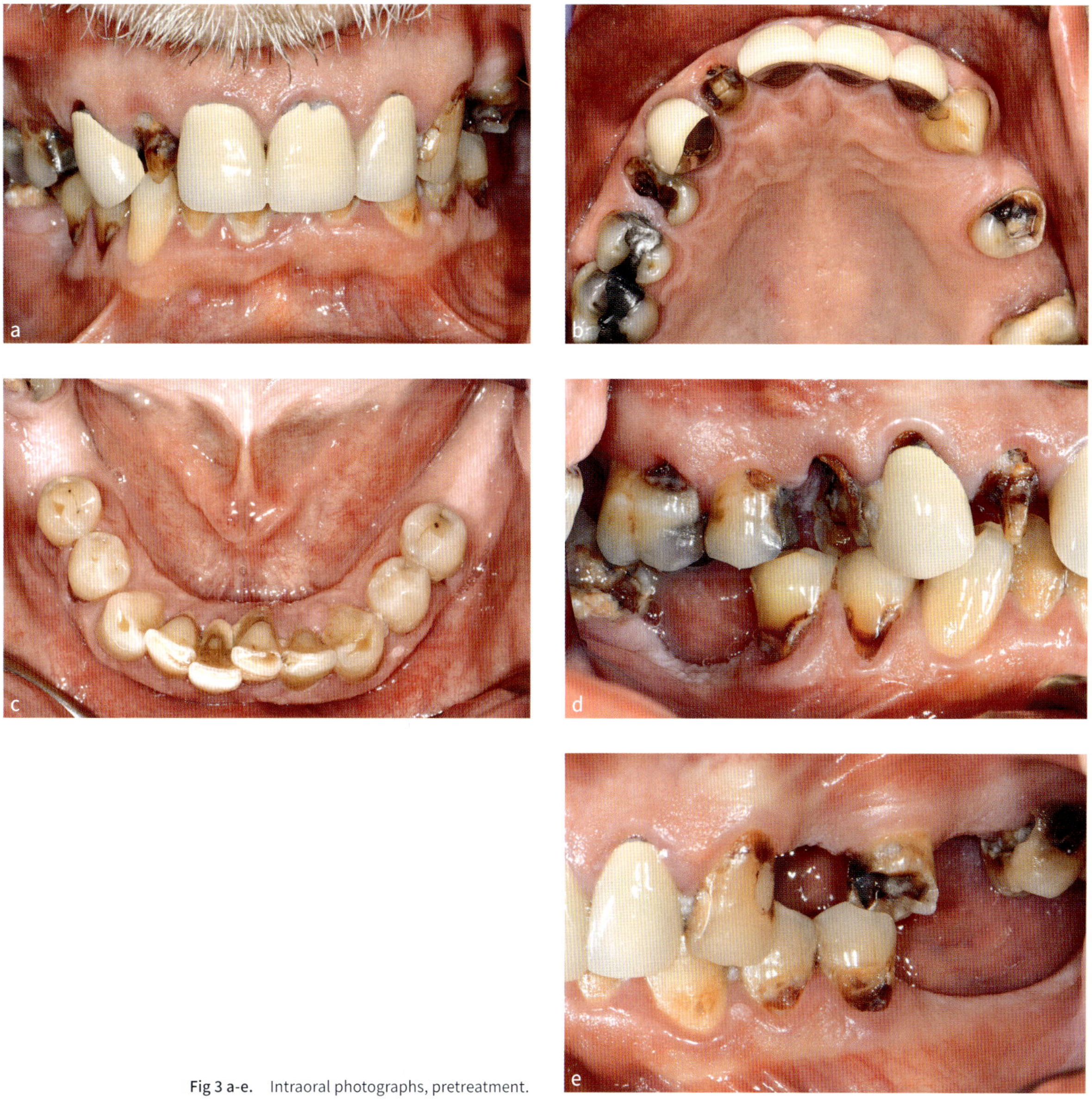

Fig 3 a-e. Intraoral photographs, pretreatment.

alerts and warnings was high (Figure 4). For the mandible, the classification was also considered complex and the estimation of risk high (Figure 5).

The patient's general risk assessment was considered to be favorable and with a low risk. He presented with no consequential medical concerns and was taking no medications. He had no history of radiation treatment, and his growth was complete. He presented with poor oral hygiene habits, although his commitment to his future oral health was strong. He demonstrated good compliance with instructions prior to the initiation of treatment, and his expectations were realistic. He demonstrated no restrictions with regard to opening or jaw movements in general, and access to both maxillary and mandibular operative fields was considered adequate. Radiographic assessment (including CBCT) identified no pathology, and he had no history of surgeries other than previous extractions, which were described as uneventful.

For the maxilla, the surgical classification was identified as a high risk of complications, specifically with regard to complexity. The treatment sequence chosen for the maxilla included extraction of the teeth and an 8- to 12-week period of healing prior to implant placement. Evaluation of the CBCT identified insufficient bone volume facial to the anterior teeth, and he therefore did not satisfy criteria for immediate implant placement. Early implant placement in the maxilla with possible facial augmentation was considered to be medium risk. The placement of more than two

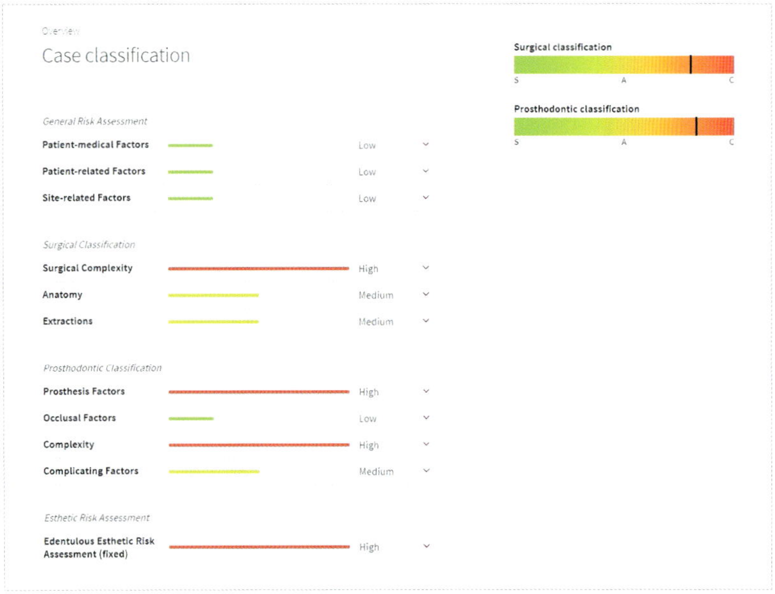

Fig 4. Overall treatment classification maxilla: Edentulous esthetic risk = high; Surgical classification = advanced to complex; Prosthodontic classification = advanced to complex.

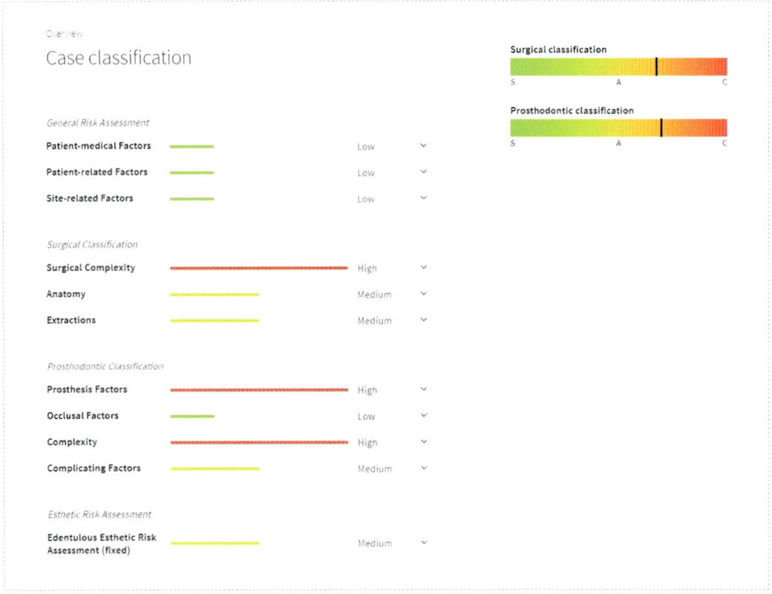

Fig 5. Overall treatment classification mandible: Edentulous esthetic risk = medium; Surgical classification = advanced to complex; Prosthodontic classification = advanced to complex.

implants planned to support a fixed prosthesis was considered high risk as a result of the importance of 3D implant position. The patient's anatomical evaluation concluded a low risk of complications, as did the extraction of the teeth.

The prosthodontic classification for the maxillary treatment was considered low risk with regard to prosthesis factors. There appeared to be adequate volume for the prosthesis and favorable interocclusal space. Further, the characteristics of the residual ridge were considered favorable. The involvement of guidance in the planned rehabilitation elevated risk to high with regard to occlusal factors, even with a user-defined scheme being achievable and in the absence of parafunction. Treatment complexity was also considered to be high risk. The need for an interim tissue-supported complete removable prosthesis, and the need for a screw-retained implant-supported provisional prosthesis, connecting more than two implants, elevated risk. The chosen early loading protocol was considered to be low risk. Complicating factors, including biologic, technical, and mechanical considerations in addition to the contour of the prosthesis intaglio, were also considered to be low risk.

The esthetic risk assessment for the edentulous maxilla and the planned fixed prosthesis was considered high. Although facial and labial support could be obtained from the teeth, and therefore represented low risk, the presence of a relatively short upper lip and wide buccal corridor were considered to elevate risk into the high category. The smile line and the jaw relationships were considered favorable.

For the mandible, the surgical classification was considered high risk. This was primarily as a result of the immediate implant placement protocol. The possible need for simultaneous grafting of minor defects was considered to be of medium risk. The placement of more than two implants planned to support a fixed prosthesis was considered to be high risk. The presenting anatomical conditions were considered to be of low risk, and factors relating to the extraction of the teeth were considered to be of medium risk.

The prosthodontic classification included four subcategories. Factors relating to the prosthesis were considered to be low risk as a result of adequate prosthetic volume and favorable ridge characteristics. The need to develop an occlusal scheme that included guidance elevated the occlusal factors to high risk. The complexity of the procedures was also considered high risk as a result of the need for an implant-supported fixed provisional restoration, the need for the fixed prosthesis to engage more than two implants, and the immediate loading protocol in conjunction with the immediate implant placement. Complicating factors were considered high risk as a result of likely mechanical and technical complications associated mostly with the need for a short posterior cantilever.

Although the overall edentulous esthetic risk was considered high, treatment of the mandible was considered to be of less significance than the maxilla. Aspects of esthetic risk associated with the mandible considered low included favorable facial and labial support being obtained from the teeth, a favorable smile line without maxillary ridge exposure, and a favorable maxillomandibular relationship. The wide buccal corridor of the patient was considered to be high risk with regard to complications.

PLANNING AND CLINICAL TREATMENT

The patient presented with no medical contraindications to treatment. He was philosophic and considered all treatment options presented to him. The patient consented to having his teeth removed and the placement of four implants in each arch to support fixed cross-arch zirconia prostheses. He elected to sequence his treatment. The first phase included having his maxillary teeth removed and the provision of an immediate interim complete removable denture.

After 8 weeks of healing, a digital volume CBCT was obtained and a digital diagnostic waxing was completed to facilitate restoration-driven implant planning for the maxilla and mandible. The diagnostic waxing identified proposed tooth position and demonstrated that adequate prosthetic space was available for fixed all-ceramic prostheses in each arch. Based on the proposed tooth position and the required restorative space, the 3D positions of four implants were identified for both the maxilla (Straumann Bone Level Implants) and the mandible (Straumann Tissue Level Implants).

The decision was made to place bone-level implants in the maxilla with distal inclination or tilting of the posterior implants. The implants were to be placed and loaded using early protocols. For the mandible, axially inclined tissue-level implants were planned to be placed immediately after tooth extraction and minor ridge reduction (Figure 6). A fixed screw-retained provisional prosthesis was planned to be positioned immediately after implant placement.

Maxillary and mandibular provisional restorations were fabricated and prepared for future intraoral indexing to provisional abutments. Templates for residual ridge reduction (mandible), guided implant placement (maxilla and mandible), and positioning of the provisional restorations were fabricated.

Guided placement of the four maxillary implants was undertaken, and the implants were allowed to heal undisturbed for a period of 8 weeks. Surgical management of the mandible was then undertaken. The mandibular teeth were extracted and the template for bone reduction positioned (Figure 7).

Excess alveolar bone was removed and the template for guided implant placement positioned (Figure 8). The mandibular implants were then positioned (Figure 9). During the surgical procedure, the implant planned for the mandibular left second preomlar site was moved to the position of the first premolar as a result of implant instability. Subsequent to placement of all implants, the guided template was removed and the primary stability of the implants verified.

Provisional abutments were placed into the mandibular implants and the provisional restoration positioned using an index fitted to the bone reduction guide and the opposing interim complete denture (Figure 10). Each provisional abutment was then luted to the provisional restoration using autopolymerizing methyl methacrylate resin. The mandibular provisional restoration and bone reduction guide were then removed and separated before the provisional restoration was finished and delivered.

Healing of the implants in the mandible was uneventful, and the patient was satisfied with the esthetic and function-

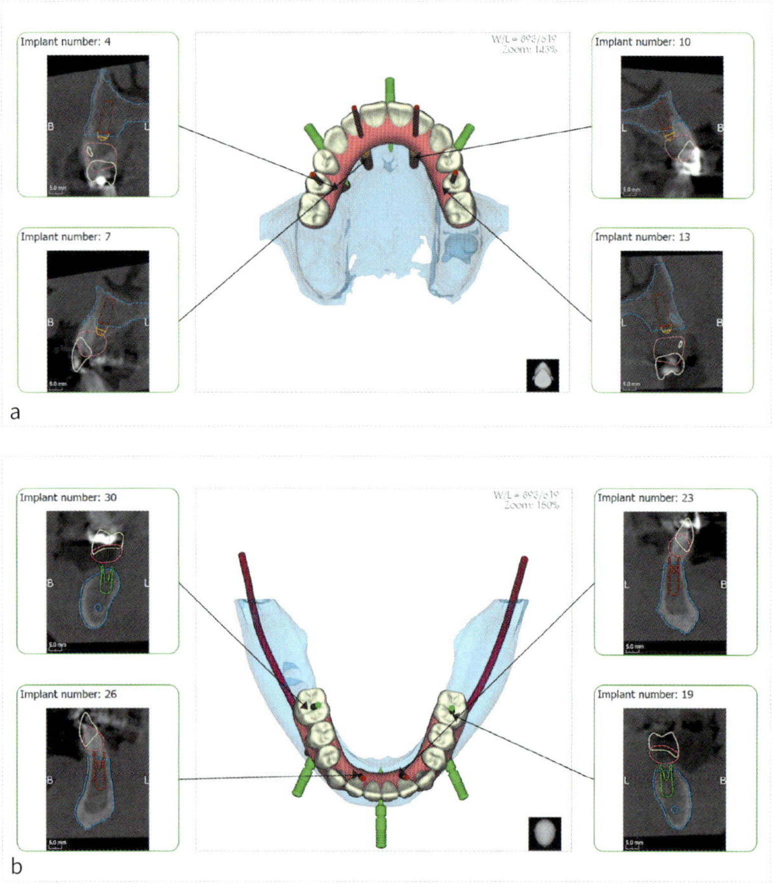

Fig 6 a-b. Implant planning.

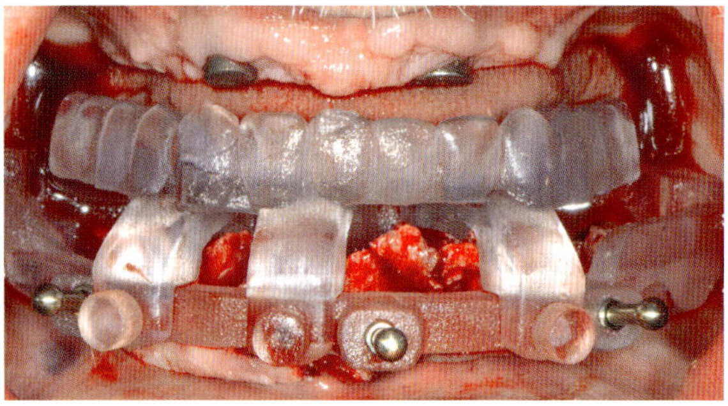

Fig 7. Mandibular tooth extractions and positioning of bone reduction template.

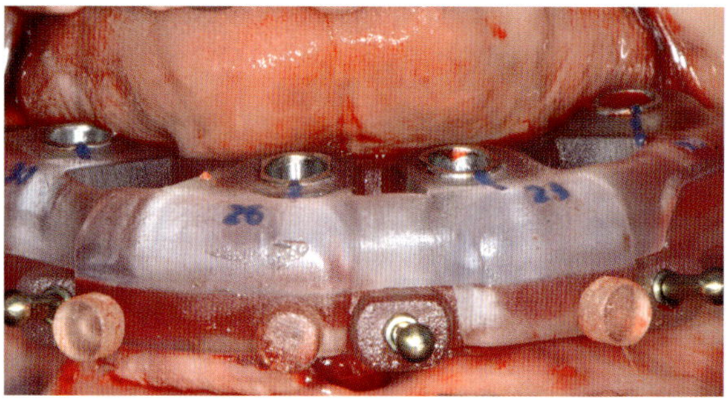

Fig 8. Template for guided implant placement.

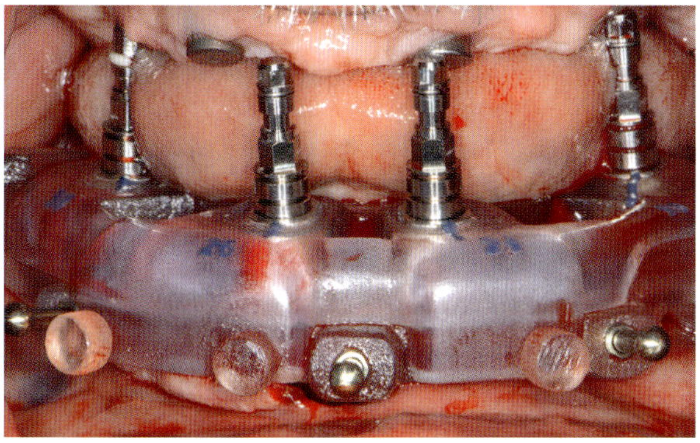

Fig 9. Placement of mandibular implants prior to repositioning of the distal left implant from second premolar to first premolar.

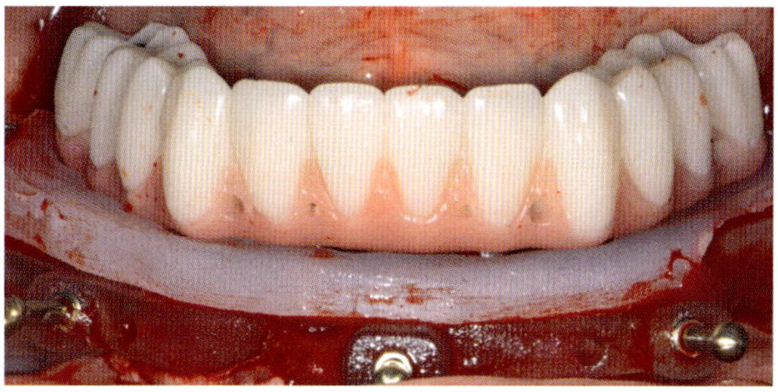

Fig 10. Positioning and indexing of the mandibular provisional restoration.

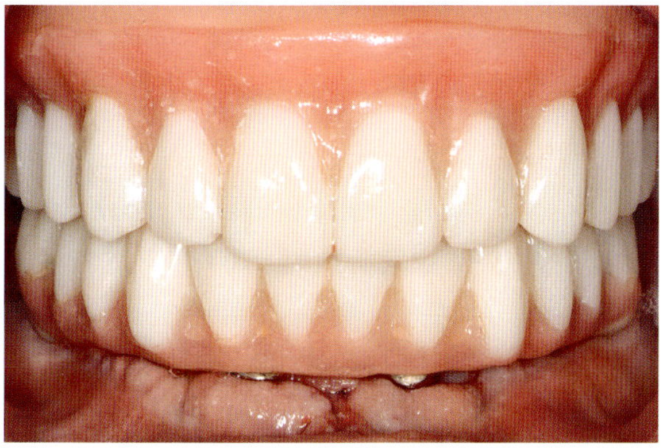

Fig 11. Two-week follow up. Mandibular fixed provisional restoration and maxillary interim complete denture.

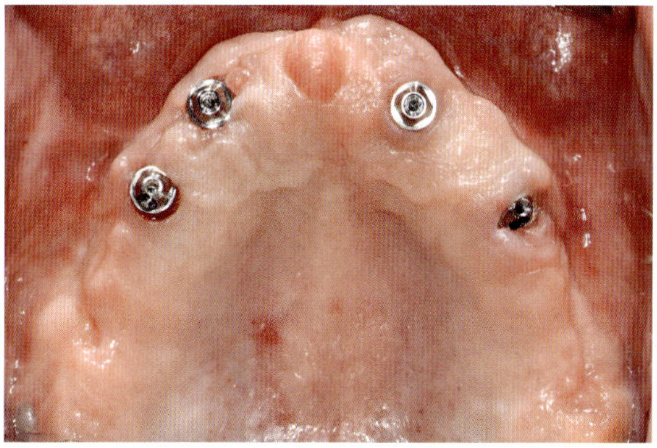

Fig 12. Maxillary SRAs.

al result. The patient returned for follow-up after 2 weeks (Figure 11).

The healing abutments on the maxillary implants were removed, and SRAs were positioned and torqued to 35 Ncm (Figure 12). Provisional titanium copings were positioned on each of the SRAs, and the tissues were protected with rubber dam. The prefabricated maxillary provisional prosthesis was positioned over the provisional abutments and connected sequentially using autopolymerizing methyl methacrylate. The position of the maxillary provisional restoration was confirmed via occlusion with the mandibular provisional while the methyl methacrylate was allowed to polymerize around each abutment. The indexed maxillary provisional prosthesis was removed, finished, and delivered. Occlusion was finely adjusted and esthetic satisfaction of the patient confirmed (Figure 13).

The patient returned after 4 weeks for evaluation. He reported no concerns with regard to function or esthetics and was completely satisfied with the outcome. He demonstrated excellent oral hygiene, and his commitment to treatment remained high. A facebow registration was obtained along with intraoral scans of the provisional restorations and digital interocclusal records. The provisional restorations were then removed from each arch and scan bodies positioned (Figure 14). Intraoral scans (digital impressions) were made of each arch. Maxillary and man-

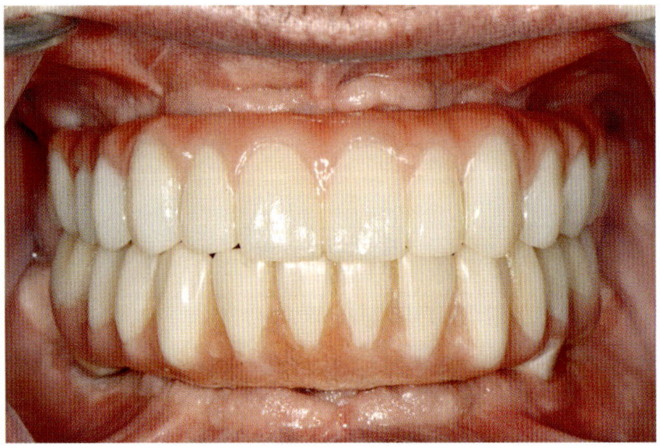

Fig 13. Frontal view of screw-retained maxillary and mandibular provisional prostheses.

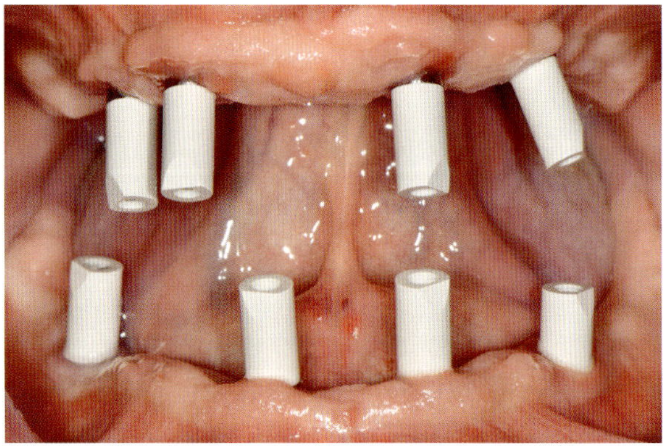

Fig 14. Scan bodies (impression copings) in place.

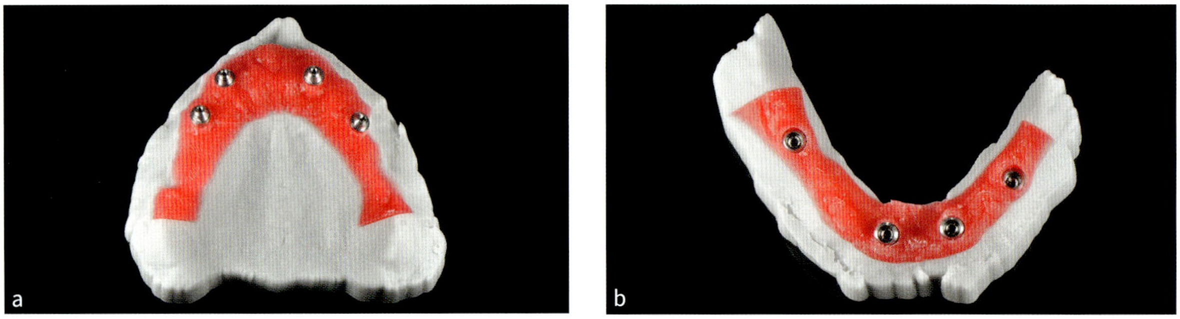

Fig 15 a-b. Printed maxillary (a) and mandibular (b) casts.

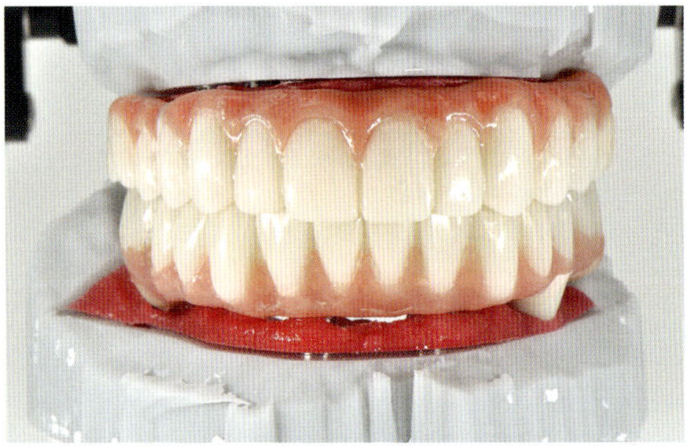

Fig 16. Articulated provisional prostheses.

dibular casts were printed and implant analogs positioned (Figure 15). The casts were articulated using the provisional prostheses, the facebow registration, and interocclusal records (Figure 16). The casts of the scanned provisional restorations were cross articulated (Figure 17).

Matrices were digitally designed and fabricated to facilitate the making of verification casts on which the final cementation of definitive prostheses will take place. Impression copings were positioned and indexed to the matrices (Figure 18). Abutment (maxilla) and implant (mandible) analogs were positioned and the verification casts poured in type IV dental stone (Figure 19). The provisional restorations were then returned to the patient.

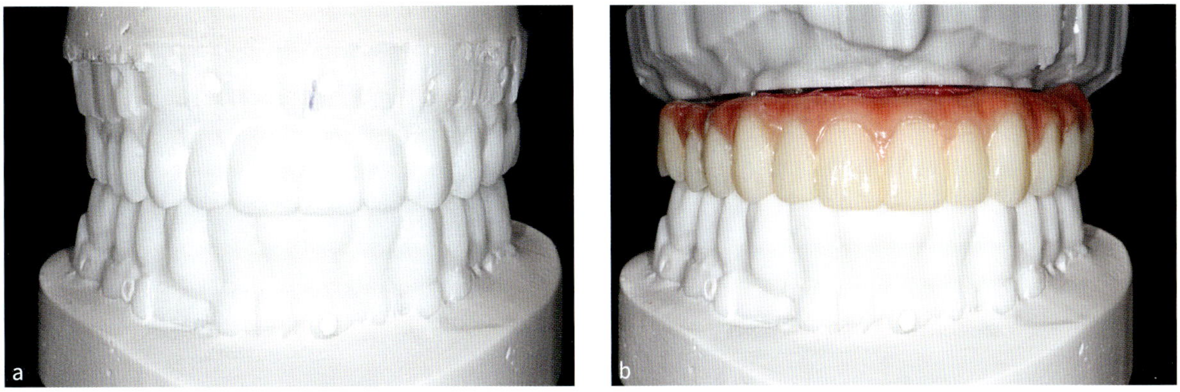

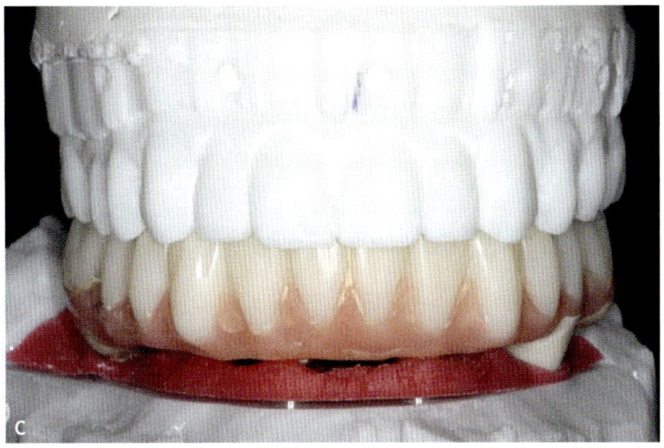

Fig 17 a-c. Cross-articulated duplicate provisional prostheses.

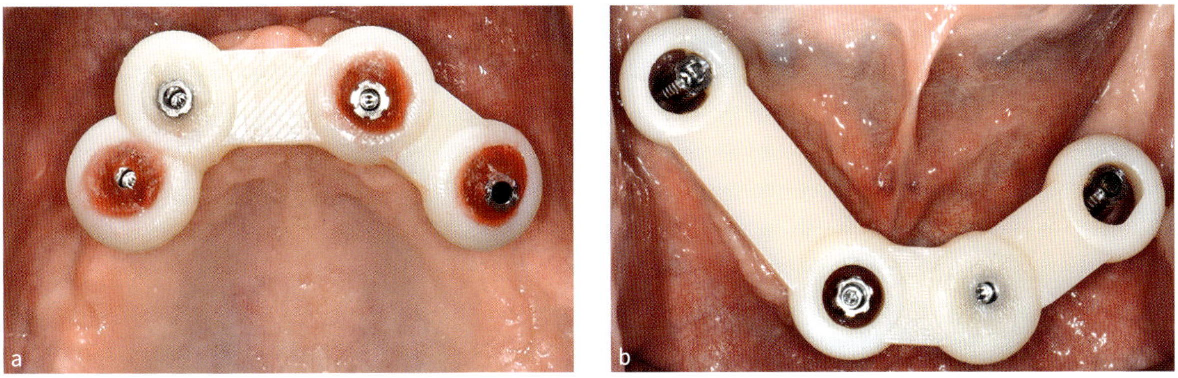

Fig 18 a-b. Indexing of maxillary (a) and mandibular (b) verification matrices.

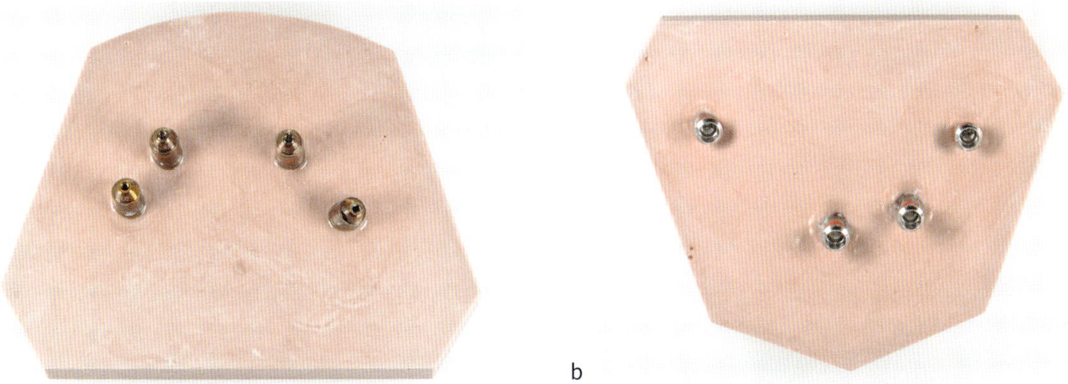

a b

Fig 19 a-b. Maxillary (a) and mandibular (b) verification casts.

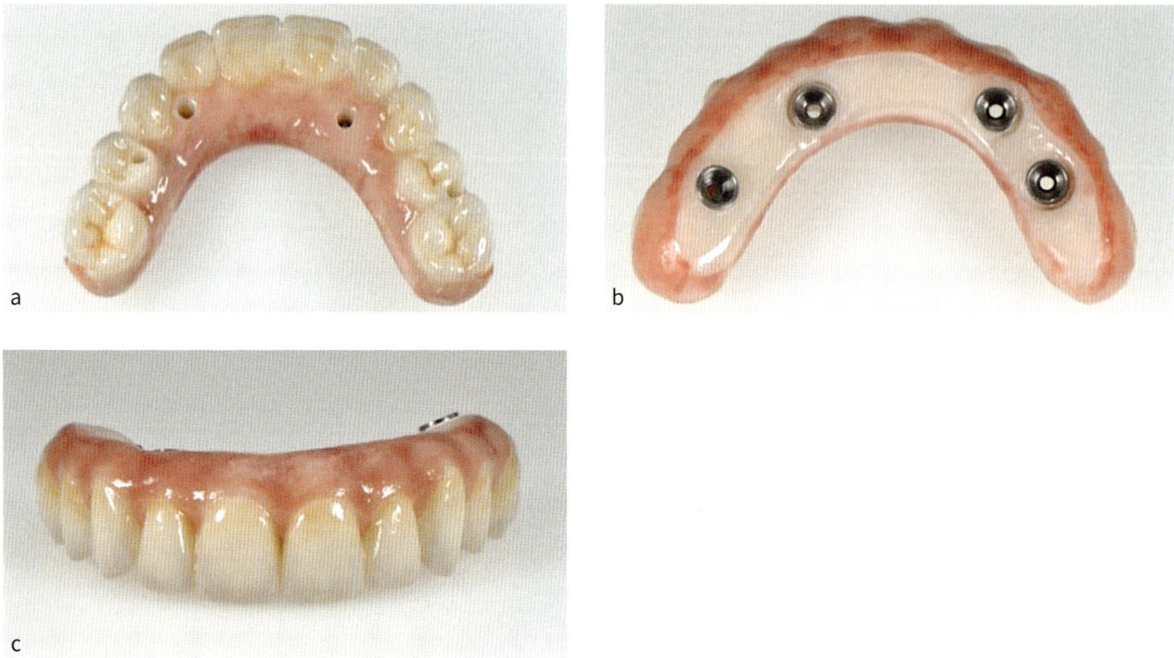

Fig 20 a-c. Definitive maxillary prosthesis.

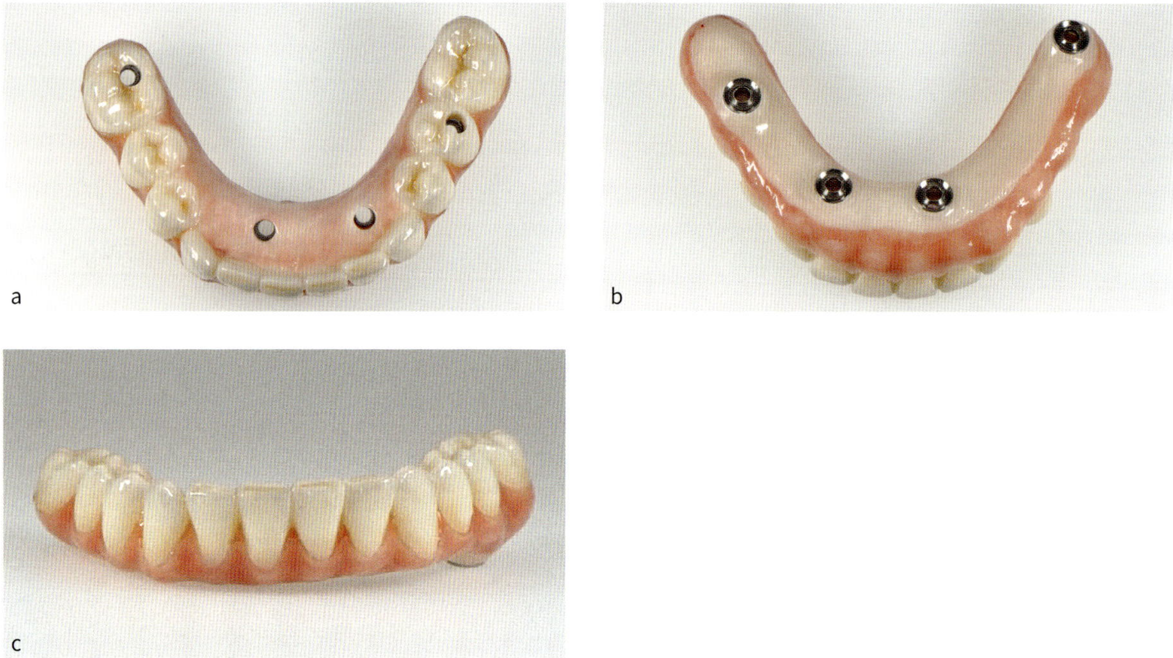

Fig 21 a-c. Definitive mandibular prosthesis.

Maxillary (Figure 20) and mandibular (Figure 21) zirconia fixed prostheses were designed, milled, and surface customized in the dental laboratory. The zirconia prostheses were luted to copings positioned on the verification casts, cleaned, and finished. The definitive prostheses were returned for delivery to the patient.

Subsequent to removal of the maxillary provisional restoration, torque was confirmed for the SRAs. The maxillary definitive prosthesis was tried in and confirmed as clinically passive prior to esthetic and phonetic evaluation by the patient. Cleansability was confirmed along with tissue adaptation. The mandibular provisional restoration was then removed and

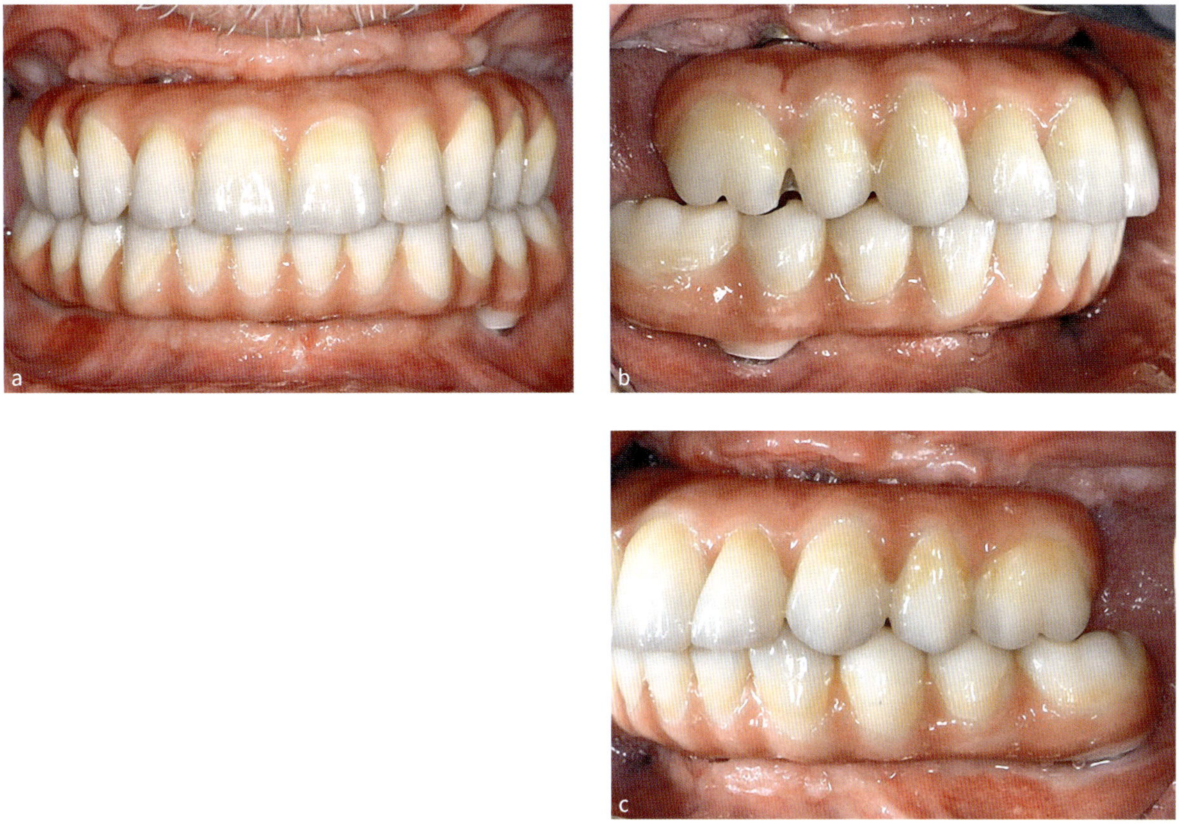

Fig 22 a-c. Definitive maxillary and mandibular prostheses.

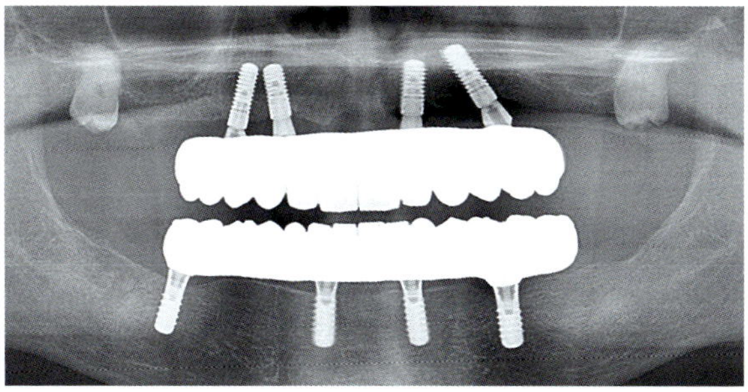

Fig 23. Panoramic radiograph at delivery appointment.

the definitive prosthesis introduced. Clinical passivity, tissue adaptation, and cleansability were confirmed. Occlusion was carefully evaluated and minor adjustments made as indicated, and the prostheses were then removed and the minor areas of adjustment highly polished. The definitive prostheses were then delivered. The maxillary retaining screws were torqued to 20 Ncm and the mandibular abutment screws torqued to 35 Ncm and access holes sealed (Figure 22). A panoramic baseline radiograph was obtained (Figure 23).

The patient has reported complete satisfaction with the treatment outcome. He has experienced no functional, mechanical, or technical complications. He is extremely satisfied with the esthetic outcome (Figure 24a, b). He is committed to supportive maintenance each 3 months for the first year and then every 6 months.

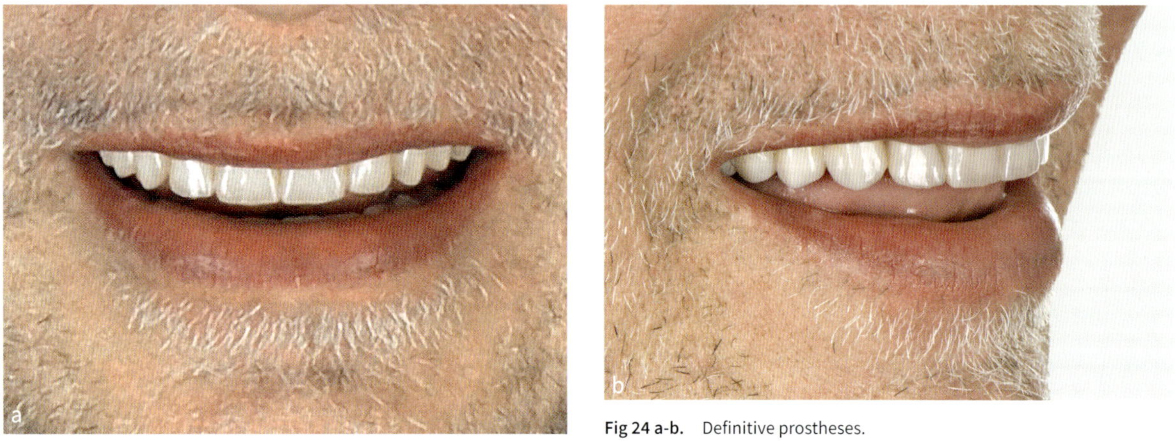

Fig 24 a-b. Definitive prostheses.

REFLECTION ON THE TREATMENT APPROACH AND OUTCOME

The mandibular treatment plan involved immediate implant placement and immediate provisional restoration of the implants. Tissue-level implants were chosen for their biomechanical superiority and because a majority of each implant would be placed in healthy bone beyond the confines of the extraction sockets. It is recognized that tapered (BLX) or apically tapered (BLT) implants offer advantages with regard to primary stability for immediately placed implants. Should the anatomical conditions have been less favorable, tapered implants would have been indicated. A new implant option combining a tapered intraosseous implant component with a polished collar (TLX) may be the future for treatments of this type.

Intraoral scanning (digital impression making) remains controversial, and accuracy can be limited for edentulous arches. This can be the result of inconsistent capture of the soft tissue, and the accuracy of implant relationships across an arch. A matrix was digitally designed and fabricated as part of this patient presentation. The matrix was not used to verify accuracy of existing casts. Rather, it was indexed intraorally to copings and confirmed to be passive before being used to fabricate verification casts upon which final cementation of the zirconia prostheses could be undertaken. The authors believe that this procedure may help overcome inaccuracies associated with digital workflow at this time, although additional research support is indicated.

Lastly, implant-supported provisional prostheses are considered essential for complex implant-based treatments. The interim prostheses serve as prototypes for both the patient and the treatment team and facilitate confirmation of esthetic and functional goals. Importantly, clinical adjustment of definitive zirconia prostheses should be minimized. In addition to being time consuming, adjustment of zirconia can introduce surface defects and result in a decrease in clinical longevity. The provisional prostheses in this report were impressed and used as a laboratory reference to aid in design and detail of the definitive prostheses.

ACKNOWLEDGEMENT

The authors would like to acknowledge the skills and commitment of our laboratory partner, Mr. Bart Hyde.

CHAPTER 6: Conclusion

A. DAWSON, W. MARTIN, W. D. POLIDO

The original 2009 edition of *The SAC Classification in Implant Dentistry* aimed to meet an undersatisfied need for a risk management tool in implant dentistry. This aim was realized, and the SAC classification is widely accepted in its field. The later development of an online SAC Assessment Tool further simplified the process, allowing easy access for clinicians to assess their own cases.

More than a decade later, the SAC classification still meets this need. The passage of time, and the further evolution of techniques and technologies in implant dentistry, indicated that a refresh for the classification was in order. However, given the success of the SAC classification and its wide acceptance, the goal of the review was to update the assessment system but also to maintain consistency with the original. The roles of the book and the online assessment tool have reversed – the review was primarily aimed at updating the online tool. This publication aims to support the tool by detailing the rationale behind the updates.

The new SAC Assessment Tool now addresses more clinical applications and provides an individualized classification outcome that focuses on the case as it presents. This should assist clinicians to:

- Identify all potential risks associated with a case and communicate those risks to their patient as part of the informed consent process.
- Select appropriate cases for their care or arrange appropriate referral for all or some of the treatment.

In its broadest sense, the SAC classification system remains a useful and modern framework to assist clinicians to develop their skills in an incremental manner, and for educators to structure implant dentistry training programs.

CHAPTER 7: References

Aarup-Kristensen S, Hansen CR, Forner L, Brink C, Eriksen JG, Johansen J. Osteoradionecrosis of the mandible after radiotherapy for head and neck cancer: Risk factors and dose-volume correlations, Acta Oncologica 2019;58(10)1373–1377.

Abrams L. Augmentation of the deformed residual edentulous ridge for fixed prosthesis. Compend Contin Educ Gen Dent 1980;1: 205–213.

Aparicio C. Zygomatic Implants: The Anatomy Guided Approach. Berlin: Quintessence, 2017.

Aparicio C, Polido WD, Zarrinkelk HM. The zygoma anatomy-guided approach for placement of zygomatic implants. Atlas Oral Maxillofac Surg Clin North Am 2021;29(2):203–231.

Aparicio C, Polido WD, Chow J, David L, Davo R, Moraes ED, Fibishenko A, Ando M, Mclellan G, Nicolopoulos C, Pikos M, Zarrinkelk H, Balshi T, Peñarrocha M. Identification of the pathway and appropriate use of four zygomatic implants in the atrophic maxilla: A cross-sectional study. Int J Oral Maxillofac Implants 2021;36(4):807–817.

Beer GM, Manestar M. Prevalence of transverse upper labial crease. Eur J Plast Surg 2017;40:401–406.

Belser UC, Buser D, Hess D, Schmid B, Bernard JP, Lang NP. Aesthetic implant restorations in partially edentulous patients – a critical appraisal. Periodontol 2000 1998;17: 132–150.

Benic GI, Hämmerle CH. Horizontal bone augmentation by means of guided bone regeneration. Periodontol 2000 2014;66:13–40.

Blanco J, Carral C, Argibay O, Liñares A. Implant placement in fresh extraction sockets. Periodontol 2000 2019;79: 151–167.

Buser D, von Arx T. Surgical procedures in partially edentulous patients with ITI implants. Clin Oral Implants Res 2000;11(suppl 1): 83–100.

Buser D, Chappuis V, Belser UC, Chen S. Implant placement post extraction in esthetic single tooth sites: When immediate, when early, when late? Periodontol 2000 2017; 73:84–102.

Buser D, Chen S. Factors influencing the treatment outcomes of implants in post-extraction sites In: Buser D, Wismeijer D, Belser UC (eds). ITI Treatment Guide, Vol 3: Implant Placement in Post-extraction Sites: Treatment Options. Berlin: Quintessence, 2008.

Buser D, Martin W, Belser UC. Optimizing esthetics for implant restorations in the anterior maxilla: Anatomic and surgical considerations. Int J Oral Maxillofac Implants 2004;19 (suppl):43–61.

Cardaropoli D, Re S, Corrente G. The Papilla Presence Index (PPI): A new system to assess interproximal papillary levels. Int J Periodontics Restorative Dent 2004;24:488–492.

Carlsson GE, Bergman B, Hedegård B. Changes in contour of the maxillary alveolar process under immediate dentures. A longitudinal clinical and x-ray cephalometric study covering 5 years. Acta Odontol Scand 1967;25:45–75.

Chackartchi T, Romanos GE, Sculean A. Soft tissue-related complications and management around dental implants. Periodontol 2000 2019;81:124–138.

Chappuis V, Araújo MG, Buser D. Clinical relevance of dimensional bone and soft tissue alterations post-extraction in esthetic sites. Periodontol 2000 2017;73:73–83.

Chen ST, Buser D. Esthetic outcomes following immediate and early implant placement in the anterior maxilla – a systematic review. Int J Oral Maxillofac Implants 2014; 29(suppl):186–215.

Chen ST, Darby IB, Reynolds EC, Clement JG. Immediate implant placement postextraction without flap elevation. J Periodontol 2009;80:163–172.

Chen L, Schärer P. Introduction. In: Naert I, van Steenberghe D, Worthington P. Osseointegration in Oral Rehabilitation: An Introductory Textbook. London: Quintessence, 1993.

Chiapasco M, Casentini P, Zaniboni M. Bone augmentation procedures in implant dentistry. Int J Oral Maxillofac Implants 2009; 24(suppl):237–259.

Chiapasco M, Casentini P. Horizontal bone-augmentation procedures in implant dentistry: Prosthetically guided regeneration. Periodontol 2000 2018;77:213–240.

Cho SC, Shetty S, Froum S, Elian N, Tarnow D. Fixed and removable provisional options for patients undergoing implant treatment. Compend Contin Educ Dent 2007;28: 604–624.

Choquet V, Hermans M, Adriaenssens P, Daelemans P, Tarnow DP, Malevez C. Clinical and radiographic evaluation of the papilla level adjacent to single-tooth dental implants. A retrospective study in the maxillary anterior region. J Periodontol 2001;72: 1364–1371.

Chu SJ, Salama MA, Salama H, Garber DA, Saito H, Sarnachiaro GO, Tarnow DP. The dual-zone therapeutic concept of managing immediate implant placement and provisional restoration in anterior extraction sockets. Compend Contin Educ Dent 2012; 33(7):524–532, 534.

Correia A, Rebolo A, Azevedo L, Polido W, Rodrigues PP. SAC Assessment Tool in implant dentistry: Evaluation of the agreement level between users. Int J Oral Maxillofac Implants 2020;35:990–994.

Cortellini P, Stalpers G, Mollo A, Tonetti MS. Periodontal regeneration versus extraction and prosthetic replacement of teeth severely compromised by attachment loss to the apex: 5-year results of an ongoing randomized clinical trial. J Clin Periodontol 2011;38:915–924.

Curtiss P, Warren P. The Dynamics of Life Skills Coaching. Prince Albert, Saskatchewan: Training Research and Development Station, Dept. of Manpower and Immigration, 1973.

Dawson A, Chen S (eds). The SAC Classification in Implant Dentistry. Berlin: Quintessence, 2009.

de Freitas RF, de Carvalho Dias K, da Fonte Porto Carreiro A, Barbosa GA, Ferreira MA. Mandibular implant-supported removable partial denture with distal extension: A systematic review. J Oral Rehabil 2012;39:791–798.

Derks J, Schaller D, Håkansson J, Wennström JL, Tomasi C, Berglundh T. Effectiveness of implant therapy analyzed in a Swedish population: Prevalence of peri-implantitis. J Dent Res 2016;95: 43–49.

Desjardins RP. Prosthesis design for osseointegrated implants in the edentulous maxilla. Int J Oral Maxillofac Implants 1992;7: 311–320.

Doyle DJ, Goyal A, Bansal P, Garmon EH. American Society of Anesthesiologists Classification. In: StatPearls. Treasure Island (FL): StatPearls, 2021.

Evans CD, Chen ST. Esthetic outcomes of immediate implant placements. Clin Oral Implants Res 2008;19:73–80.

Felton DA, Kanoy BE, Bayne SC, Wirthman GP. Effect of in vivo crown margin discrepancies on periodontal health. J Prosthet Dent 1991;65:357–364.

Furze D, Byrne A, Alam S, Brägger U, Wismeijer D, Wittneben JG. Influence of the fixed implant-supported provisional phase on the esthetic final outcome of implant-supported crowns: 3-year results of a randomized controlled clinical trial. Clin Implant Dent Relat Res 2019;21:649–655.

Gallucci GO, Guex P, Vinci D, Belser UC. Achieving natural-looking morphology and surface textures in anterior ceramic fixed rehabilitations. Int J Periodontics Restorative Dent 2007;27:117–125.

Gallucci GO, Hamilton A, Zhou W, Buser D, Chen S. Implant placement and loading protocols in partially edentulous patients: A systematic review. Clin Oral Implants Res 2018;29(suppl 16):106–134.

Gawande A. The Checklist Manifesto: How to Get Things Right. New York: Metropolitan Books, 2009.

Gobbato L, Paniz G, Mazzocco F, et al. Significance of crown shape in the replacement of a central incisor with a single implant-supported crown. Quintessence Int 2013;44: 407–413.

Hämmerle CH, Chen ST, Wilson TG Jr. Consensus statements and recommended clinical procedures regarding the placement of implants in extraction sockets. Int J Oral Maxillofac Implants 2004;19(suppl):26–28.

Heitz-Mayfield LJ, Huynh-Ba G. History of treated periodontitis and smoking as risks for implant therapy. Int J Oral Maxillofac Implants 2009;24(suppl):39–68.

Januário AL, Barriviera M, Duarte WR. Soft tissue cone-beam computed tomography: A novel method for the measurement of gingival tissue and the dimensions of the dentogingival unit. J Esthet Restor Dent 2008;20:366–374.

Jerjes W, Hopper C. Surgical experience, workload and learning curve vs postoperative outcome. Eur J Oral Implantol 2018;11 (suppl 1):S167–S178.

Kan JY, Rungcharassaeng K, Umezu K, Kois JC. Dimensions of peri-implant mucosa: An evaluation of maxillary anterior single implants in humans. J Periodontol 2003;74: 557–562.

Kaufmann R, Friedli M, Hug S, Mericske-Stern R. Removable dentures with implant support in strategic positions followed for up to 8 years. Int J Prosthodont 2009;22:233–242.

Kim Y, Oh TJ, Misch CE, Wang HL. Occlusal considerations in implant therapy: Clinical guidelines with biomechanical rationale. Clin Oral Implants Res 2005;16:26–35.

Kois JC. Predictable single tooth peri-implant esthetics: Five diagnostic keys. Compend Contin Educ Dent 2001;22: 199–208.

Kruger J, Dunning D. Unskilled and unaware of it: How difficulties in recognizing one's own incompetence lead to inflated self-assessments. J Pers Soc Psychol 1999;77: 1121–1134.

Kwok V, Caton JG. Commentary: Prognosis revisited: A system for assigning periodontal prognosis. J Periodontol 2007; 78:2063–2071.

Lambert PM, Morris HF, Ochi S. Positive effect of surgical experience with implants on second-stage implant survival. J Oral Maxillofac Surg 1997;55(12 suppl 5):12–18.

Levine RA, Huynh-Ba G, Cochran DL. Soft tissue augmentation procedures for mucogingival defects in esthetic sites. Int J Oral Maxillofac Implants 2014;29(suppl):155–185.

Lin WS, Eckert SE. Clinical performance of intentionally tilted implants versus axially positioned implants: A systematic review. Clin Oral Implants Res 2018;29(suppl 16):78–105.

Lindhe J, Socransky SS, Nyman S, Westfelt E. Dimensional alteration of the periodontal tissues following therapy. Int J Periodontics Restorative Dent 1987;7:9–21.

Malo P, de Araújo Nobre M, Lopes A, Moss SM, Molina GJ. A longitudinal study of the survival of All-on-4 implants in the mandible with up to 10 years of follow-up. J Am Dent Assoc 2011;142:310–320.

Mankoo T. Maintenance of interdental papillae in the esthetic zone using multiple immediate adjacent implants to restore failing teeth – a report of ten cases at 2 to 7 years follow-up. Eur J Esthet Dent 2008;3:304–322.

Markus SJ. Interim esthetic restorations in conjunction with anterior implants. J Prosthet Dent 1999;82:233–236.

Martin AJ, Buschang PH, Boley JC, Taylor RW, McKinney TW. The impact of buccal corridors on smile attractiveness. Eur J Orthod 2007;29:530–537.

Martin W, Chappuis V, Morton D, Buser D. Preoperative risk assessment and treatment planning for optimal esthetic outcomes. In: Buser D, Chen S, Wismeijer D (eds). ITI Treatment Guide. Vol 10: Implant Therapy in the Esthetic Zone: Current Treatment Modalities and Materials for Single-tooth Replacements. Berlin: Quintessence, 2017:23–46.

Mattheos N, de Bruyn H, Hultin M, et al. Developing implant dentistry education in Europe: The continuum from undergraduate to postgraduate education and continuing professional development. Eur J Dent Educ 2014;18(suppl 1):3–10.

Matuliene G, Pjetursson BE, Salvi GE, et al. Influence of residual pockets on progression of periodontitis and tooth loss: Results after 11 years of maintenance. J Clin Periodontol 2008;35:685–695.

Mitrani R, Adolfi D, Tacher S. Adjacent implant-supported restorations in the esthetic zone: Understanding the biology. J Esthet Restor Dent 2005;17:211–223.

Mitrani R, Brudvik JS, Phillips KM. Posterior implants for distal extension removable prostheses: A retrospective study. Int J Periodontics Restorative Dent 2003;23:353–359.

Papaspyridakos P, De Souza A, Vazouras K, Gholami H, Pagni S, Weber HP. Survival rates of short dental implants (≤6 mm) compared with implants longer than 6 mm in posterior jaw areas: A meta-analysis. Clin Oral Implants Res 2018;29(suppl 16):8–20.

Patras M, Martin W. Simplified custom impression post for implant-supported restorations. J Prosthet Dent 2016; 115:556–559.

Payne AG, Tawse-Smith A, Wismeijer D, De Silva RK, Ma S. Multicentre prospective evaluation of implant-assisted mandibular removable partial dentures: Surgical and prosthodontic outcomes. Clin Oral Implants Res 2017; 28:116–125.

Pinsky HM, Taichman RS, Sarment DP. Adaptation of airline crew resource management principles to dentistry. J Am Dent Assoc 2010;141:1010–1018.

Polido WD, Aghaloo T, Emmett TW, Taylor TD, Morton D. Number of implants placed for complete-arch fixed prostheses: A systematic review and meta-analysis. Clin Oral Implants Res 2018;2 9(suppl 16):154–183.

Polido WD, Misch CM. An update on vertical bone augmentation. ITI Forum Implantologicum 2021;17(2):118–131.

Pollini A, Goldberg J, Mitrani R, Morton D. The lip-tooth-ridge classification: A guidepost for edentulous maxillary arches. Diagnosis, risk assessment, and implant treatment indications. Int J Periodontics Restorative Dent 2017;37: 835–841.

Renouard F, Amalberti R, Renouard E. Are "human factors" the primary cause of complications in the field of implant dentistry? Int J Oral Maxillofac Implants 2017;32: e55–e61.

Renouard F, Rangert B. Risk Factors in Implant Dentistry: Simplified Clinical Analysis for Predictable Treatment. Paris: Quintessence, 1999.

Renouard F, Rangert B. Risk Factors in Implant Dentistry: Simplified Clinical Analysis for Predictable Treatment, ed 2. Paris: Quintessence, 2008.

Richter WA, Ueno H. Relationship of crown margin placement to gingival inflammation. J Prosthet Dent 1973;30: 156–161.

Roccuzzo M, Bonino F, Aglietta M, Dalmasso P. Ten-year results of a three arms prospective cohort study on implants in periodontally compromised patients. Part 2: Clinical results. Clin Oral Implants Res 2012;23:389–395.

Roccuzzo M, Bonino L, Dalmasso P, Aglietta M. Long-term results of a three arms prospective cohort study on implants in periodontally compromised patients: 10-year data around sandblasted and acid-etched (SLA) surface. Clin Oral Implants Res 2014;25: 1105–1112.

Roccuzzo M, Grasso G, Dalmasso P. Keratinized mucosa around implants in partially edentulous posterior mandible: 10-year results of a prospective comparative study. Clin Oral Implants Res 2016;27:491–496.

Sailer H, Pajarola G. Oral Surgery for the General Dentist. Stuttgart: Thieme, 1999.

Salvi GE, Brägger U. Mechanical and technical risks in implant therapy. Int J Oral Maxillofac Implants 2009;24(suppl):69–85.

Salvi GE, Zitzmann NU. The effects of anti-infective preventive measures on the occurrence of biologic implant complications and implant loss: A systematic review. Int J Oral Maxillofac Implants 2014;29(suppl):292–307.

Sanavi F, Weisgold AS, Rose LF. Biologic width and its relation to periodontal biotypes. J Esthet Dent 1998;10:157–163.

Schnitman PA. The profile prosthesis: An aesthetic fixed implant-supported restoration for the resorbed maxilla. Pract Periodontics Aesthet Dent 1999;11:143–151.

Schropp L, Wenzel A, Kostopoulos L, Karring T. Bone healing and soft tissue contour changes following single-tooth extraction: A clinical and radiographic 12-month prospective study. Int J Periodontics Restorative Dent 2003; 23:313–323.

Schulte W. Implants and the periodontium. Int Dent J 1995; 45: 16–26.

Sculean A, Gruber R, Bosshardt DD. Soft tissue wound healing around teeth and dental implants. J Clin Periodontol 2014;41 (suppl 15):S6–S22.

Sendyk DI, Chrcanovic BR, Albrektsson T, Wennerberg A, Zindel Deboni MC. Does surgical experience influence implant survival rate? A systematic review and meta-analysis. Int J Prosthodont 2017;30(30):341–347.

Shahdad S. Patient Dental Factors. International Team for Implantology, 2015. https://www.iti.org/academy/theory-and-principles/learning-module/-/module/patient-dental-factors/211. Accessed 15 October 2021.

Shahdad S. Site-Specific Clinical Examination. International Team for Implantology, 2015. https://www.iti.org/academy/theory-and-principles/learning-module/-/module/site-specific-clinical- examination/214. Accessed 15 October 2021.

Shahmiri RA, Atieh MA. Mandibular Kennedy Class I implant-tooth-borne removable partial denture: A systematic review. J Oral Rehabil 2010;37:225–234.

Stein RS. Pontic-residual ridge relationship: A research report. J Prosthet Dent 1966;16:251–285.

Stellini E, Comuzzi L, Mazzocco F, Parente N, Gobbato L. Relationships between different tooth shapes and patient's periodontal phenotype. J Periodontal Res 2013; 48:657–662.

Stilwell C. Occlusion on Fixed Implant Prostheses. International Team for Implantology, 2015. https://www.iti.org/academy/theory-and-principles/learning-module/-/module/occlusion-on-fixed-implant-prostheses/229. Accessed 15 October 2021.

Takei HH. The interdental space. Dent Clin North Am 1980; 24: 169–176.

Tallgren A. The reduction in face height of edentulous and partially edentulous subjects during long-term denture wear. A longitudinal roentgenographic cephalometric study. Acta Odontol Scand 1966;24:195–239.

Tallgren A. The effect of denture wearing on facial morphology. A 7-year longitudinal study. Acta Odontol Scand 1967;25:563–592.

Tan WL, Wong TL, Wong MC, Lang NP. A systematic review of post-extractional alveolar hard and soft tissue dimensional changes in humans. Clin Oral Implants Res 2012; 23(suppl 5):1–21.

Tarnow DP, Cho SC, Wallace SS. The effect of inter-implant distance on the height of inter-implant bone crest. J Periodontol 2000; 71:546–549.

Tarnow D, Elian N, Fletcher P, et al. Vertical distance from the crest of bone to the height of the interproximal papilla between adjacent implants. J Periodontol 2003;74 :1785–1788.

Taylor TD. Fixed implant rehabilitation for the edentulous maxilla. Int J Oral Maxillofac Implants 1991;6:329–337.

Tjan AH, Miller GD, The JG. Some esthetic factors in a smile. J Prosthet Dent 1984;51:24–28.

Van der Weijden F, Dell'Acqua F, Slot DE. Alveolar bone dimensional changes of post-extraction sockets in humans: A systematic review. J Clin Periodontol 2009;36: 1048–1058.

Vig RG, Brundo GC. The kinetics of anterior tooth display. J Prosthet Dent 1978;39:502–504.

Vorster C. Additional Diagnostic Investigations. International Team for Implantology, 2015. https://www.iti.org/academy/theory-and-principles/learning-module/-/module/additional-diagnostic-investigations/216.v Accessed 15 October 2021.

Weber HP. Structured Assessment and Treatment Planning. International Team for Implantology, 2015. https://www.iti.org/academy/theory-and-principles/learning-module/-/module/structured-assessment-and-treatment-planning/207. Accessed 13 October 2021.

Weber HP, Morton D, Gallucci GO, Roccuzzo M, Cordaro L, Grutter L. Consensus statements and recommended clinical procedures regarding loading protocols. Int J Oral Maxillofac Implants 2009; 24(suppl):180–183.

Weisgold AS. Contours of the full crown restoration. Alpha Omegan 1977;70:77–89.

West CP, Huschka MM, Novotny PJ, et al. Association of perceived medical errors with resident distress and empathy: A prospective longitudinal study. JAMA 2006;296: 1071–1078.

Wismeijer D, Buser D, Belser U (eds). ITI Treatment Guide. Vol 4: Loading Protocols in Implant Dentistry: Edentulous Patients. Berlin: Quintessence, 2010.

Wismeijer D, Chen S, Buser D (eds). ITI Treatment Guide. Vol 6: Extended Edentulous Spaces in the Esthetic Zone. Berlin: Quintessence, 2012.

Zancopé K, Abrão GM, Karam FK, Neves FD. Placement of a distal implant to convert a mandibular removable Kennedy class I to an implant-supported partial removable Class III dental prosthesis: A systematic review. J Prosthet Dent 2015;113:528–33.e3.

Zitzmann NU, Marinello CP. Fixed or removable implant-supported restorations in the edentulous maxilla: Literature review. Pract Periodontics Aesthet Dent 2000;12:599–609.

Zitzmann NU, Marinello CP. Treatment plan for restoring the edentulous maxilla with implant-supported restorations: Removable overdenture versus fixed partial denture design. J Prosthet Dent 1999;82:188–196.

The SAC Classification in Implant Dentistry